H 01251

616.5 H8

D1643877

This book is to be returned on or before
the last date stamped below. 616.5

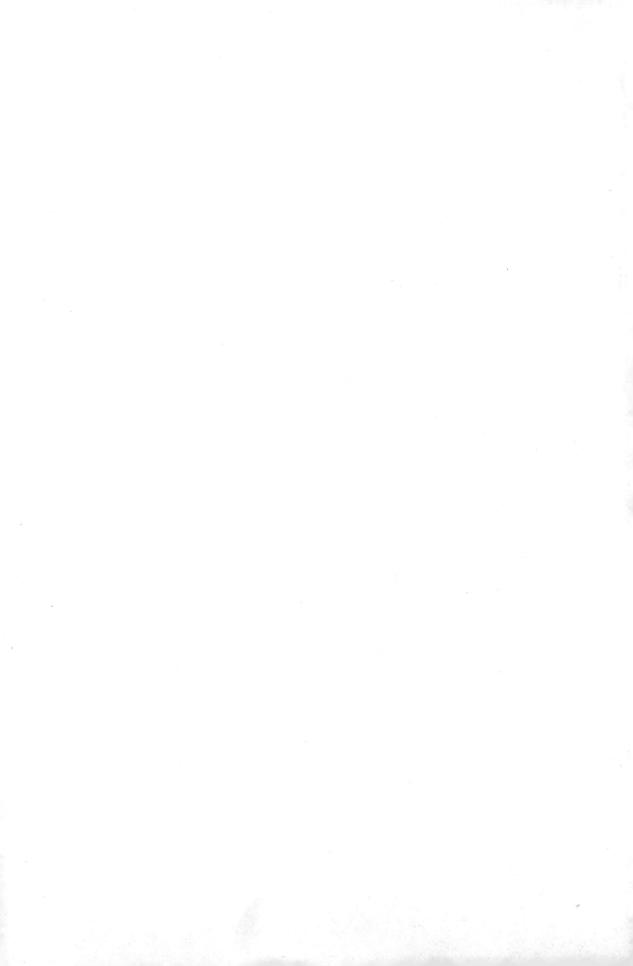

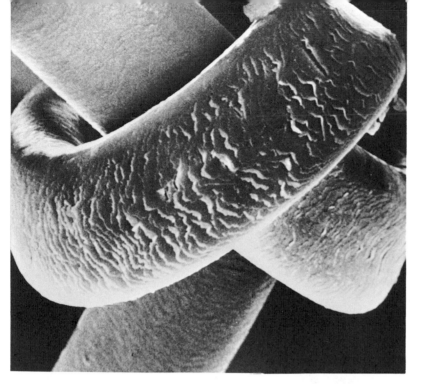
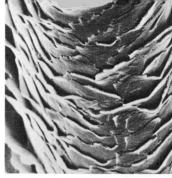
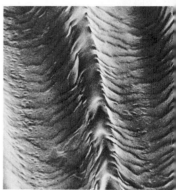
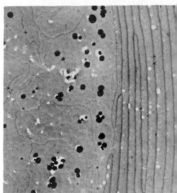
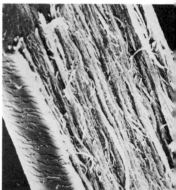
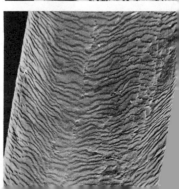

HAIR STRUCTURE AND CHEMISTRY SIMPLIFIED

BY A. H. POWITT, B.SC., A.S.T.C. (APPLIED BIO.)
AUTHOR OF "LECTURES IN HAIR STRUCTURE AND CHEMISTRY"
Milady Publishing Company (A Division of Delmar Publishers Inc.)
3839 White Plains Rd., Bx., N.Y. 10467-5394

1990 Printing

Copyright © 1972, 1977
Milady Publishing Company
(A Division of Delmar Publishers Inc.)

ISBN 0-87350-388-0

PREFACE

The *routine* performance of hair work in the salon or shop may very quickly take on the aspects of the *mechanic* performing his work.

The professional artisan, on the other hand, acquires a complete knowledge and understanding not only of "why" certain techniques are performed but also the chemical actions and reactions which may be expected from the cosmetic products employed. It is this knowledge and understanding which differentiates between the true "professional" and the "basic mechanic."

In recent years there have been a number of significant changes in "hair-care" methods and techniques. Many new cosmetic products have been developed for professional use that require careful handling and controlled application.

It has therefore become important that the "professional artisan" acquire a good basic understanding of the chemistry of the skin, the hair and of the products employed in their care. It is vital that persons engaged in performing professional grooming services develop an understanding of the proper "use" of cosmetic products instead of their "misuse."

This text is designed to make professional hair and skin services readily understandable through a clear presentation of the relative facts pertaining to the chemistry and structure of hair and skin. It is offered in an attempt to insure the safe and effective use of all professional products.

While the techniques of performance may differ greatly in terms of cosmetic brand, the chemical principles, which apply, are exactly the same. This text was not designed to, nor does it intend to, discuss the techniques of application. Therefore, the scientific data presented is pertinent for all students and all schools regardless of the brand name of the supplies used in training.

WORDS USED INTERCHANGEABLY

A number of terms are used interchangeably to conform with common usage within the industry.

1. The words "practitioner" and "artisan" have a professional connotation and are used interchangeably throughout the text.
2. The words "salon" and "shop" are interchanged as these terms are stressed from one region to another.
3. The words "lightener" or "lightening" are interchanged with "bleach" or "bleaching" to indicate the removal of color from the hair.

INTRODUCING SCANNING ELECTRON MICROSCOPE PHOTOGRAPHY

Many of the photos presented in this text, by courtesy of the Gillette Company Research Institute, Rockville, Maryland, are the product of the latest and most scientific method of studying skin and hair.

The instrument employed in the process is the Scanning Electron Microscope (SEM). This remarkable device permits direct viewing of surfaces in "three dimensions," as compared with the "flat-surface," shallow depth of field view, common to photos made with optical microscopes.

The method introduces a very unique technique of thinly coating the object to be photographed, first with carbon and then with gold palladium. After coating they are examined in the Scanning Electron Microscope and appropriate photos taken.

As part of this text these photos present very interesting and extremely instructive views of the hair and skin under various conditions.

CONTENTS

THE SCIENCE OF PROFESSIONAL HAIR CARE

MEANING OF SCIENCE

You have perhaps heard and read a great deal about science and scientists in the newspapers, popular magazines, on radio and on television. Science is doing a great deal both to explain and to change the world we live in today. Science is a word derived from the Latin verb "scire" which means "to know." But, science is not simply concerned with knowing facts and memorizing them as if we were preparing for some quiz show or to demonstrate how much knowledge we have managed to cram into our brains. Science is something more than this and, we will take a brief look to see what it really is.

SCIENCE MEANS KNOWING OR GETTING FACTS

Science has been defined as the accumulated and accepted knowledge which has been systematized and formulated with reference to the discovery of general truths or the operation of general laws.

Science is first of all concerned with finding out unknown facts about the world and ourselves. Three basic steps are employed for this purpose:

1. Observation
2. Reasoning
3. Experimentation

OBSERVATION   Many facts are available to us if we keep our eyes and ears open. Much knowledge can be gained by paying close attention to the task we are doing. The great scientist, Louis Pasteur, once remarked that "chance favors the prepared mind." This means that the more we know about a subject the more likely we are to recognize something new or important about it.

The more training and experience you have, the more you can expand and extend your knowledge. Practice careful observation at all times. Remember that each head of hair is different and provides you with yet another opportunity for fresh experience and knowledge.

REASONING   We can gain new information through the powers of reasoning. Reasoning is an important tool of mankind, but it is handicapped if it is not supported by fact or observation.

Many of the old wives' tales about our hair are firmly believed because they sound reasonable. But this is because they have not been put to the real test of reasoning. Are these tales supported by facts or are they formed by guesswork and foolish imagination?

It is inevitable that man uses his powers of reasoning to widen his understanding. Remember that we are constantly looking for reasons to explain those facts we already know.

Necessity of Changed Ideas

As more knowledge becomes available, we often see how faulty was our previous reasoning. The intelligent person adjusts to these changes brought about by science and does not cling to blind, unproven beliefs.

EXPERIMENTATION   We can sometimes test our reasoning by carefully setting up a test situation. We can then examine the changes that take place while we control them or merely watch them as they occur. This is called a scientific experiment.

Experiments in the School and Shop

Practitioners are limited in the amount of experimenting they can do because of the great risks involved to the patron's hair and scalp.

Nevertheless, the successful person is always a careful, modest experimenter. Each new style or different texture of hair must be approached as a challenge, if we are to master it.

Experiments performed on swatches of hair, that have been cut from the head, can provide a great deal of valuable knowledge without endangering the patron's hair or health. However, great care must be exercised because, in hair coloring and other chemical services especially, unless you are extremely competent, the effects of experimentation on the head could end in disaster. The more ability the artisan has, the more expert and rewarding will be the results of the experiment or trial. But experiments need to be carefully planned and controlled, to minimize the element of doubt about their result and the danger of permanent damage.

SCIENCE IS CONCERNED WITH CAUSE AND EFFECT

CAUSE OF EVENTS   Science is not interested in facts only. A scientist is not a person who goes around getting information as if he were a walking encyclopedia. Much more important than the facts are such questions as—what caused them or what effect do they produce themselves?

It is the opinion of scientists that for every event (that we can see, hear or measure) there must be a cause. In other words, things do NOT happen without a reason.

ANCIENT EXPLANATION OF CAUSE   The ancients believed that the world was governed by demons or mischievous spirits. These superstitious beliefs led to meaningless rituals and hocus-pokus. These people thought they could not succeed in anything unless the spirits were won over with gifts, incense or magic charms.

MODERN VIEWPOINT   We know that superstition is absurd, because we have learned to recognize the necessary connection between cause and effect. Although we know this now, it does not mean that our difficulties are easily or automatically solved. With all our wisdom and experience, we are still unable to solve many problems that baffle mankind, e.g., baldness is an effect that is easily recognized. But, what is the cause of this baldness?

Science accepts the fact that there must be a cause and possibly a cure for baldness. But without knowing the real cause it is almost impossible to discover a permanent baldness cure. All we can do in the meantime is to proceed by trial and error. The reason why there are so many conflicting claims for the treatment of baldness is that, without certain knowledge, we cannot discredit the so-called "cures" that are sold for treating baldness and other scalp disorders.

IMPORTANCE OF CAUSE AND EFFECT   Since the dawn of history, man has tried to see into the future. Man's interest in what the future holds for him is probably the reason why science has gripped his imagination. First, we have to separate the real cause from its effect. This finding will then make our forecasts sounder and of more certain value to the practitioner. For example, scientists can determine effects of products by testing various substances on animal hair, swatches of human hair, wool or fur.

VALUE TO THE PRACTITIONER   If the solutions used in hair treatments are properly tested in the laboratory (or by special shops before release to the public) then we will know their effect before we put them on a patron's hair. An example of this is the fact that we know from previous tests that *ALL* types of porous hair require a specially weakened permanent waving solution. If the hair we are about to wave is in a weakened condition, we can expect with some certainty that it also will require a weaker solution.

SCIENCE AND COMMON SENSE

THE PRACTICE OF SCIENCE   is open to everybody. Nowadays, a scientific approach to life is almost automatic. It is much wiser to use scientific methods to solve our problems than to rely on blind guesswork. We want to seek the truth to explain certain happenings and no longer rely on superstition, prejudice, or ignorance for our explanations.

SCIENCE AND COMMON SENSE IN THE SHOP   In the shop, for example, you have been asked to lighten (bleach) a patron's hair. You find that after carrying out the proper procedures, the results are poor. Naturally, you want to find out what the trouble is and how you can avoid it the next time. If your reasons were *unscientific* they might be as follows:

The Unscientific Answer

1. This lightener does not work because it is raining today.
2. The patron was upset today; therefore, it did not work.
3. It does not work because this is my bad day. (This is a common excuse.)

Science does not allow bad luck to explain our failures, but claims it is more likely to be a matter of carelessness or poor technique.

The Scientific Answer

A more sensible and scientific approach would be to consider one of the following possibilities:

1. Someone left the cap off the hydrogen peroxide bottle and it was not up to proper strength.
2. The bottle may have been exposed to heat or direct sunlight. (Hydrogen peroxide must always be kept in a cool, dark place.)
3. The peroxide bottle could have been accidentally filled with water.
4. The hair was very resistant and more lightening time should have been allowed.
5. Fresh lightener should have been reapplied. (Lighteners stop working after a time and so should be renewed.)

CONSTANT NEED FOR CARE

One of the first things you must do if things go wrong is to recheck the manufacturer's directions.

For example: Research by the shampoo manufacturers shows that a great many practitioners are unaware of the correct way to shampoo the hair. They use an excessive amount of shampoo, fail to massage the hair properly, and then leave far too much shampoo in the hair through improper rinsing. Failure to follow the manufacturer's directions in shampooing often causes poor results in services that follow.

VALUE OF SCIENCE

IMPROVES OUR KNOWLEDGE By using the methods of science we can often discover the reasons why things go wrong. By being able to predict scientifically, we learn to avoid mistakes and also to improve our results. It is basic that the more facts known about the skin, hair and cosmetic chemistry, the more likely the professionals will be able to do better work.

RESEARCH Science continually assists industry by carrying out research into new products and techniques. Most research work is specialized and requires a highly qualified staff. The equipment is costly and besides, there is always far too much to do in the shop for the practitioner to even attempt it.

DEVELOP SAFE, WORKABLE PROCEDURES Behind text materials and manufacturers' instructions lies a tremendous amount of investigation and preliminary experimentation. Products themselves are tested and retested before they are placed on the market for public or professional use. Many progressive firms give special, on-the-spot instructions about their products by trained representatives. The artisan is well advised to take advantage of these valuable services.

For example: Practitioners are foolish if they ignore the manufacturer's advice with relation to the use of shampoos. They fail to appreciate the importance of the shampoo and its influence upon the success or failure of services which follow. These individuals complain about poor results, claiming that modern shampoos ruin the hair. In reality, the responsibility should be placed where it belongs, on the careless application of the shampoo by the user.

IMPROVES OUR STANDARD OF LIVING Science aids the practitioner further by reducing the costs of production and thus helping to increase profits and to raise the standard of living.

This means that people have more time and money to spend on their personal appearance. Many special services were once only available to very few because of their high cost. Since the introduction of the modern products (which were developed by science) almost everyone in the community can now afford regular visits to the shop for professional service.

SUMMARY:
1. Better methods mean lower costs.
2. Lower costs mean lower prices.
3. Lower prices mean more business.
4. More business means more skilled professionals as the demand increases.
5. All of these mean more income for the practitioner.

LIMITATIONS OF SCIENCE

SCIENCE IS NO CURE-ALL Merely knowing what went wrong cannot repair or cover up bad technique. If the hair is badly damaged or destroyed, nothing can restore it to its former condition. The practitioner takes the final responsibility for the materials used. The solutions, even if carefully prepared under scientific control, are not fool-proof; much depends on the skill of the professional during application.

SCIENCE MAKES NO EXTRAVAGANT CLAIMS Scientific methods are slow and methodical. Scientists realize how little we really know about the hair and the changes that can take place in it. Therefore, they hesitate to make extravagant claims of hair treatment success.

LEARNING THEORY AND PRACTICAL KNOW-HOW

THE PROBLEM OF WHAT TO LEARN   Many people are confused over the issue of what a professional should know and how it should be taught. The real truth of the matter is that no method can stand strictly on its own. A rare combination of knowledge, application, direction and business sense is required to be a success in any field.

There is a long, hard road that leads from the inexperienced novice to the final, polished artisan. It is beyond doubt, however, that the more you know about your job, the more likely you are to reach this goal of professional and financial success.

Hair care is an art, completely dependent upon the personal skill of the individual. As such, it cannot be learned completely from a book or simply by watching another person, but requires personal training and ability.

SCIENCE AND THE PRACTITIONER   Science provides us with information that tells us WHY we should do certain things. But, science does NOT tell us HOW to do them. A mere study of theory could not make a competent practitioner and neither could an untrained individual expect to automatically become an able artisan.

As hair care grows and develops, we will be forced to depend greatly upon science to provide answers to many of the problems which will arise. Professional standards will be elevated only through a close, cooperative effort between the scientist and the professional.

Both the practitioner and the scientist, therefore, will be required to understand the underlying nature of the important problems facing the industry. In the past, the scientist has concentrated all of his efforts upon technical difficulties. However, many of the practitioner's problems are human or economic as well. Professional success cannot be assured by mere specialization in hair-care techniques. The fields of economics, commerce and management present many obstacles which scientific knowledge alone will not overcome.

ADDITIONAL SOURCES OF INFORMATION

Scientists are not at all satisfied with their present knowledge of the hair. Much study will inevitably lead to future discoveries which will bring many major changes in the techniques, materials and equipment used in the practice of professional hair work.

The successful practitioner will be required to adjust to these changes by keeping informed of the latest discoveries and newest trends that science and industry bring out.

1. Keeping in close touch with your manufacturers and their technical representatives.
2. Attending demonstrations, conventions, shows and special schools that pass on new developments to professional artisans.
3. Reading current or up-to-date information in trade or general magazines, textbooks, newspapers and other media.

CONCLUSION

It is important to understand how most of us may use science in our everyday lives. This knowledge can improve our methods and increase our efficiency and the understanding of our work in the shop. Success in the shop requires more than good technical skills and ability. It requires, also, an inquiring mind and a willingness and eagerness to learn and to keep up with the very latest developments in professional hair work.

The future success of hair care practice may depend on the cooperative effort of scientific developments and artistic application.

CHAPTER 2

SCIENCE OF LIVING THINGS

Introduction

The science of professional hair care is a study of the nature of the skin and hair and of those products which are of value in their treatment. Both skin and hair are products of living things and, therefore, a study of them must include a brief investigation of the properties of all living things.

STRUCTURE OF LIVING THINGS

Scientists have found that living things are organizations of countless millions of tiny structures (visible only under a microscope) called "cells." Organs are composed of tissues which are composed of cells and, although they exhibit a great variety of form, a similar basic organization exists. All cells have many similar characteristics.

CELLS

Cells, indeed, are the building blocks of living things, just as bricks are the building blocks of houses. Similar cells, arranged in various patterns, form the features or structures of the human body.

Scientific studies reveal that not only is the human body composed of millions of cells but that these are specialized cells which perform all the functions required for living. In performing shop or salon services the artisan must keep in mind the ultimate effect of each treatment on the cells of the human body.

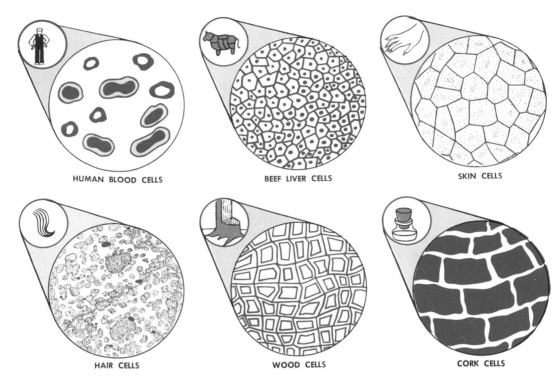

HUMAN BLOOD CELLS   BEEF LIVER CELLS   SKIN CELLS

HAIR CELLS   WOOD CELLS   CORK CELLS

SIZE For the most part, cells are microscopic in size. It is important to consider that cells are the basic unit of all living matter and that living cells differ from each other in size, shape, structure and function. In human beings, the cells are highly specialized and perform all the vital functions of the body.

VARIATION IN SHAPE OF CELLS

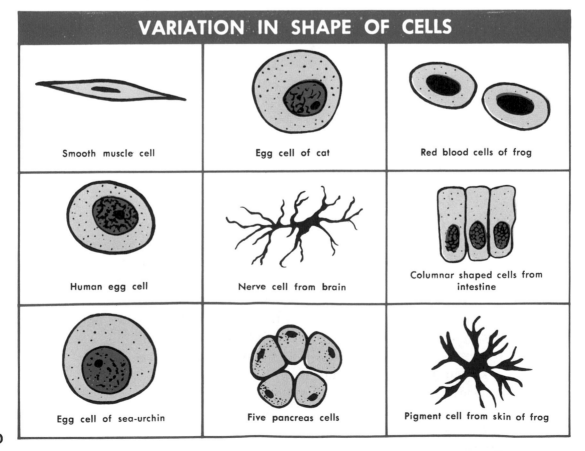

Smooth muscle cell	Egg cell of cat	Red blood cells of frog
Human egg cell	Nerve cell from brain	Columnar shaped cells from intestine
Egg cell of sea-urchin	Five pancreas cells	Pigment cell from skin of frog

CELL STRUCTURE

Most cells possess similar structures. The scientific concept of a cell is a small mass of living substance called "protoplasm." In the center part of the cell can be seen a small body, circular in outline. This is the nucleus; the portion outside the nucleus is the cytoplasm, and both are composed of protoplasm. Also found outside the nucleus is a small circular body called "centrosome," also composed of protoplasm.

Therefore, an examination of the cell under the microscope reveals the following main parts:

1. Protoplasm which, in turn, consists of (a) the cytoplasm, (b) the nucleus, and (c) the centrosome.
2. The cell membrane.

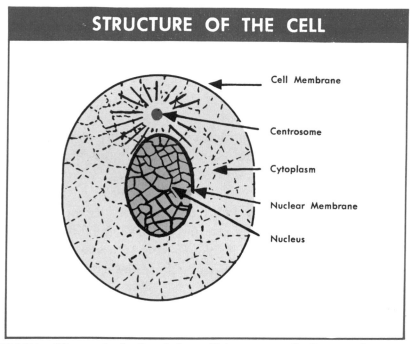

STRUCTURE OF THE CELL

Cell Membrane

Centrosome

Cytoplasm

Nuclear Membrane

Nucleus

CYTOPLASM The main body of the cell is composed of a translucent, somewhat jellylike substance. This colorless, watery substance, cytoplasm, contains the proteins, fats, carbohydrates, water and mineral salts necessary for growth, reproduction and self repair. Most of the activities of the cell are carried on by the cytoplasm, under the control of the nucleus.

NUCLEUS The metabolic, reproductive and other living functions of the cell are regulated by the nucleus. The nuclear matter is protoplasm, differing somewhat chemically from that of the cytoplasm. The nucleus plays a major role in directing the functions of the cell. In addition, it is of vital importance in the process of cell division, the reproductive process wherein the genes pass along the exact characteristics of the parent cell. Since cells have a limited life and must be replaced continuously, this reproductive procedure is essential to the life and well-being of the body.

CENTROSOME   Near the nucleus, at the time of cell division, a small body called the "centrosome" appears. The centrosome, together with the nucleus, organizes and controls the reproductive process of the cell.

CELL MEMBRANE   At the surface of liquids, where they are in contact with air, a film is present, possessing the property known as "surface tension." This film or membrane permits soluble substances to enter and leave the protoplasm. This cell membrane regulates the passage of oxygen and food compounds into the cytoplasm and the exit of carbon dioxide and nitrogenous waste products.

FUNCTION OF CELLS

As the human body is made up of countless millions of cells, the functions of these living "building blocks" are essential to maintain life. As long as the cell receives an adequate supply of food, oxygen and water, eliminates waste products and is surrounded by a favorable environment (proper temperature and absence of poisons and pressure), it will continue to grow and remain healthy. When these requirements are not fulfilled, the cell will stop growing and may eventually die.

CELLS NEED OXYGEN   Cells require a constant supply of oxygen to enable them to perform their work. A few minutes' interruption in this vital supply and the cells themselves will be injured or may die.

CELLS NEED NOURISHMENT   In addition to oxygen, living cells require a supply of nourishment. However, certain cells have the ability to store sufficient food materials to keep the body operating for some time in emergencies. Food eaten at regular intervals throughout the day is stored for use as it is required.

CELLS MUST GET RID OF WASTE   Living cells accumulate waste products which must be eliminated if the cells are going to operate normally. Carbon dioxide is one example of the various waste materials produced by the cells of our bodies and this is breathed out by way of the lungs. Other cell wastes are carried away in either a liquid or solid form and then excreted.

For this purpose, the body needs a constant reserve of water which must be replenished at fairly frequent intervals; otherwise, the cells may die of dehydration.

CELLS MUST REPRODUCE   Most cells have only a short life and so they must be replaced continuously; otherwise, the number of cells would steadily decrease and threaten the life of the body. In certain parts of the body there is a further need to produce a constant supply of additional cells forming new growth. These cells function to produce protective tissues, such as skin and hair.

When the cell reaches maturity, reproduction takes place by either direct or indirect division.

DIRECT DIVISION   This is a simple procedure whereby the cell elongates and the nucleus and cytoplasm divide in half, formiing two separate cells. This method of reproduction occurs among bacteria, but rarely takes place in human tissues.

BACTERIAL CELL REPRODUCTION

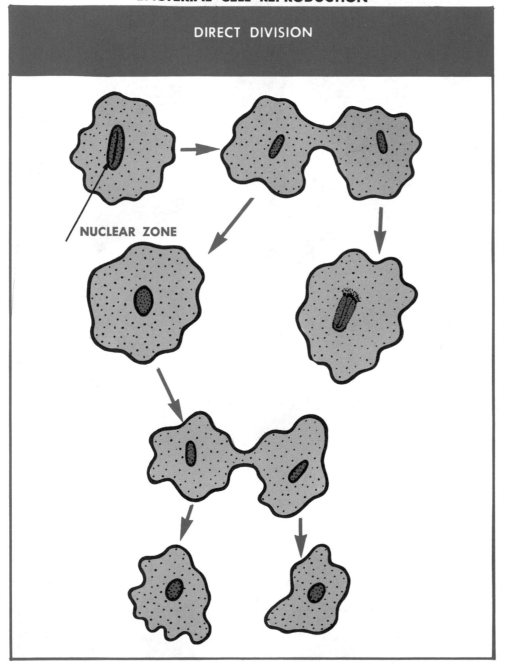

DIRECT DIVISION

NUCLEAR ZONE

INDIRECT DIVISION   This is a more complex process whereby a series of changes occurs in the nucleus before the cell divides in half. In this procedure, the centrosome plays an important role in maintaining the characteristics of the original cell. This method of reproduction occurs in human tissues including hair and skin.

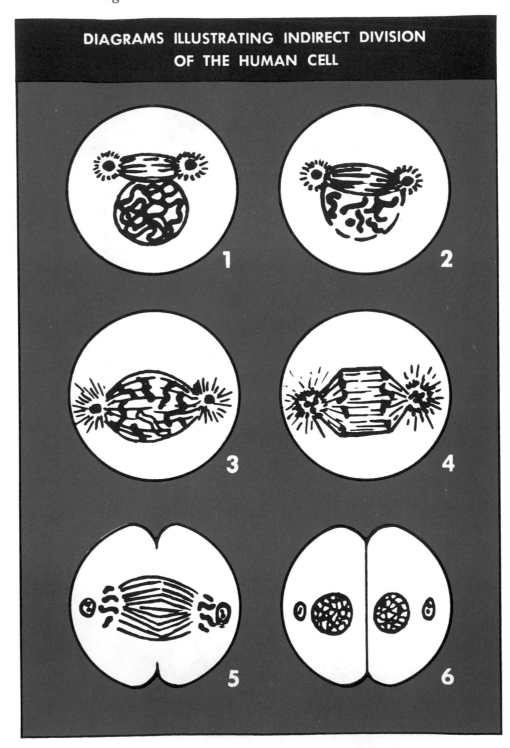

DIAGRAMS ILLUSTRATING INDIRECT DIVISION OF THE HUMAN CELL

CHAPTER

3

THE SKIN

Introduction

The skin is a most essential structure of the body, not merely a covering. It is, in fact, the largest organ of the human body. The total skin area of an average adult is 18.2 square feet, and the weight is approximately six pounds. Its unbelievable complexity is partially indicated when we consider the fact that each square inch contains numerous hair follicles, as well as:

10,000 nerve endings	34 feet of nerves
30 sebaceous (oil) glands	200 sudoriferous (sweat) glands
8 feet of blood vessels	12 million cells

The epidermis of the skin serves to protect the delicate tissues of the body from injury. This protective ability of the skin is due to the fact that it is made of a substance called KERATIN.

COMPOSITION

Keratin is a rather hard, horny protein with remarkably resistant properties. Being a protein, it contains the following elements:

Carbon	Nitrogen
Hydrogen	Phosphorus
Oxygen	Sulphur

The presence of sulphur* gives it a degree of chemical and biological resistance. No other tissue of the body contains as much sulphur as is found in keratin.

* *"Sulphur" and "sulfur" will be used interchangeably.*

FORMS OF KERATIN

Keratin is found in two main forms; soft and hard.

SOFT KERATIN   Soft keratin contains about 2% sulphur, 50% to 75% moisture and a small percentage of fats.

Location

It is found in the skin, especially in the layer of the epidermis, where it occurs in the form of flattened cells or as dry scales.

HARD KERATIN   Hard keratin, as found in hair, has a sulphur content of 4% to 8%, a lower moisture and fat content and is a particularly tough, elastic material.

Features

It forms continuous sheets (fingernails) or long endless fibers (hair). Hard keratin has no tendency to break off or flake away. It remains as a continuous structure.

DIFFICULTIES WITH KERATIN

Because of the close chemical and physiological relationship of soft and hard keratin, it is very difficult to treat these materials independently. This poses certain problems for the practitioner.

IN PERMANENT WAVING, hard keratin (hair) must be softened and yet the soft keratin (epidermis of the scalp) must be unaffected by the chemical solutions being used on the hair.

DANDRUFF, composed of soft keratin (scales) must be washed away. Soft keratin (skin) and hard keratin (hair) must not be damaged by anti-dandruff treatments.

Courtesy: Gillette Company Research Institute, Rockville, Maryland

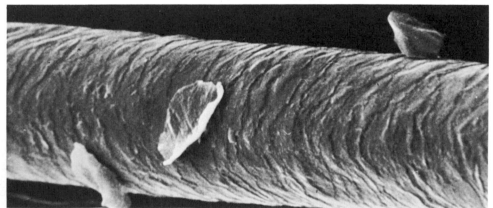

Normal hair with dandruff flakes adhering to hair fibers.

LIGHTENING AND TINTING   In these processes the hard keratin (hair) must be altered in color yet the soft keratin (skin) must be protected.

THE SKIN AS AN INDICATOR

The skin may be used as a simple mirror which reflects the general state or physical condition of the individual. The color, appearance and functioning of the skin are rough guides to our health and fitness. Physical condition is often reflected in the skin in the following manner:

1. Clear rosy cheeks usually mean robust health.
2. Yellow or sallow skin can indicate jaundice, hepatitis or malaria.
3. Pallid or very pale skin is typical of malnutrition or sickness.
4. Blotchy skin often tells of a poor diet or disturbance of the glands.

The skin also reacts immediately to traces of food or foreign matter to which the body may be allergic. The patch test, used in hair tinting, is designed to indicate this type of allergic reaction.

There are numerous other areas where physical conditions are shown by the skin. For example, the first signs of a vitamin deficiency would appear on the skin.

A very close connection between the brain and the skin is revealed by nerve and fever rashes, as well as other skin irritations.

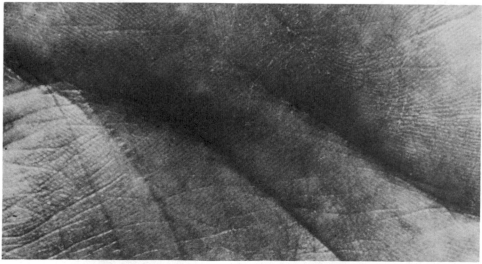

Palm of hand showing characteristic ridges and grooves in the skin.

STRUCTURE OF THE SKIN

APPEARANCE When magnified, even a cursory examination reveals that the surface of the skin is not smooth but is covered with many ridges and grooves. If the palms and fingers of the hands and the soles and toes of the feet are closely examined there can be seen a regular pattern of these furrows.

These finger or toe prints are different in each person and have proven very useful for identification, e.g., newborn babies are often registered by palm or footprints in large hospitals and criminals are identified by the study of fingerprints. The surface of the skin is also broken by the pores of the sweat glands and by the hair follicles (or pockets).

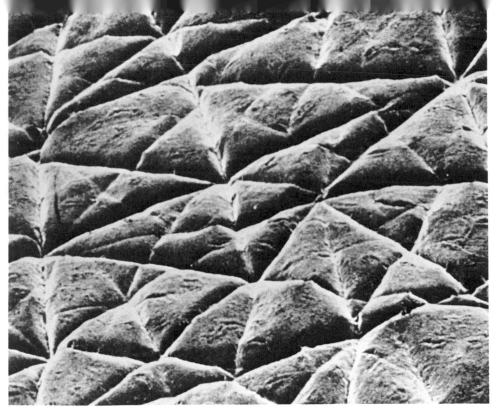

Photo of the skin on the back of the hand of a young female, magnified 60 times. Notice the triangular appearance of the major divisions of the skin surface.

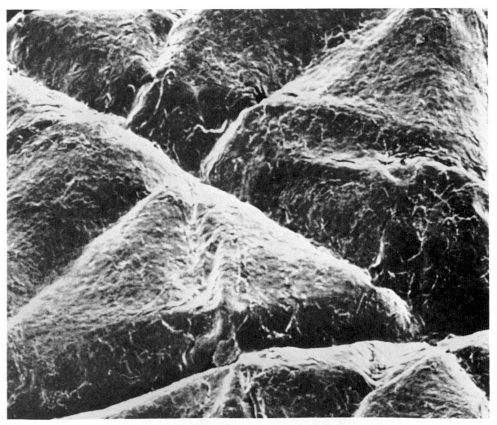

The same skin section, magnified 176 times. Notice the edges of the individual stratum corneum cells adhering tightly to the skin. *Courtesy: Gillette Company Research Institute, Rockville, Maryland*

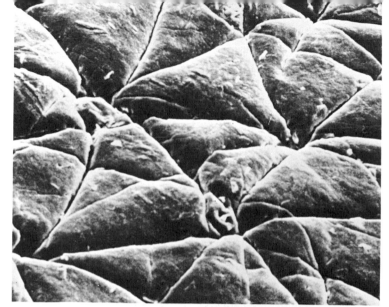

Cheek of a young female, magnified 210 times. Notice that the surface looks more plump and more rounded than the back of the hand photos. This probably is the result of more moisture in the skin. Follicle openings can be seen in the center of the photo.

Elbow skin from a young female, magnified 60 times. Notice how the overall architecture of the skin differs from previous skin photos. This indicates that skin from different areas have very different structures.

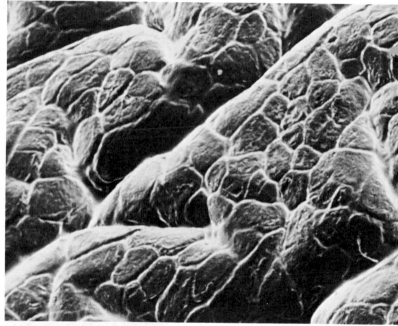

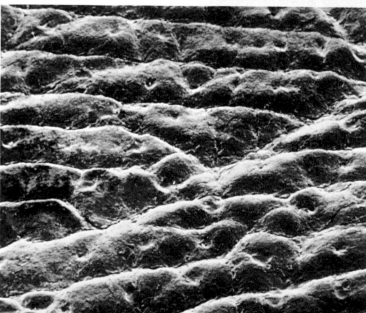

The skin from the palm of the hand, magnified 60 times. Small indentations of ridges are sweat gland openings.
Courtesy: Gillette Company Research Institute, Rockville, Maryland

DIAGRAM OF A SECTION OF THE SCALP

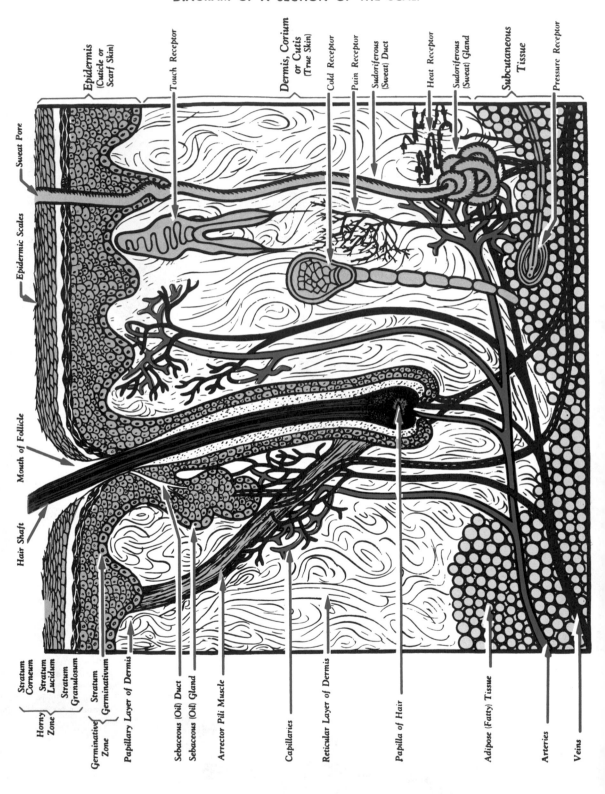

Epidermis (Cuticle or Scarf Skin)

Touch Receptor

Dermis, Corium or Cutis (True Skin)

Cold Receptor

Pain Receptor

Sudoriferous (Sweat) Duct

Heat Receptor

Sudoriferous (Sweat) Gland

Subcutaneous Tissue

Pressure Receptor

Sweat Pore

Epidermic Scales

Mouth of Follicle

Hair Shaft

Stratum Corneum

Stratum Lucidum

Stratum Granulosum

Horny Zone

Stratum Germinativum

Germinative Zone

Papillary Layer of Dermis

Sebaceous (Oil) Duct

Sebaceous (Oil) Gland

Arrector Pili Muscle

Capillaries

Reticular Layer of Dermis

Papilla of Hair

Adipose (Fatty) Tissue

Arteries

Veins

BLOOD SUPPLY   From ½ to ⅔ of the total blood supply of the body is found supplying the dermis of the skin with nourishment and warmth. These blood vessels can expand or contract in width through such stimuli as heat and cold.

THICKNESS   Generally the skin is $\frac{1}{12}$ to ⅕ of an inch thick except on the soles of the feet and the palms of the hands. On the soles of the feet it is likely to be over ¼ of an inch thick. The thickness of the palms of the hands depends primarily on occupation, since people performing manual labor have thicker and more calloused skin than people doing less physical work.

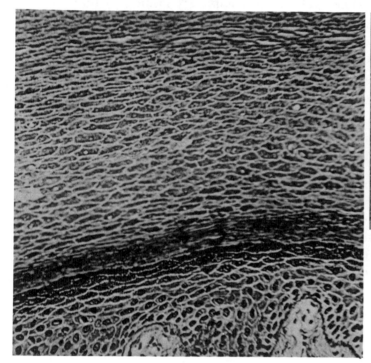
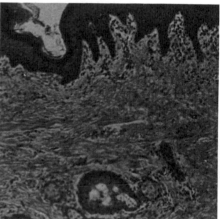

Sections of skin showing thickened epidermis (left—sole of feet) compared to normal epidermis (top—back of hand).

LAYERS OF THE SKIN

In order to properly carry out its particular functions the skin is composed of two different layers.

1. *Epidermis*
   This is also known as the "scarf skin."
2. *Dermis*
   This is also known as the corium or "true skin."

EPIDERMIS

DESCRIPTION   The epidermis rests upon the dermis and is the outer layer of the skin. This portion is in direct contact with the outside world. When we look at our skin, this is the layer which we can see and readily recognize. The epidermis is like a plastic, flexible envelope (which is also self-reproducing) covering and protecting the entire human body.

DEVELOPMENT OF NEW CELLS   At the base of the epidermis (immediately adjacent to the dermis) is a special row of cells called the germinative layer. This germ layer is constantly forming new cells by cell division. The older cells are pushed ever upwards by the younger cells coming underneath them. They eventually arrive at their destination which is the outermost part of the skin. This process of movement, from the germinative layer to the outermost part of the epidermis, takes about one month, during which time changes take place in the cell structure.

CHANGES IN CELLS   The epidermis is completely lacking in blood vessels, but the lower layers of cells (being closer to the blood vessels of the dermis) obtain some of their nourishment from the dermis. Therefore, the bottom rows of cells are still alive for a time even though the epidermis has no blood supply of its own.

Slowly, as these layers of cells move farther away, they gradually die. The cells become flattened, the nucleus disappears and the cell loses nearly half of its moisture content.

LOSS OF EPIDERMIS   These flattened cells arrive at the surface of the skin where they flake off as powdery scales. Friction or contact with foreign objects will speed the removal of these scales.

Where the skin is covered for long periods (e.g., by a plaster cast or adhesive bandage) the scarf skin appears as whitish, fleshy, flakes when the covering is removed, due to an accumulation of scales under the covering. This excessive skin formation and flaking, when it occurs on the scalp, is referred to as "dandruff."

DERMIS

DESCRIPTION   The dermis or lower part of the skin is protected by the epidermis above it. The structure of the dermis is quite different from that of the epidermis. We have seen how the cells of the epidermis are constantly changing their position as they are pushed outwards towards the surface. No such change takes place in the dermis.

The dermis, moreover, is extremely well supplied with nerves, blood vessels and lymph vessels. It also contains large numbers of hair follicles, sweat (sudoriferous) and oil (sebaceous) glands.

SPECIAL FEATURES   Lying directly underneath the dermis is found a layer of "fat" cells. These special cells can store great quantities of fat (swelling as they do so). They are plentiful at certain places on the body (e.g., hips). Since the fat is used as a reserve supply of energy, when dieting, the size of these cells decreases and as a result we lose weight and size.

FUNCTIONS OF THE SKIN

In the introduction to this chapter, it was noted that the skin is not just an inert, passive covering of the body. In addition to its role as a reflector of our health and inner emotional state, the skin also performs a number of vital specific functions. The primary function of the skin is to protect the body against harmful materials entering it and from vital material leaking out.

SKIN FUNCTIONS:
1. Protection
2. Absorption
3. Sensitivity
4. Regulation of Body Temperature
5. Secretion
6. Excretion

PROTECTIVE FEATURES

The skin, because of its position on the body, is the first physical contact we have with the world around us. It is obvious that the skin must, therefore, be a protective wrapping for the entire body.

Its outer layer, the epidermis, is composed of relatively hard, resisting cells that protect the lower, delicate tissues against:

WARNING OF INJURY

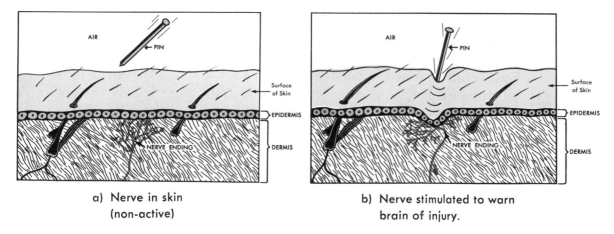

a) Nerve in skin (non-active)

b) Nerve stimulated to warn brain of injury.

MECHANICAL ATTACK

THICKENING OF SKIN The skin is subjected to much friction from the objects it comes into contact with in our daily lives. Certain areas of the skin (soles of the feet, palms of the hands) are specially thickened in order to provide for more protection; they come into contact with these objects more frequently. If the friction or pressure is too great, the skin may develop corns or bunions to warn us or even to prevent us from doing whatever it is that is causing such injury.

ACTION OF NATURAL OILS As a further means to prevent loss of the skin cells by friction, the skin possesses special glands called sebaceous glands, which, by secreting oils, are able to make the surface of the skin more slippery and thus serve as a protective coating. Sebum assists in the defense mechanism of the skin because of its ability to retard the growth of bacteria and fungi. These functions can be materially assisted by regular skin hygiene, especially on the scalp.

BACTERIAL ATTACK

HEALING OF CUTS IN THE SKIN An unbroken skin offers an excellent first line of defense against the entry of germs into the body. The epidermis, because of its remarkable property of reproduction, is able to quickly heal minor cuts and abrasions, thus preventing attack by bacteria. When a deep wound occurs, the doctor assists the skin by stitching the wound together so that healing will proceed at a faster pace. However, in this case, as damage to the skin has been more severe and a part of it destroyed, the new skin is usually non-pigmented and is known as scar tissue.

ACTION OF NATURAL OILS Certain bacteria and fungi can exist on the outside of the skin, but they are held in check by the sebum or natural oils from the sebaceous glands. Sebum is especially effective in preventing skin invasion by dangerous organisms.

CHEMICAL ATTACK

The skin is also exposed to the attack of certain chemicals, such as cold wave solution, which can destroy the epidermis. Due to the tough nature of its structure, it is able to resist destruction much more readily than other delicate tissues of the body.

WATER Another problem to be considered is the effect of water on the skin. The skin, itself 50–75% moisture, is able to maintain this level only by the secretion of sebum which coats its surface. This layer of oil slows down the evaporation of the water in the skin and prevents excess moisture from penetrating into it. But if the natural oils are removed by any means whatsoever, especially from the hands, this protection is lost.

Let us examine the case where the hands are excessively exposed to cold, drying winds. As the oil barrier is lost, the skin cannot prevent its cells from becoming dry and scaly (chafed). If further exposed to drying winds, cracking and bleeding takes place. This is more frequently noticed in winter than in summer, because the cold usually restricts the flow of blood to the dermis and the evaporation of the skin moisture cannot be balanced by a greater flow of blood and lymph.

PROTECTIVE ACTION OF SEBUM

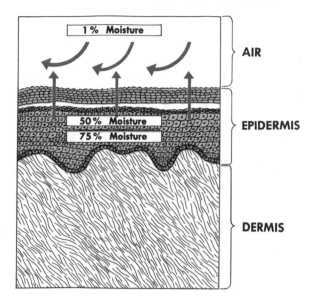

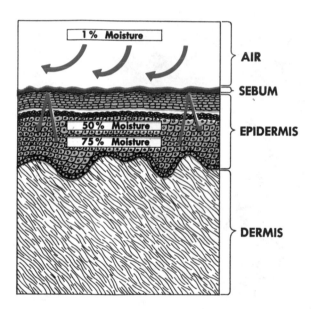

Summer increases the rate of sweating and this enables the skin to be kept naturally moist and prevents drying and chafing. On the other hand, if the skin is kept constantly in water, after the removal of oils, the skin soaks up some of the water and expands. This causes wrinkling and softening of the skin accompanied by discomfort.

PREVENTION OF CHEMICAL ATTACK Practitioners should take particular care of their hands because of their greater exposure to chemical attack. They should use protective creams in order to supplement the action of the natural oils.

NATURAL OPENINGS IN SKIN Although we have discussed the skin as an intact outer layer of the body, it is in fact penetrated by hair follicles with their sebaceous (oil) glands and by the pores of the sudoriferous (sweat) glands. These openings, although normally resistant to bacterial attack (except in certain cases where they show as pimples, boils, blackheads or acne), will allow the entry of special drugs and chemicals into the body. These chemicals may be absorbed in order to combat infections of the skin (e.g., antiseptic creams and ointments) or they may be used as skin conditioners to help overcome dryness or damage (e.g., vitamin and hormone creams).

Sweat from pores on palm of hand

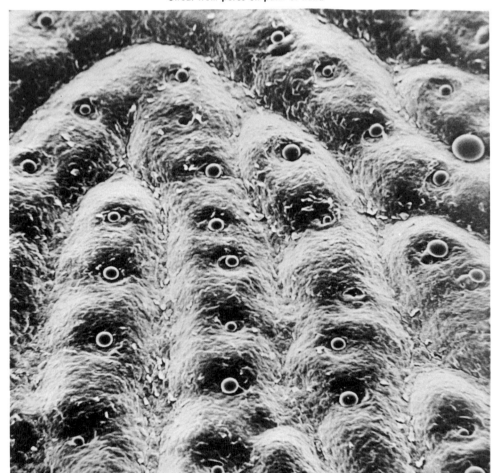

Courtesy: Isleworth Laboratory, Unilever Limited, Middlesex, England

SKIN FOODS The virtue of using skin "foods" in this manner is doubtful. No evidence suggests that the skin receives nutrition by absorption. But it is well recognized that the use of cosmetics containing oils, closely related to natural oils, benefit the epidermis by keeping it smooth and soft.

PHYSICAL AGENTS Various physical agents may also be absorbed by the skin and these include sunlight, x-rays and infra-red rays. Caution must be exercised to be certain that the amount of sunlight being absorbed is carefully controlled.

The epidermis contains a black pigment called melanin. An increase in the amount of this pigment is caused by exposure to the sun. This increase is known as "suntan." As tanning of the skin can be quite painful upon initial exposure, it is advisable to expose oneself to the sunlight for short periods only, until the pigment has been increased sufficiently to prevent sunburn. The use of an artificial "screen" in the form of a suntan preparation will assist the skin during the initial unprotected period. Otherwise, painful sunburn and blisters may occur.

PROTECTION FROM SUNS RAYS

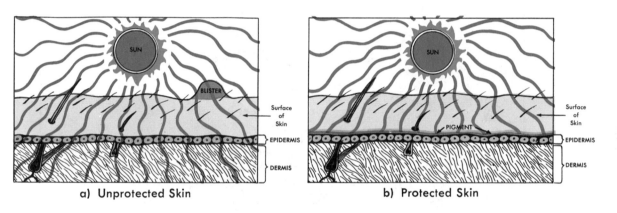

a) Unprotected Skin   b) Protected Skin

A certain amount of sunlight is of benefit for the maintenance of our general state of good health and vigor. However, excess exposure will cause skin to become leathery and may even lead to skin cancer.

SENSITIVITY

NERVES The skin is usually the first tissue or organ to come into contact with our outside world. For the purpose of keeping us well informed of our environment it is extremely well equipped with special cells, called nerves.

STRUCTURE The endings of each variety of these nerves are of a different construction and are able to pick up special signals and transmit them to the brain. The nerve endings react specifically to:

        a) pressure or touch;
        b) pain;
        c) heat;
        d) cold.

ACTION Each ending can send only one type of signal or sensation to the brain. For example, the ending for "heat." If we accidentally touch a hot stove, this nerve ending is activated and a message is sent quickly to the brain. A reflex action occurs and we automatically withdraw our hand from the stove preventing further injury.

Other sensations, such as the sense of smoothness, itching, tickling, etc., are considered to be the result of a combination of two or more of these specific nerve endings in action.

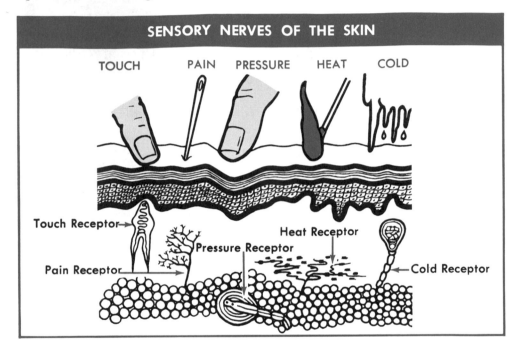

SENSORY NERVES OF THE SKIN

TOUCH   PAIN   PRESSURE   HEAT   COLD

Touch Receptor
Pain Receptor
Pressure Receptor
Heat Receptor
Cold Receptor

REGULATION OF BODY TEMPERATURE

Besides acting as a protective covering for the body, the skin is concerned with the regulation of body temperature. This it is able to do by a variation in the:

a) fatty layer
b) circulation of blood
c) evaporation of perspiration

FATTY LAYER This layer occurs below the dermis and is able to assist in the preservation of heat. In man its importance is not great, because man protects himself by artificial means, using warm clothing or heating devices. However, in some warm-blooded animals, especially those living in cold conditions, such as whales or walruses, it is vital to preserving life.

CIRCULATION OF BLOOD The dermis is well supplied with blood which passes through special blood vessels, the walls of which can be constricted or expanded, under the control of the nervous system.

Results of blood vessel constriction:

In cold weather the body attempts to conserve heat by exposing less blood to the skin surface. When the vessels are constricted, less blood flows to the skin and the decrease is shown by the following effects:

If the flow is restricted only to a minor extent, the skin appears bluish, and, because there is insufficient warmth being brought by the blood to the skin, the hands, feet, face and ears feel cold and uncomfortable. If the flow is completely shut off, the skin turns white. This extreme measure occurs under very cold conditions and is an attempt by the body to keep warm blood flowing to the more vital organs at the expense of the extremities. Warm clothing is essential under these conditions and the fingers, toes and ears, must be well protected.

Results of blood vessel expansion:

In summer, the position is reversed and there is often an abundance of warmth to be spread around the body. The blood vessels in the skin expand and more blood flows to the skin. The circulation of air over the skin picks up this extra heat that the body no longer requires and the body is cooled. We can assist this process by wearing light clothing during hot weather. One has only to consider the uncomfortable feelings of heat in an over-crowded room, especially if the windows happen to be closed, to realize how much body heat is given off through the skin, by all of the people present. The skin shows this extra circulation of blood by appearing pink or flushed.

Other effects:

In addition to these effects of the outside environment, various psychological factors may influence and control the circulation, particularly to the face. A sudden decrease of blood will cause the pallid, pale look of fear or fright. On the other hand, a sudden rush of blood to the face will cause blushing.

EVAPORATION OF SWEAT (Perspiration) It should be realized that control of the blood circulation only offers a gradual or slow method of regulating body temperature. When performing vigorous exercises, or when the temperature of the air approaches or exceeds that of the body, this method loses its effect.

Another extremely important method of controlling excess heat in the body is by the function of sweating. The evaporation of sweat serves to cool the skin and creates a drop in temperature.

Sweat (Sudoriferous) glands

The skin contains many small structures with openings (pores) leading to the surface of the skin. They are known as sweat (sudoriferous) glands. Under the control of the nerves, these sweat glands produce a substance known as sweat or perspiration.

There are about 2½ million of these glands in the skin and they excrete mainly water which, by evaporation, leads to a loss of heat from the body. In a normal, healthy person such a loss is automatic unless the surrounding air is extremely hot or humid. In this case, where evaporation is insufficient to prevent a sharp rise in temperature, heat distress may occur. In the very young or old person this distress may be fatal, unless artificial means such as bathing, cold towels, air conditioning or fans assist the sweating mechanism to decrease body temperature.

SWEAT GLAND

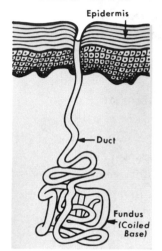

Epidermis

Duct

Fundus (Coiled Base)

Action of sweating

The cooling action of the evaporation of perspiration from the skin can be compared with the cooling effect that wind has on us when we emerge from the water after bathing. But, when we dry ourselves we immediately notice a rise in skin temperature which is pleasant if the air is cool, but uncomfortable if the air is hot.

Because of the nervous system's control over the sweat glands, sweating sometimes take place due to causes other than the temperature. Instances of this are sweating caused by fear or fright, and certain disorders of the body, such as fevers and malaria.

SECRETION

DEFINITION A secretion is defined as something produced by certain glands of the body that is useful to another part of the body.

FUNCTION OF SEBUM The secretion of the sebaceous gland, sebum, is of immense benefit to the skin and hair by coating them with a film of oil. This coating of oil is able to perform the following duties.

1. *It acts as an external lubricant* and keeps the surface of both the skin and hair smooth, giving them a characteristic slippery surface.

2. *It forms a slightly oily coating over skin and hair* and thus helps to prevent the excessive evaporation of moisture. If skin moisture is removed by excessive washing, or by strong solvents, the skin and hair very soon become dry and weakened.

This is especially true of the skin which contains from 50% to 75% moisture and requires the maintenance of this level to stay soft and supple. If excessive evaporation takes place it results in the shrinkage of the cells of the skin, with subsequent painful cracking or chafing when the skin is exposed to cold, dry winds.

EXCRETION

DEFINITION An excretion, on the other hand, is a substance that is produced by certain glands, but in itself is of no further use to the body.

SWEAT   Sweating is a function of the skin which is of prime importance to the maintenance of body health. The excretion or sweat produced, however, is of no use (except in the side effect of cooling the body) and in fact may become an embarrassment.

Sweat is mainly water (99.5%) with 0.5% being organic compounds and minerals. There are two types of sweat glands which function in the human body. The first type of sweat glands has the primary function of the production and secretion of water. The second type of sweat glands produces and secretes materials or chemicals which can lead to, so-called, body odors.

Contrary to popular belief, the axillae (armpits) become wet, not because of excessive sweating, but because the sweat evaporates from this region only with difficulty. Men as a rule tend to sweat more profusely than women.

BODY ODOR   Sweat occurs as a colorless fluid having a peculiar but not unpleasant odor (however, certain foods in the diet, such as garlic, spices, cheeses or asparagus can be detected in the perspiration). Bacterial decomposition soon sets in and the odor may then become obnoxious.

DEODORANTS AND ANTI-PERSPIRANTS   Control of body odor is exercised by body cleanliness (bathing), which removes sweat, together with the use of deodorants and anti-perspirants.

HOW THEY WORK:

1. By combining with the odor already produced to make it less unpleasant.
2. By reducing the number of bacteria on the skin.
3. By decreasing the amount of perspiration formed on areas where it is applied (anti-perspirant).

CARE OF THE SKIN

CONTROL OF SKIN HEALTH   Though the health of the skin is primarily under internal control, we do have direct access to its entire surface. This means we can do more to maintain it in good health than we can with most of our internal organs. But the skin is a very sensitive organ and if exposed to harsh cleansers or strong chemicals will soon show widespread damaging effects.

The sensible use of mild soap and warm water together with various cosmetics can do wonders in improving the skin. Cleansing and nourishing creams, lotions, skin conditioners and face powders have both a psychological and practical value in maintaining both its appearance and health.

DRY SKIN

The skin is normally protected by its tough character and natural oil (sebum). Dry skin is caused by a lack of this oil or by too little water being found in the skin. This complaint is common in people past their middle twenties. If your skin is dry, you should be careful not to use strong detergents or soaps, especially in the winter. Skin creams are helpful in correcting the low level of oils on the surface of the skin.

OILY SKIN

On the other hand, oily or greasy skin is often a problem in the teens. More frequent washing and avoiding oily lotions or cosmetics may improve the condition. Careful control of the diet, avoiding sweet and oily foods may often help clear up or improve the condition. The scalp, too, needs frequent shampooing, as an oily skin usually means an oily scalp.

But persons with an oily skin have compensation. Their difficulties are over by the time they reach their late twenties. The activity of the sebaceous glands then returns to normal.

EFFECTS OF AGE

As a person gets older, still other complications of the skin may arise. Causes of wrinkling and aging of the skin are not yet wholly understood even by expert dermatologists or skin specialists. These effects are connected with hormone changes and a breakdown of fat cells and the elastic tissue of the skin. New hormone creams, constantly being introduced, may be helpful in improving a dry or wrinkling skin.

ACTION OF SUNLIGHT

The rays of the sun also cause wrinkling of the skin. A heavy skin tan accelerates skin breakdown. Suntan lotion can screen out harmful rays and will help to prevent this damage. The skin around the eyes is the first to show wear. To avoid unnecessary squinting in strong glaring sunlight it is wise to wear sun glasses.

EFFECTS OF OVERWEIGHT

To prevent stretching the skin unduly, it is better to maintain a constant average weight. Excessive gain and loss in weight may create flabby skin around the neck and face.

CONCLUSION   In conclusion, it is fairly safe to say that what is best for your general health, happiness and appearance, is also best for your skin. However, great care must be exercised to maintain the health and appearance of this very vital body organ.

HAIR, ITS FUNCTION AND RELATED STRUCTURES

FUNCTION OF HAIR

Hair has a number of separate and distinct functions to perform. They are adornment, protection and warmth.

ADORNMENT

We are accustomed to the part that hair plays in the appearance and well being of the individual. On arising in the morning and at various intervals during the day, our composure and peace of mind is maintained by minor attentions to the hair. Very few of us would care to disregard elementary hair care and hygiene and appear in public with untidy, unmanaged and dishevelled hair. People seldom feel at ease unless they are sure of their appearance by having a quick check at frequent times during the day.

EXPRESSION OF PERSONALITY Individual grooming of the hair is often used as an indicator of personality. The professional must be careful to choose a hairstyle that is in harmony with the personality or wishes of the patron. We sometimes tend to overlook the fact that in our modern society the dictates of custom and mode of behavior also govern the fashions and practices associated with our hair.

DIFFERENT HAIR PRACTICES Certain groups have their own special attitudes toward the hair. An East Indian sect will not comb out or clean their hair and so it becomes long and matted. Other religious bodies follow the practice of growing long beards and hair.

INDICATIVE OF RANK In some primitive societies the hair is often an indicator of certain rank or ceremony. American Indians are well-known for the distinctive ways of wearing their hair. The Australian aborigine wails and tears at the hair when a close member of the tribe dies. In New Guinea the males make a great display of their headdress and wear many ornamental objects in it. In islands of the Pacific the warriors have huge bushy hairdos of which they are very proud. Some of these natives have, in the past few years, adopted the practice of lightening the hair and so becoming the envy of the less fortunate men of the village.

These customs are the opposite of our usual habits because we find it is the females who usually have the gaudy, colorful hair fashions in our community. But a look at the pages of history shows that this was not always the case. Once, it was the man who powdered and perfumed his long locks.

Another practice took place in the days of knighthood and chivalry when the hero cherished the few strands of hair that his lady fair had given him before he went off to defeat his enemies. The lock of hair served not only as a keepsake but was supposed to give some magical powers of protection to the holder.

BIOLOGICAL DIFFERENCES Biologically, there is a difference in the length of hair between the sexes. If the hair is left uncut, the female usually has the longer hair of the two. We have no real explanation for this. Humorously, it has been claimed the reason may well be that when our cavemen forefathers sought a wife, women with longer flowing hair were more easily caught.

COMMERCIAL IMPORTANCE OF HAIR Today we have a situation in which the care of the hair is of ever growing importance to our economy. Millions of dollars are spent annually on our hair and its care. The beauty and barber industries employ thousands of workers and indirectly are partly responsible for the ever increasing productivity of the country, because if we look and feel better, we also work much better.

PSYCHOLOGICAL VALUE OF ADORNMENT Lastly, we must not overlook the benefits of the good mental health and well-being of the community. This is assisted by the work of the artisan who gives professional attention to the decorative properties and condition of our hair.

PROTECTION

The most important task of hair is to assist the skin in protecting certain areas of the body. In fact, hair may be regarded as a specialized form of skin which, for the purpose of protection, has a more effective structure.

THE BRAIN The value of hair protection can be quickly recognized. The brain can be regarded as the most delicate and essential organ of the body.

A thick head of hair serves as a cushion to a possible bump on the head and possible injury to the brain. The brain is also protected by the hard bony framework of the skull.

Over the ages, man has experienced a general reduction in body hair. However, this is not true in the case of the scalp. This suggests that scalp hair still has a very important protective purpose. This fact was realized by primitive natives and many of their massive hairstyles were worn by the males to help them ward off the effects of an otherwise fatal blow.

EYES   The eyes are protected by the hairs of the eyelashes and those of the eyebrows.

ACTION OF EYELASHES   The eyelashes are extremely sensitive and cause a reflex shutting of the eyelids whenever a foreign object comes within contact range.

ACTION OF EYEBROWS   The eyebrows serve to divert water, sweat, oils, or chemical substances from running down the brow and into the eyes from the scalp. For this reason it is unwise to completely pluck the eyebrows.

EARS AND NOSE   The ears and nose have special hairs which line the delicate passages of these organs. Particles of dust in the air which may enter are trapped by these protective hairs.

Regular movements of the internal hairs by beating carries the debris away from the internal organs, thus keeping them clean and functioning properly.

BODY   The body is protected from friction, caused by muscular movements and the wearing of clothing, by having hairs in the areas where that movement usually takes place. For example, the hairs under the armpits are to prevent the danger caused by rubbing of the arms and the body together at this joint. They also assist in the evaporation of sweat from this area by increasing the surface air contact with the droplets of sweat.

WARMTH

PREHISTORIC FUNCTION OF HAIR   It may be another fundamental purpose of hair to help keep us warm. Certainly, prehistoric man is thought to have possessed a great deal of hair that almost completely covered his body, thus giving protection from the cold, wind, rain and sun. Later on he borrowed the feathers and skins of animals for this purpose.

Because of the wearing of clothing (taking away one of the functions of hair), man continually loses hair. It may well be as a result of this continuing loss that in the distant future, hair may cease to exist and both males and females will be completely bald. The hair on the scalp reminds us of this property of warmth each time the hair is shaped (cut). We feel the cold winds, particularly on the back of the neck. However, the skin becomes adjusted to this very quickly and in a few days we hardly notice the difference. Clothing itself has displaced the biological need for protection and warmth that the hair formerly provided for mankind.

THE HAIR FOLLICLE

ORIGIN OF THE FOLLICLE The growth of hair is caused by the development of small pockets in the skin, which are called follicles.

Quite some time before birth, certain changes take place in the epidermis. At first, small pits or depressions develop in the outer layers. These depressions gradually grow deeper into the underlying dermis. Finally they develop the form of mature follicles.

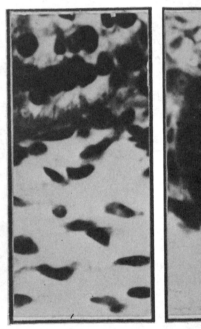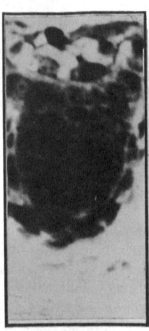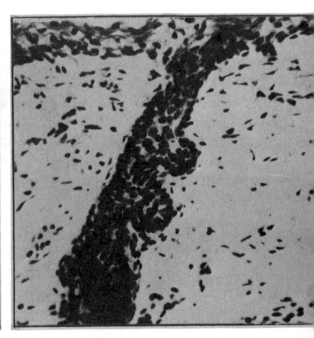

FORMATION OF FOLLICLE
Three stages in the development of hair follicles in the scalp approximately six months before birth.—Courtesy: *Structure & Function of Skin—Academic Press*

IMPORTANT FEATURES You will note that there is *NO* break or hole in the epidermis in the formation of the follicle. This important outside layer of the skin dips down into the bottom of the follicle and remains as a protective covering. Thus there is no actual break in the skin at all.

However, the epidermis of the follicle lacks the dry, scaly nature seen on the upper, outer layers. If we pluck a living hair out of its follicle, some of the follicle wall tears away. This is what you see as a whitish blob of soft tissue at the bottom of the hair shaft.

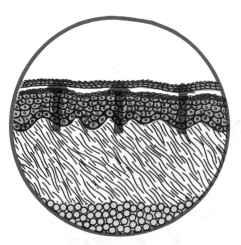

1—Undeveloped Skin

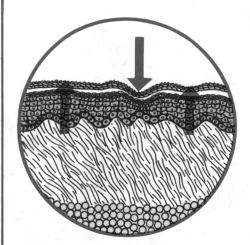

2—Beginnings of follicle

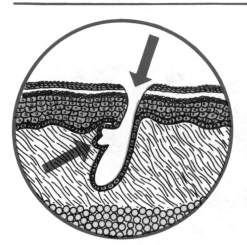

3—Formation of sebaceous gland

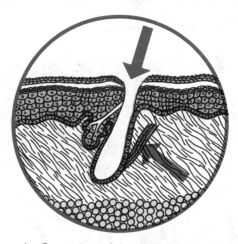

4—Formation of Arrector Pili Muscle

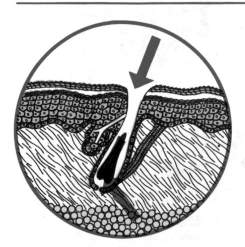

5—Formation of Papilla

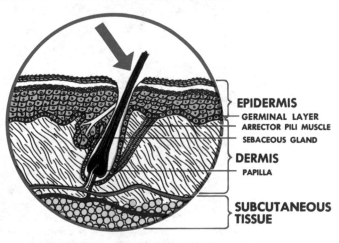

6—Growth of young hair

EPIDERMIS
GERMINAL LAYER
ARRECTOR PILI MUSCLE
SEBACEOUS GLAND

DERMIS
PAPILLA

SUBCUTANEOUS TISSUE

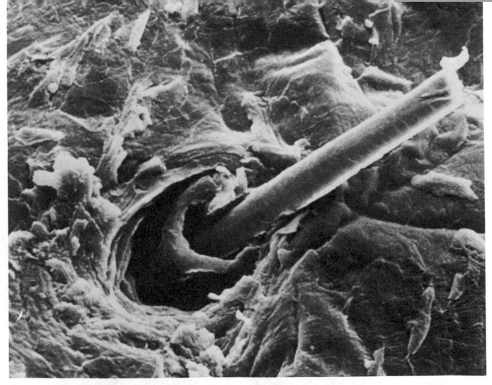

Single hair growing from follicle, magnified 600 times. This is an excellent view of the follicle opening and the sheath around the base of the hair.

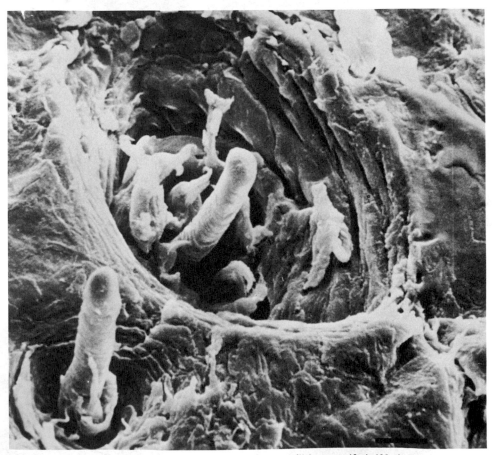

Multiple hairs growing from what appears to be a single follicle, magnified 630 times. Notice follicle architecture which is clearly shown in the center. *Courtesy: Gillette Company Research Institute, Maryland*

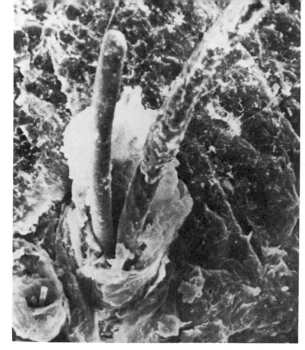

Photo of human skin, magnified 360 times, showing two hairs emerging from what appears to be a single follicle. Also notice two fine hairs emerging from follicle in lower left corner.

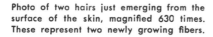

Photo of two hairs just emerging from the surface of the skin, magnified 630 times. These represent two newly growing fibers.

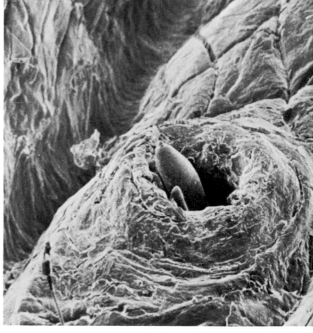

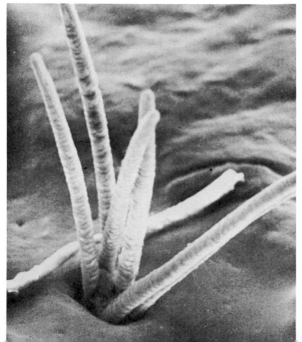

Multiple hairs growing from what appears to be a single follicle, magnified 780 times, obtained from the forehead of a young male.

Courtesy: Gillette Company Research Institute, Rockville, Maryland

DISTRIBUTION OF FOLLICLES   Nearly the entire surface of the skin is covered with thousands and thousands of these follicles. Most of them remain inactive and never produce hairs. On the other hand, some are very active, particularly on the scalp. Other follicles may only produce hairs at a definite period in our lives, e.g., beard follicles of adult males. Still others will produce hairs in certain abnormal situations, e.g., on the face of women suffering from a disturbance of the glands.

STRUCTURE OF THE FOLLICLE   Let us examine the features of a mature, active scalp follicle.

1. It is a complete pocket in the skin formed by a downgrowth of the epidermis.
2. At the bottom of the follicle is found a small upgrowth of the dermis called the papilla.
3. The follicle does not dip directly downwards at right angles to the surface of the skin. It is sloped at some angle.

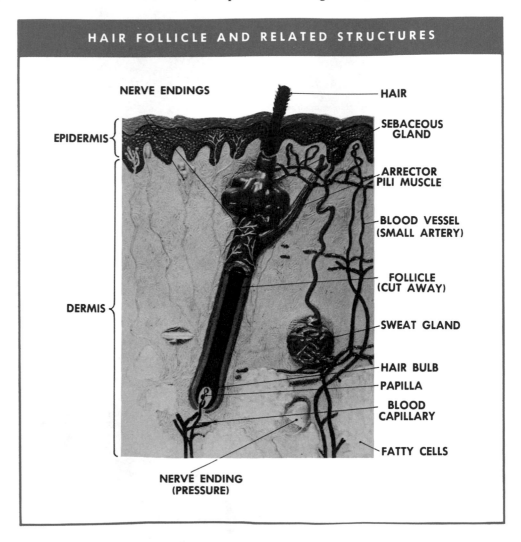

HAIR FOLLICLE AND RELATED STRUCTURES

NERVE ENDINGS
HAIR
SEBACEOUS GLAND
EPIDERMIS
ARRECTOR PILI MUSCLE
BLOOD VESSEL (SMALL ARTERY)
FOLLICLE (CUT AWAY)
DERMIS
SWEAT GLAND
HAIR BULB
PAPILLA
BLOOD CAPILLARY
FATTY CELLS
NERVE ENDING (PRESSURE)

4. Around the follicle is found a network of nerves. These are directly connected to the brain. If a live hair is plucked from the follicle these nerves transmit a message of pain.

5. On one side, the follicle has a small muscle (the arrector pili muscle) attached to it.

6. The follicles are not scattered evenly on the scalp but are grouped together. These groups contain from 2 to 5 hairs each.

7. Around the mouth of the follicle the skin dips down to form a small depression. These hollows are clearly visible in the grooves on the surface of the skin.

8. Sometimes the mouths of two separate follicles come together. Compound hairs can be seen and it appears that two hairs grow from the same follicle. However, each hair still has its own individual papilla at the bottom of each follicle.

STRUCTURE OF THE PAPILLA

1. This is an upgrowth of the dermis at the bottom of the follicle.

2. It is shaped like an inverted light globe or like a door knob, the neck of the papilla (at the base) being the narrowest section.

3. It is richly supplied with small blood vessels and these supply the growing hair with nourishment.

4. The outer portion of the papilla comes in contact with the germinal matrix and transfers nutrients to the germinative cells. These cells are able to change their supplies of food materials into keratin and thus form the hair.

5. Unfortunately, the papilla sometimes degenerates and the follicle is unable to continue producing hair. Thinning of hair and baldness is caused by a condition of the papilla.

6. The hair bulb is firmly clamped or anchored over the papilla. This, and the narrowness of the follicle, prevents the hair from being pulled out easily.

7. The papilla is an essential structure of the follicle and hair owes its very existence to its activity.

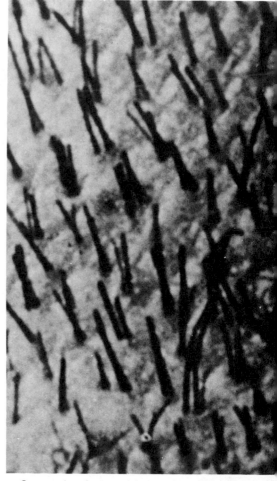

Compound and grouped hairs.—*Courtesy of Hair and Scalp—Edward Arnold*

Note:

The hair is not like a plant growing in the soil with an independent life of its own, but is a special part of the skin which is growing outwards.

ARRECTOR PILI MUSCLE

This is a primitive type of muscle found associated with the hair follicle. It is attached to the wall of the follicle and to the lower layer of the epidermis.

Contraction of this muscle pulls the hairs more upright. At the same time the whole follicle is raised a little and now is at a higher level than the surrounding skin. This action of the muscle causes what is commonly known as "goose-pimples."

Goose-pimples are triggered by cold or fright. Since man has lost most of his body hair, this is now a rather ineffective way of combating coldness. The hairs are trying to create a blanket of warm, still air around the body in a manner similar to birds that fluff out their feathers on a cold day.

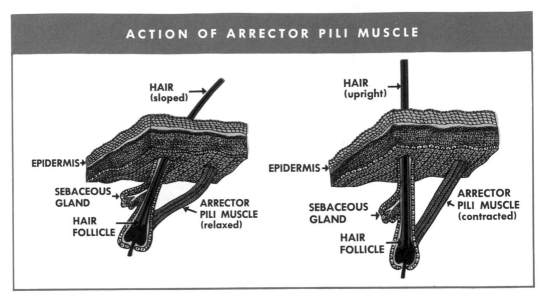

ACTION OF ARRECTOR PILI MUSCLE

Often this is accompanied by shivering. This is another uncontrollable activity which in itself is an attempt by the body to generate warmth by continuous contractions of the muscles.

In the case of shock or fear, goose-pimples show the complete interaction of the nervous system and the hair follicle.

SEBACEOUS GLANDS

The wall of the follicle is specially modified to form the sebaceous (oil) gland. This gland manufactures a special natural oil (sebum) which is essential to the maintenance of a normal skin and hair condition.

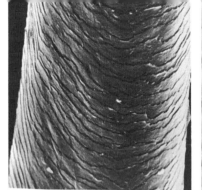
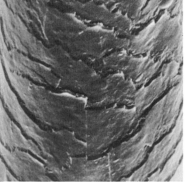

Normal hair magnified 2500 times.   Normal hair magnified 5000 times.
Courtesy: Gillette Company Research Institute, Rockville, Maryland

THE STRUCTURE
OF THE HAIR

Introduction

The hair is a special arrangement of hard keratin. It develops by the reproduction of cells from the germinal layers of the skin in distinctive structures known as follicles. As the cells move up the follicle, toward the skin surface, the amino acids (building blocks of all protein) they contain, join together to create the principal three components or parts of the hair fiber. On close examination of the visible part of the hair fiber, it is found that these components or parts are arranged into three separate and distinct layers:

1. Cuticle
2. Cortex
3. Medulla

Each one of these layers has its own functions as indicated by the following.

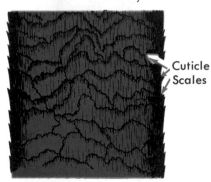
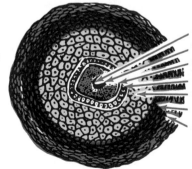

Cuticle
Scales

Medulla of Hair
Cortex of Hair
Cuticle of Hair
Inner or Epidermic Coat
Outer or Dermic Coat
Inner Root Sheath
Outer Root Sheath

**MAGNIFIED VIEW OF
HAIR CUTICLE**

**CROSS SECTION OF THE
HAIR AND FOLLICLE**

CUTICLE

DESCRIPTION   This is the layer on the outside of the hair shaft. It consists of hard, flattened, horny scales which overlap one another to the extent that five to seven scales are found in the length of one scale. In other words, at any point along the hair shaft *the cuticle can be as many as seven scales in thickness,* however, extreme cases have been found with as many as eleven layers.

This gives a very strong, flexible arrangement, similar to that of the scales of a fish. The cuticle layer permits the waving of hair, but does not, by any means, cause this waving by itself.

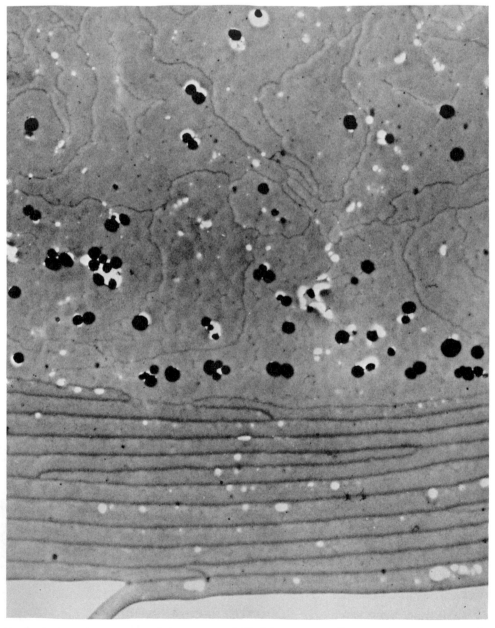

A photo of cuticle layers around the cortex, magnified 14,800 times. Eleven cuticle layers can actually be counted overlaying the cortex. The dark black spots represent melanin granules in the fibers of the cortex.   *Courtesy: Gillette Company Research Institute, Rockville, Maryland*

IMBRICATIONS   The free ends of these overlapping, sloping, flat scales (called imbrications) point upwards and outwards in the direction of hair growth. If a strand of hair is rubbed lengthwise between the finger and thumb, you will find that the fingers will slide freely in the direction of the hair ends. This is because the imbrications, pointing toward the tip of the hair, facilitate movement in this direction. Greater resistance is encountered when attempting to slide the fingers toward the root.

The arrangement of protruding scaly edges also allows for the easy removal, by brushing, of undesirable material such as: flaking skin or scalp cells, dirt particles, etc., which otherwise would accumulate on the scalp surface.

THE FUNCTION of the cuticle is to protect the more delicate cortex from injury. If the cuticle is damaged by excessive lightening, permanent wave solutions or harsh chemicals, the cortex is exposed to injury.

If steps are not taken to avoid further damage to the cuticle, the cortex could be destroyed or weakened. The cuticle is unusually resistant to chemical breakdown, but it cannot withstand careless treatment.

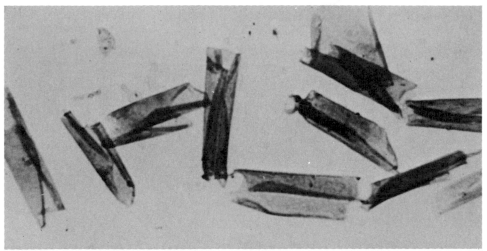

Cuticle scales after removal from hair shaft.—*(Courtesy: Unilever Limited)*

SPLIT ENDS   At the ends or tips of the hair shaft the cuticle is often dislodged or broken away. The cortex is thus open to the drying effects of air, leading to frayed and split ends, which look unsightly and ragged. For this reason alone it is advisable to keep the hair trimmed in an effort to prevent this type of cuticle damage to the hair.

SPLIT HAIR ENDS

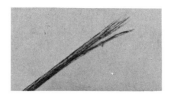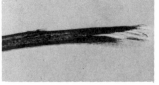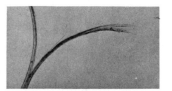

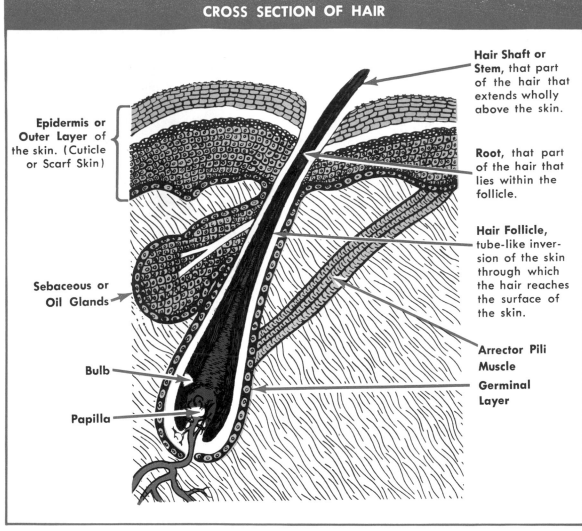

Epidermis or Outer Layer of the skin. (Cuticle or Scarf Skin)

Sebaceous or Oil Glands

Bulb

Papilla

Hair Shaft or Stem, that part of the hair that extends wholly above the skin.

Root, that part of the hair that lies within the follicle.

Hair Follicle, tube-like inversion of the skin through which the hair reaches the surface of the skin.

Arrector Pili Muscle

Germinal Layer

ADDITIONAL POINTS OF INTEREST

The cuticle scales act as tiny reservoirs in which the supply of sebum is maintained. If the cuticle was smooth this vital oil would be easily washed or rubbed off. The natural sheen of healthy hair is primarily due to this coating of sebum on the cuticle and its complete loss could cause hair to become dull and drab.

Because of the projecting nature of the scales and their oil coating, they catch much dirt, debris, broken scales and other foreign matter. Frequent shampooing is necessary to keep the hair clean and hygienic. Removal of excess oils and dirt assists the proper penetration of permanent wave solutions, tints, or other hair products into the cortex.

The cuticle is also used as a base for the deposit of hair sprays, lacquers, conditioners, fillers and other hair cosmetics.

The type of cuticle scales can vary widely from loose, open scales to tight, firm scales. The degree of porosity depends, to a large extent, on the nature of the cuticle surface. Whether the hair is porous or resistant depends on the type of cuticle it has.

CORTEX

The cortex is the most important layer of the hair and makes up from 75% to 90% of its bulk. In fact it may be said that practically all the well-known behavior of human hair is due to this most important layer.

The physical properties of the hair which depend upon the cortex are:

1. Strength
2. Elasticity
3. Pliability
4. Direction and manner of growth
5. Size or diameter.
6. Texture and quality.

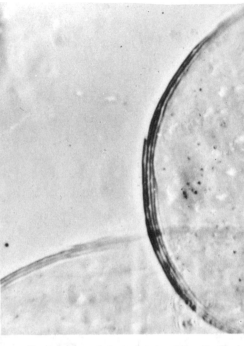

Cross-section of human hairs (magnified 500 times) showing cortex with overlapping scales of cuticle.—(Courtesy of Wool Industries Research Council)

THE NATURAL COLOR of the hair is due to the pigment in the cortex. For a natural looking tint it is necessary therefore to get cosmetic coloring matter into this layer.

THE NATURAL WAVE of the hair comes from physical changes in the cortex. These changes take place in the follicle before the hair is fully developed. Permanent waving, on the other hand, involves chemically induced changes in the cortex of mature hair. Curling, and all forms of hairstyling, depend for their results on artificial alterations to the structure of the cortex.

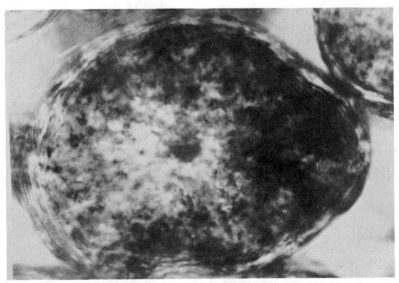

Cross-section of a straight hair. Note pigment in cortex and medulla. (Magnified 300 times.)

THE PHYSICAL STRUCTURE of the cortex is very complicated. It is made of many millions of parallel fibers of hard keratin, often referred to as polypeptide chains. These parallel fibers are twisted around one another, something very much like heavy rope in appearance.

STRENGTH Because of the nature of the cortex it gives the hair great strength and elasticity. In fact, it is claimed that human hair is stronger than copper wire of the same diameter. A single strand of hair, in good condition, will support a weight of approximately 5 to 7 ozs.

The rate and direction of growth of hair is controlled by cell division at the papilla in the follicle.

Courtesy: Gillette Company Research Institute, Rockville, Maryland

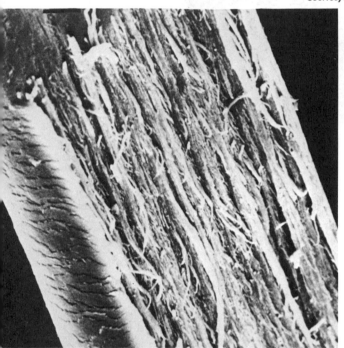

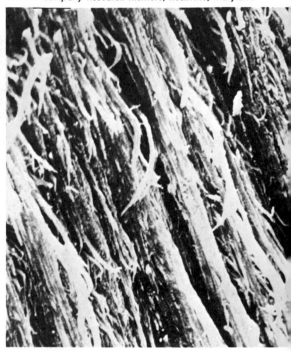

Hair fiber with part of the cuticle stripped off exposing the cortex, magnified 1470 times. Cortical fibrils can be clearly seen. Notice the vast difference in architecture of the interior of a fiber as compared to the surface.

This is a photo of the same hair structure magnified 4200 times. This gives a closer view of the cortical fibers.

EFFECTS OF LACK OF KNOWLEDGE At no other stage in history has the condition of the hair in the community been worse than it is today. Many unthinking and untrained persons try to do things to their hair for which it is wholly unsuited. Materials are available to supply the whims of everyone who desires changes in the hair. However, knowledge is required to insure their proper application and usage and to avoid a breakdown in hair structure.

The practitioner must know what can be done and what must NOT be done to the cortex and cuticle of the hair if permanent damage is to be avoided. It is the proper application of professional knowledge and skill which will help to eliminate or minimize damage to or loss of hair.

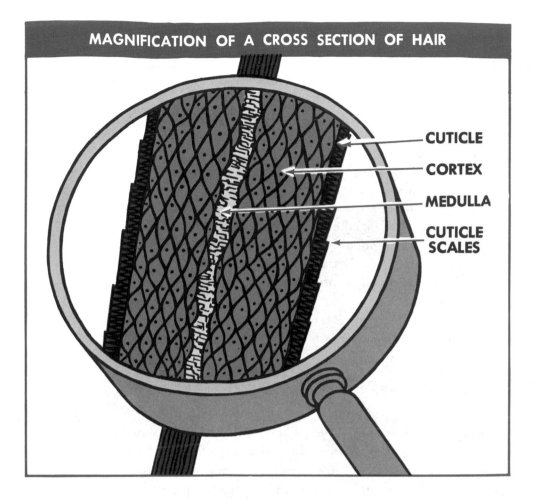

MAGNIFICATION OF A CROSS SECTION OF HAIR

CUTICLE

CORTEX

MEDULLA

CUTICLE
SCALES

MEDULLA

This is the middle layer of the hair. It is made up of a column of cells, two or four rows wide.

The medulla is not always a continuous part of the hair but it is frequently broken or even entirely absent from the hair shaft. This condition is often found in hair and it is suspected that the state of health and the taking of certain medicines has a direct bearing on its absence.

The purpose or function of the medulla is unknown. Hair does not seem to suffer when it is missing. It is made of soft keratin, whereas the cuticle and cortex are formed of hard keratin. Pigment of the hair is often found in this layer as well.

CONCLUSION

We have discussed the differing structures of the two main parts of the hair (cortex and cuticle). The reason for these differences is that each layer has to perform separate and distinct functions. These distinctions in function have resulted in the separation into two structures which are composed of different arrangements of hard keratin.

In the case of the hair we have a fine example of a biological marvel known as the "division of labor."

THE "DIVISION OF LABOR" means more than a mere specialization of structure or order. It also tells us that there is a certain interdependence between the cuticle and the cortex.

Examples:

1. The cuticle is tough and will resist wear or friction but has no strength.
2. The cortex has great strength but is not tough or able to resist wear or friction.
3. The cuticle protects the cortex, but does not hold it together. The cortex holds together very well, but is easily damaged.
4. *The cuticle allows waving and setting* to take place, but *only the cortex is able to be waved or set.*
5. The cuticle allows the hair to be stretched, but only the cortex is elastic.
6. The cortex requires a certain amount of moisture to remain soft and pliable, but only the porosity of the cuticle permits moisture to be absorbed or dried out.

THE RESPONSIBILITY OF THE PROFESSIONAL

The practitioner must always remember that the hair is designed for natural purposes and no other. There is a certain amount of freedom provided for, as the hair has an unusual but very effective design to allow for a wide margin of stress and strain. But the lesson of science is that we cannot afford to ignore the natural properties of the hair. Hair simply does not exist solely for the convenience of the cosmetologist or barber.

Hair has no power of self-repair as in the case of the skin. If the hair is damaged, little can be done to restore it except to cut off the damaged portion or apply treatments which have been found to be somewhat beneficial.

CHAPTER 6

THE NATURE
OF HAIR PROTEIN

THE COMPLEXITY OF HAIR

The structure of the hair is an important study, but it is only within recent years that science has been able to discover the real facts about its complicated nature. Although hair is, of course, a very well-known substance, it is rather difficult to examine closely. For one thing, it varies greatly from one person to another and even each individual may show variations in structure along a single hair fiber. Nevertheless, there are now known certain common features of hair, for it is a type of protein called *HARD* KERATIN.

PAPILLA

The outer layer of the cells of the papilla are continually producing new cells by a process called "cell division." The outer layer of the cells of the papilla is called the "germ" layer and is the same layer that is present at the bottom of the epidermis of the skin. However, the germ layer of the epidermis forms only SOFT KERATIN. The germ layer of the papilla is concerned with forming HARD KERATIN.

Since most of the hair consists of the cortex layer, the greatest number of the cells of the germ layer of the papilla are concerned with forming the hard keratin of the cortex. The continual production of these cells which will form the cortex, results in an upward and outward growth of hair. The most recent cells are closest to the papilla while the older cells are furthest from the papilla.

PROTEINS

Proteins are complicated organic compounds essential for life. As organic substances, proteins contain the elements carbon, hydrogen and oxygen, and, in addition, they supply the element nitrogen to the body. As nitrogen is essential for cell structures, a daily intake of food protein is vital.

AMINO-ACIDS

The basic units or building blocks of proteins are called amino-acids. There are about twenty of the amino-acids known to science. The structure and formula of each amino-acid is known and each has been named (several of them are glycine, tyrosine, cystine and cysteine).

"A GRADE" PROTEINS   Certain proteins contain the element sulphur. Proteins with a high level of sulphur are called "A grade" proteins. Examples of foods rich in A grade proteins are meats, eggs, fish and milk.

The wide range of proteins available indicates the complexity of this vital food material. Despite the seemingly wide differences in appearance, structure, smell and taste, all proteins are made of the same basic units, amino-acids.

"B GRADE" PROTEINS   However, not all proteins have every one of these amino-acids present. "B grade proteins are deficient in certain amino-acids which have the element sulphur in their structure.

Even when all amino-acids are present, the percentage of each may vary from one source to another. For example, not all meats, such as pork, beef, lamb, chicken, game, etc., are identical in amino-acids.

Even in the same meat range, different cuts contain varying amounts of the same amino-acids. Whether the cut is young and tender or old and tough will also change the amino-acid content.

SIMPLE PROTEIN

Not only is the amount of each amino-acid important, but the arrangement of the individual amino-acids themselves fix the nature of that protein.

Each amino-acid is joined end-on-end by chemical bonds called peptide or end-bonds. Furthermore, the amino-acids are joined together in a definite order. The determination of this exact order is a problem confronting the modern biochemist. So far, only simple proteins (such as insulin) have had their precise amino-acid arrangement fully investigated.

However, the strings of amino-acids, chemically joined together by peptide bonds (which are found in all proteins) are called polypeptides (poly = many). These polypeptides may simply form into long, coiled chains containing many hundreds of amino-acids. "Simple" proteins like this are found in milk, raw eggs or blood. *Simple proteins are water-soluble* and are easily broken down in the digestive system of the body.

PROTEINS

SIMPLE PROTEIN (Highly Magnified)

PEPTIDE BOND

SULFUR AMINO-ACID
(Cysteine)

AMINO-ACIDS

EXAMPLES FOUND IN
EGGS, MILK, BLOOD, ETC.

COMPLEX PROTEIN (Section)

PEPTIDE BOND

POLYPEPTIDE
CHAIN

SULFUR BOND
(Cystine)

EXAMPLES FOUND IN
MEAT, CHEESE, FISH, ETC.

DIGESTION

DIGESTION

SULFUR AMINO-ACID
(Cysteine)

(Cystine)

BLOOD CIRCULATION

SUMMARY

PROTEINS ARE MADE FROM MILLIONS OF SMALL RESIDUES CALLED AMINO-ACIDS (Approximately 20 Types). THE AMINO-ACIDS ARE JOINED LENGTHWISE BY PEPTIDE OR END BONDS TO FORM LONG CHAINS OF POLYPEPTIDES.

POLYPEPTIDE CHAINS MAY BE:

1. SIMPLE SPIRAL OR ROUND CHAINS. THESE ARE EASILY DIGESTED, RELEASING CONTAINED AMINO-ACIDS.

2. COMPLEX CHAINS BOUND TOGETHER BY CROSS BONDS OF CYSTINE OR SULFUR TYPE.

PROTEINS MAY CONSIST OF:

A GRADE TYPE (fish meat, eggs, milk, etc.) THAT CONTAIN HIGH LEVELS OF SULFUR AMINO-ACIDS (Cystine & Cysteine).

B GRADE TYPE (beans, peas, cereals, nuts, etc.) CONTAIN LOW LEVEL OF SULFUR AMINO-ACIDS.

53

COMPLEX PROTEIN

More complicated proteins form when adjacent spirals of polypeptides are cross-linked by other bonds. The strongest link occurs when sulphur-amino-acids (such as cysteine or cystine) are opposite to one another on adjacent polypeptide chains.

CYSTINE or sulphur bonds give added strength to the properties of that protein and the cross-bonds give them a tougher texture.

During digestion of food proteins, certain protein-splitting enzymes are secreted by the digestive system. These enzymes split the peptide bonds, thus releasing the amino-acids of the protein.

These amino-acids are water-soluble and therefore can be easily absorbed by the body. The amino-acids pass into the blood circulation for distribution throughout the body.

Regardless of the type of protein in the diet, the body reduces it completely into the individual amino-acids. For this reason different diets can still provide us with the necessary amino-acids.

Another class of proteins is found which cannot be broken down. These exceedingly complicated proteins are known as "fiber" proteins. They consist of countless numbers of polypeptide chains twisted around and around into long fibers.

FIBER PROTEINS

Fiber proteins possess exceptional numbers of cross-bonds. In fact half the weight of fiber proteins is due to these cross-bonds.

Examples of fiber proteins are human and animal hair, natural silk and the horns of some animals.

Although the keratin of human hair is a protein, it cannot be formed by consuming other fiber proteins for they are not digestible to humans. The amino-acids needed for the formation of hair can only come from edible proteins.

Furthermore, these edible proteins must be especially rich in sulphur to supply the cross-bonds needed for fiber proteins, such as hair keratin.

FORMATION OF HARD KERATIN IN HAIR

A—Amino-acids leave the bloodstream

The formation of hair begins with the digestion of proteins in the diet. These proteins are broken down to release their amino-acids into the bloodstream. *These amino-acids eventually reach the blood capillaries in each papilla and the follicle cells surrounding the germinal matrix.*

The wall of the blood capillary has minute cracks thru which fluids are constantly seeping. These fluids bathe the cells with a supply of nourishment and amino-acids. The red and while cells remain in the blood vessel and continue around in the circulation.

FORMATION OF HARD KERATIN IN HAIR

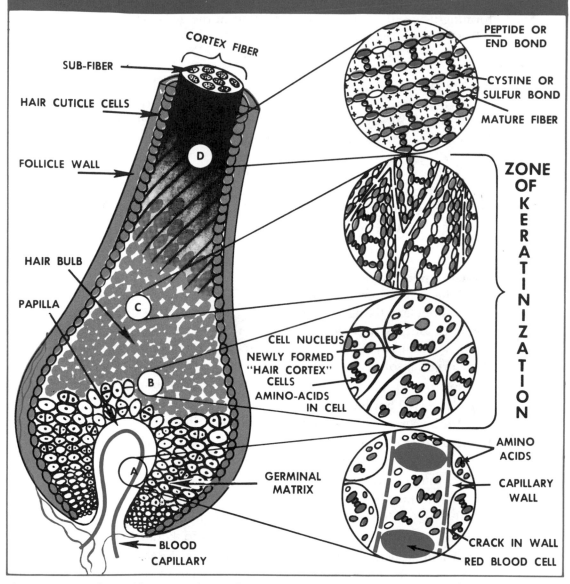

A. Amino acids in blood circulation leave the capillaries thru minute cracks in vessel walls.

B. Hair cortex cells are constantly formed in the germinal matrix of the hair bulb. Selected amino acids (rich in sulfur) from A enter these new cells and are randomly scattered within cell contents.

C. In each cell (pushed up from B) amino acids are orientated into one direction. These amino acids are then joined together (by peptide or end bonds) in short strings of keratin. Cystine or sulfur cross bonds link adjacent keratin strings together. Cell nucleus and wall disappear. Hydrogen bonds assist crosslinkage as cortex loses moisture. (Not shown on diagram).

D. Hard Keratin from C results from complete coupling of keratin chains into a twisting complex structure. Hydrogen bonds are now present. These twisted bundles are called sub-fibers. The sub-fibers are also twisted around each other to form the cortex fiber.

The cell fluids eventually reach the outer layer of the papilla. This layer of special cells is part of the epidermis and is in contact with the germinative area or germinal matrix.

The function of the germinal matrix is to continually divide, thus forming new cells. This repeated division in the germ area pushes the older cells slowly up the follicle.

B—The Germinative Area

When first formed, these new cells are similar to those of the germinal matrix itself. As such, they contain a nucleus and a well-defined cell membrane. Their cell contents are quite fluid (more than 75% of the cell is water).

Inside the cell contents are found the amino-acids which have seeped from the blood capillaries. There is also some evidence to suggest that more amino-acids enter the cells from the follicle wall and, quite possibly, enter into the formation of the cuticle layer.

C—Early phase of keratinization

The cells of growing hair, when first produced, are soft and liquid filled. They are living cells, containing amino-acids scattered within their contents. But, as they slowly move up the follicle they begin to change in appearance and by the time they have travelled 1/3 of the way, they have lost their original soft, cell-like look.

Further up the follicle we find still older cells, but these have changed considerably. They have become part of the cortex layer.

In the cortex part of the hair the nucleus dies and the cell wall or membrane disappears. The contents of the former cells shrink in volume as the water is removed to a much lower level than in the hair bulb (finally down to 10% in the mature hair).

In the first formed cells of the cortex, next to the germ layer of the papilla, the amino-acids are scattered throughout the contents of the cell. Gradually they join together to form the hard keratin type of chains of amino-acids. Then, as the cell walls disappear (in the zone of keratinization) these chains link up crosswise with chains of adjacent cells into a spiral. The result is a long fiber. In the hair cortex, it is no longer possible to see the original cells, although they can be isolated by special methods. In addition, large numbers of cystine or sulphur cross-bonds join these parallel polypeptide chains together. As the moisture level drops, other bonds, called hydrogen or physical bonds, gradually appear.

The hard keratin of the cuticle forms in a different manner than the cortex, since it makes a loose, scaly covering around the hair. However, the hard keratin of the cuticle has few of the features of the cortex.

The cells in the cuticle layer also lose moisture and become harder and scalier, but, unlike those cells in the cortex, remain somewhat separated.

D—Mature fiber

This part of the hair fiber has reached the upper extent of the zone of keratinization. In other words, the amino-acids from the germ layer are fully converted to keratin. Keratin is the hard fiber protein of hair. All visible sign of the original cells has gone. Special enzymes can separate these cells which show as elongated structures.

However, in the normal cortex we find *it is made of countless billions of long polypeptide chains* as arranged in a characteristic fiber.

The polypeptide chains are joined together by large numbers of cross-bonds. Both sulphur and hydrogen bonds form links that give the polypeptide chains a very strong arrangement.

SUB-FIBERS

These strengthened polypeptide chains are called keratin. The keratin chains are twisted around each other into many bundles called sub-fibers. These sub-fibers are in turn twisted around each other to form hard keratin. The cortex can be likened to a series of coil-springs all twisted around each other. The number of sub-fibers in the hair cortex is not known but it is very large. Around the cortex in the mature hair fiber are found the flattened, hardened scales of the cuticle cells. These scales exist as overlapping layers which protect the cortex without restricting its flexibility.

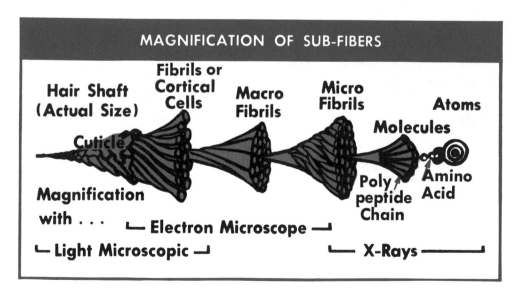

Thus the cuticle layer is somewhat like a column of paper ice-cream buckets. They give protection, but still retain their individual movement for extending when the hair is stretched.

The remarkable properties of hair are due to the combined action of both cortex and cuticle. A knowledge of their individual structures is essential to the proper understanding of hair.

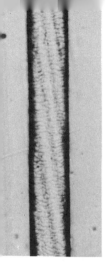

Arrangement of twisted chains of hard keratin sub-fibers in hair cortex.

BONDS OF THE HAIR CORTEX

In the performance of hair services, the practitioner must alter or change the structure of the hair cortex in many ways. It is only by taking a look at the detailed nature of the hard keratin that an understanding of these important changes can be achieved.

END-BONDS OR PEPTIDE BONDS

Each amino-acid is joined to another by peptide bonds, forming a chain as long as the hair. They are the strongest bonds in the cortex, and most of the strength of hair is due to their properties.

End-bonds are chemical bonds, and if even a few are broken, the hair will be weakened or become damaged. If many of these bonds are broken, the hair will break off.

Once end-bonds are broken there is no way of reforming them. If serious damage has occurred, the only thing that can be done is to wait until that section of hair grows out to a sufficient length to be trimmed off.

AGENTS BREAKING END-BONDS
1. *Chemical*
   Strong alkalies and acids, strong waving solutions or lighteners.
2. *Physical*
   Excessive stretching or cutting.

CROSS-BONDS

It is the presence of cross-bonds or links that has given hard keratin its unique properties. Hair contains more cross-bonds than any other protein. Hair can resist decay better than any other protein and it is also undigestible in man solely because of these cross-bonds. There are two types that are of major concern in hair work:

1. Sulphur bonds
2. Hydrogen bonds

SULPHUR BONDS (OR CYSTINE BONDS)

POSITION The end-bonds hold the long chains of amino-acids together, but if there was no attachment between the parallel chains, these chains would simply fall apart once the growing hair had left the protection of the hair follicle. Special amino-acids (cysteine) in the long chains contain SULPHUR atoms which project outward from the rest of the chain.

At certain places on the chains such atoms are exactly opposite other sulphur atoms on the neighboring chain. When this happens the two projections of sulphur atoms form a cross-bond between them. This means that the one chain of amino-acids can be joined at many places and in many different directions by the action of these sulphur bonds.

TYPES OF BONDS IN HAIR

PHYSICAL NATURE

NATURE	EXAMPLES	IMPORTANCE	AGENTS AFFECTING PHYSICAL BONDS	
			BREAKING	REFORMING
MAGNET NAIL (Attracted to Magnet by Physical Bonds.)	**A** HYDROGEN BONDS (Cross Bond in Hair)	KEEPS POLYPEPTIDE CHAINS OF CORTEX TOGETHER. ADDS BODY TO HAIR. NUMBER OF BONDS CAN BE ALTERED BY SIMPLE TREATMENTS.	WATER DILUTE ALKALIES SPECIAL CHEMICALS CAUSES CORTEX TO SWELL USED IN SETTING LOTIONS	DRYING MILD ACIDS CAUSES CORTEX TO SHRINK

CHEMICAL BONDS

NATURE	EXAMPLES	IMPORTANCE	AGENTS AFFECTING CHEMICAL BONDS	
			BREAKING	REFORMING
BRICKS MORTAR (Forms Chemical Bond)	**B** SULFUR BOND (Cross Bond)	GIVES STRENGTH TO NATURAL WAVES. NUMBER OF BONDS DEPENDS ON SULFUR IN HAIR.	COLD WAVE SOLUTIONS HEAT WAVE SOLUTIONS Causes hair to soften	NEUTRALIZERS OXIDATION Causes hair to harden into new waves
	C PEPTIDE BOND (End Bond)	SUPPLIES STRENGTH AND ELASTICITY TO CORTEX. NUMBER OF BONDS DEPEND ON THICKNESS OF CORTEX.	DIGESTIVE JUICES OR ENZYMES STRONG ACIDS OR ALKALIES, ETC. OVER-STRETCHING	GERM LAYER CELLS IN PAPILLA (Newly formed hair) NONE (Mature hair fiber)

NATURE   Sulphur bonds are fairly strong chemical bonds and their number depends on the type of hair itself. For example:

Average hair contains 4–5% sulphur.

Natural red hair contains up to 8% sulphur.

Thus, some types of natural red hair have twice as many sulphur bonds as does the average hair. Because of this higher sulphur content, red hair is resistant and is more difficult to treat.

Sulphur bonds are very important in hair care treatments because they give hair its resistance to being permanently waved or straightened. However, by the use of certain chemical solutions, the sulphur bonds may be broken and then reformed. This breaking and reforming of the sulphur bond within the cortex causes the softening and hardening of the hair. Waving or straightening can be achieved in the process.

AGENTS BREAKING SULPHUR BONDS

Special chemical solutions are required, as in waving solutions (ammonium thioglycolate), chemical hair relaxers (sodium hydroxide).

AGENTS REFORMING SULPHUR BONDS

Permanent wave neutralizer, hydrogen peroxide, oxygen from air (all oxidizers).

HYDROGEN BONDS

POSITION   Hydrogen bonds (H) are very weak bonds and reflect change and interaction in the hair fiber. Since they are also a type of cross-bond, they help the sulphur bond keep the parallel or adjacent chains of amino-acids together, thus giving "body" to the hair.

Although a single H-bond is very weak, *there are many more present in the hair than any other bond.* Thus, hydrogen bonds are very important in the study of hair.

NATURE   Hydrogen bonds are typically involved only with physical changes that take place in the hair, as in setting, waving or curling of the hair. Their nature is that of electrostatic forces of attraction existing between positive and negative charges. In order to distinguish their nature from those of the sulphur and peptide bonds, this text will often refer to them as physical bonds.

AGENTS BREAKING HYDROGEN BONDS

Water, dilute alkali, neutral and acid lotions.

AGENTS REFORMING HYDROGEN BONDS

Drying and dilute acids.

OVERALL PICTURE OF HAIR STRUCTURE

CORTEX

1. Hair cortex is made from millions of tiny amino-acids which serve as basic building blocks.
2. These amino-acids are joined end-on-end by the end-bonds (peptide bonds) to form chains.
3. The chains are held together because of the holding power of the cross-bonds.
4. The chains do not simply parallel along the hair shaft but are twisted around one another.
5. The parallel twisted protein chains combine or unite into fibrils (long, rope-like structures).
6. In addition, the sub-fibers are twisted around one another (like a piece of ordinary string which has a similar type of structure. In string however, there are only 3 sub-fibers, but the same twisted pattern is present as in the hair cortex). The cortex is made of many twisted, amino-acid chains, secured together by various bonds. This arrangement gives strength to the hair but still allows stretching and waving.

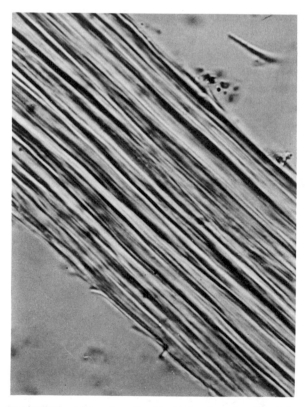

Longitudinal section of cortex illustrating long keratin chain structure.—(Courtesy of Wool Industries Research Council)

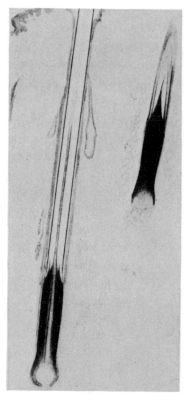

Hair follicles showing soft keratin of hair (dark) and hard keratin (white).

CUTICLE

The detailed pictures, now available, show that the cuticle is a thin wrapping of scales around the cortex. These scales serve to give protection, yet allow the hair to stretch and bend easily.

MEDULLA

The medulla does not appear to be important, for it is made of cells which contain soft keratin, which is not found in either cuticle or cortex.

OTHER FEATURES

FREE AMINO-ACIDS There still remains a great deal to be discovered about human hair. For example, between the chains of keratin in the cortex are "free" amino-acids. Recently, it has been shown that these "free" amino-acids hold the moisture within the cortex at a desirable level (10%). Together with the sebum they function as moisturizers or moisture retainers.

Moisture is required to lubricate the chains and so allow the hair to bend and be pliable. If these free, unattached, amino-acids are removed by excessive shampooing, the hair cannot retain its desired level of moisture within the cortex. *Some hair treatments now include free amino-acids or treated protein substances* to replace the amino-acids washed from the hair by various chemicals.

SALT BONDS and several other bonds occur between the polypeptide chains, but they are not as important as the sulphur or hydrogen bonds.

In some cases of unusual reaction to chemical treatment of the hair these may have to be considered. But, most of the changes that take place in the hair can be explained in relation to the sulphur and hydrogen bonds.

IMPORTANCE OF CROSS-BONDS As previously indicated, half of the weight of the hair is found in chemical bonds that hold the chains together. These cross-bonds have been found to be very important in the study of the overall properties and structure of the hair. The changes that take place in the cortex during waving and setting are explained by a detailed study of these cross-bonds.

CHAPTER 7

REQUIREMENTS AND PROPERTIES OF HAIR

SOURCE OF NUTRITION

The average scalp hair growth of ½ inch per month will produce in excess of 250 feet of hair a day (if all the growth on the scalp was concentrated at one follicle). This growth requires a considerable organization and exercise of other structures and organs in the body.

For normal hair growth we require a constant supply of nourishment. The food we eat is the primary source of nutrition, and it is the fuel required to "drive" the living cells. It is important, therefore, that we know more about food and its effect upon the body.

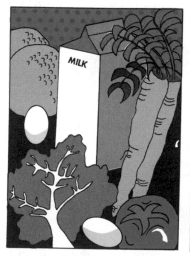
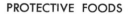

PROTECTIVE FOODS

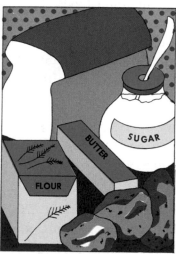

ENERGY FOODS

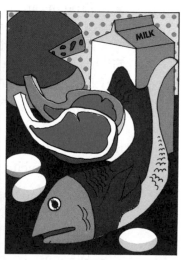

BODY BUILDERS

FOOD

NATURAL FOODS, such as fresh fruit and vegetables, usually contain many different substances required by the body.

REFINED FOODS, such as refined sugar or polished rice, on the other hand, are not well balanced and the amount of these in the diet must be carefully regulated for good health.

CARBOHYDRATES

Function

More than 50% of our diet is carbohydrate. This supplies us with most of the energy we require to live. An excessive carbohydrate intake is stored as fat in certain areas of the body (e.g., hips). The prime aim of dieting is to reduce the amount of excess food consumed, particularly carbohydrates.

Examples of carbohydrates:

Pastry, flour, bread, cakes, potatoes, cereals, sugar, sweets and chocolate, are all predominantly carbohydrates.

FATS

Function

Fats are also high energy foods. They are closely related to the carbohydrates. Excess amounts of carbohydrates and fats are both stored as fat in the fatty layer of the dermis.

Examples of fats:

Butter, cream, ice cream, cod liver oil, peanut butter, olive oil, margarine, etc. (Baked and fried foods are also high in fats, but steaming and grilling reduce the fat content.)

PROTEINS

Function

Proteins are very important foods. They contain nitrogen, which is an essential requirement for cell growth and repair.

The hair needs a constant supply of high grade protein in the diet. High grade protein contains rich amounts of nitrogen and sulphur, both of which are essential to the growth of healthy hair.

Energy level

Proteins are low energy foods and some modern diets are based on a high level of them. This high protein diet helps to reduce the consumption of the fat producing foods, such as carbohydrates and fats.

Examples of proteins:

High grade (or A grade—lean meat, fish, eggs, cheese, milk, etc.
Low grade (or B grade) —peas, beans, vegetables, etc.

We must have good quality protein foods because both the skin and hair are themselves made of a special protein—KERATIN.

OTHER DIET REQUIREMENTS

We need most of our food for energy and to maintain body heat. If we do not eat sufficient food to provide for energy, then the hair will also be deprived of nourishment. The hair growing thin and sparse could be the result of a scarcity of this food in the diet. This may occur in the following cases:

SICKNESS When illness, injury and worry prevent us from being our real selves, then our appetites also suffer.

OLD AGE Elderly people tend to take insufficient care of their general health and of their eating habits and so their hair and skin are inclined to suffer. The skin becomes thinner and scalier and the hair loses condition and becomes drier.

MINERALS

Small amounts of mineral salts are required by the body. These essential minerals are:

Calcium—required for strong bones and teeth.

Common salt—essential for life.

Iodine—minute amounts are required daily, as lack of iodine in the diet can lead to:

1. Lowered health.
2. Thinning and loss of hair.
3. Goiter and other disabilities that require medical care.

SULPHUR Sulphur is required for proper growth of hair and is only available through high quality proteins.

VITAMINS

NATURE OF VITAMINS Vitamins are chemical substances essential for healthy life. They are found in very small quantities in certain foods. As they were discovered, they were named A, B, C, etc.

FUNCTION Each one is required to perform certain functions in the body. For example:

1. Vitamin B is important in order to maintain the normal condition of the skin. Skin conditioners and creams are usually rich in Vitamin B, in an attempt to furnish nourishment to the skin.
2. Lack of the other vitamins can cause "run-down" conditions of the body, with subsequent ill-effects on hair growth and appearance.

LIQUIDS

Water is required to help maintain the supply of blood and body fluids. The average water loss from the body is about 4½ pints daily and this must be replaced. Water is supplied by milk, tea, coffee, fruit, etc., in addition to drinking water.

ROUGHAGE

Vegetable fiber is needed to prevent constipation. Fruits and vegetables are the natural sources of this indigestible matter. Certain cereals, high in bulk, are also helpful.

DIGESTION OF FOOD

Digestion converts the food we eat into a form that can supply nourishment to the skin and hair.

ACTION OF CHEWING Digestion begins by careful chewing of the food, mixing it with the saliva.

FINAL DIGESTION After swallowing, the food passes into the stomach for partial digestion and on into the intestines. The breakdown of the food continues here and the completely digested food particles finally pass into the blood stream.

BLOOD CIRCULATION Circulation of the blood distributes nourishment to all parts of the body. The papilla of each growing hair is well supplied by numerous, very small blood vessels known as capillaries.

Any abnormal condition of the blood such as anemia or leukemia, will, of course, affect the condition of the cells of the body. Among other widespread effects, this can also reduce hair growth.

LYMPH CIRCULATION Only a few cells actually line the blood vessels and so gain their nourishment directly. The bulk of body cells rely on the lymph or fluid portion of the blood, for their constant supply of nourishment.

Accumulating cell wastes are also swept away by this lymph circulation, thus preventing poisoning of the cells. This waste is returned to the blood and is filtered out by the kidneys.

GROWTH OF HAIR

EXTERNAL NOURISHMENT There is no evidence to support the view that hair may be "fed" from the outside by direct application of "hair foods." The external or visible hair is quite dead and so, despite its hungry condition, it is unable to accept or use this nourishment. The "hungry" condition is really due to excess porosity and this hair needs conditioners, not "foods."

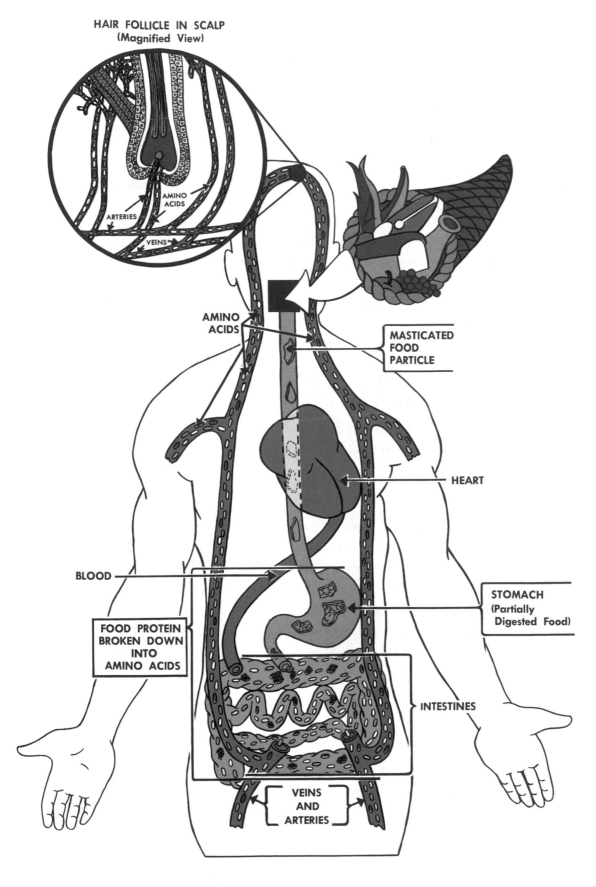

HAIR FOLLICLE IN SCALP
(Magnified View)

AMINO ACIDS

ARTERIES

AMINO ACIDS

VEINS

AMINO ACIDS

MASTICATED FOOD PARTICLE

HEART

BLOOD

STOMACH
(Partially Digested Food)

FOOD PROTEIN BROKEN DOWN INTO AMINO ACIDS

INTESTINES

VEINS AND ARTERIES

INTERNAL NOURISHMENT For proper, healthy growth, hair relies on the constant supply of nourishment received by means of the blood and lymph systems and on such additional factors as:

HEALTH We have to carefully guard our health and obtain sufficient sleep. Sickness and the taking of certain drugs can seriously affect the condition of the hair.

DIET Proper amounts of food, including fresh fruits and vegetables, are essential.

HEREDITY Depending on certain factors handed down from our parents, the hair may be sparse or dense, thick or thin, weak or wiry, straight or curly, etc.

NERVES Excessive worry and mental strain can seriously interfere with the natural health of our hair. Long periods of emotional tension are among the most common causes of varying disorders of the hair.

AGE As we get older our body processes slow down and this in turn produces ill effects on the skin and hair.

1. The skin becomes dryer and thinner.
2. The hair becomes sparser.

RESTORATION OF GROWTH

To restore the growth of hair it is necessary to regain health and achieve freedom from anxiety and nervous strain. This would be the first step.

Some success is possible by attempts to artificially stimulate circulation. These may have two effects:

1. To supply additional nourishment to the hair.
2. To remove excess cell wastes that are "poisoning" the living papilla and thus slowing down the production of the germinative cells that make up the hair.

Various methods are:
1. Massage
2. Hot towels (heat)
3. Regular brushing

Some limited "cures" are possible by drug hormone treatments and surgery. One such method involves transplanting active follicles to bald areas of the scalp.

PROPERTIES OF HAIR

INSOLUBILITY   Hair is composed of a protein material called hard keratin. This keratin is rather tough and resists the action of many agents that are harmful to the skin and tissues (soft keratin). Examples of harmful agents would be solvents such as kerosene, alcohol, benzene.

THE EFFECT OF SOLVENTS   No common solvents will destroy the hair, e.g., alcohol is commonly used in hair sprays because it evaporates from the hair, leaving a moisture resistant film without harming the hair.

Solvents will, however, remove natural sebum or hair conditioners and so the hair may soon become dry and brittle. For this reason, it is not advisable to use them as shampoos, as was the practice before the modern shampoo was discovered.

CHEMICAL PROPERTIES OF HAIR

Hair is the most resistant structure of the body to chemical attack but, of course, strong alkalies or acids can dissolve or weaken it. Chemicals such as permanent wave solutions, tints or lighteners (bleach) can also cause serious damage if applied carelessly.

ELEMENTS FOUND IN HAIR

COMPOSITION   Hair contains the following elements:

Oxygen	Nitrogen
Hydrogen	Sulphur
Carbon	Phosphorus

The exact composition varies widely with the type of hair, depending to a large extent on age, race, sex and color.

SULPHUR CONTENT   The resistant properties of the hair are apparently due to its relatively high sulphur content (4% to 8%). The skin has much less sulphur content than hair and is therefore softer and more prone to chemical attack.

Hair containing the highest amounts of sulphur (natural red hair) is the strongest type of hair. This hair is hard to wave but will hold the resultant wave much more strongly than other types of hair.

ORGANIC NATURE   Hair is an organic substance and will burn or singe readily. It also gives off a strong characteristic odor due to the protein or nitrogen present.

EFFECTS OF WATER

Water has no chemical effect on hair,
but it does have great physical effects.

WETS HAIR Hair is wetted by water, but not as readily as it might seem. The air trapped between the scales of the cuticle may act as a barrier, as does natural sebum and other substances found on the hair shaft, all offering resistance to the water.

The softer the water the more effective it is in wetting the hair. Most hair products have wetting agents in them to make the hair less resistant to water. On the other hand, salts found in hard water are inclined to be damaging to the hair because they remain in and on the hair after drying.

SOFTENS AND SWELLS HAIR Water can be used as a shaping agent and it may swell the hair as much as 14% in diameter in the process. The swelling causes a loosening of the internal structure, allowing it to adjust internally to the new shape provided by the artisan's efforts. This results in a temporary styling that will last only as long as the moisture content of the hair is kept low. A hair style does not hold well on a damp or humid day.

ALTERS ELASTICITY *Dry hair* has a *low stretch limit* (how much it can be stretched without causing damage). *Wet hair* has a *high stretch limit.*

CHANGES STATIC ELECTRICITY Dry hair has a maximum static electrical charge which causes "flyaway." Wet hair has a minimum static electrical charge which causes limpness.

STATIC ELECTRICITY IN HAIR

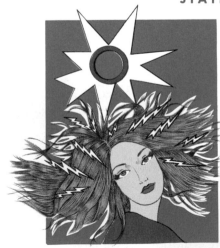 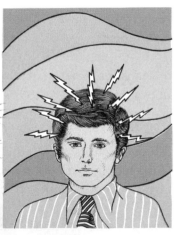 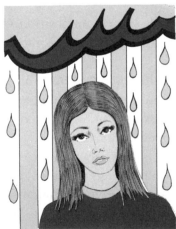

a. Excess (Dry and "fly-away)   b. Normal (Normal and   c. Nil (Limp and heavy)
manageable)

CONTROLS MANAGEABILITY OF HAIR Hair normally contains 9% to 10% moisture, and even when it looks quite dry it still contains 4% to 5% moisture. This moisture is required to lubricate the cortex and therefore has an important role in the properties of the hair.

High moisture content

Hair is much easier to comb, wind or style when it is in a dampened, softened condition. Hair can soak up to 33% moisture when it is fully saturated with water, but in this state it has a clingy, limp, heavy, unattractive appearance.

Low moisture content

Dry hair, on the other hand, has a "flyaway," harsh, lifeless or brittle feel and is quite unmanageable. Hair, even when very dry in appearance, still contains up to 5% moisture.

PHYSICAL PROPERTIES OF HAIR

The physical properties of the hair are related to its elasticity, feel, texture, porosity, quality, "body" and manageability. These properties are of extreme importance to the professional in all phases of setting, waving, lightening, tinting, etc.

CONDITION AND POROSITY

The condition of the hair depends to a large extent on its previous treatment. A thorough understanding of the condition of the hair is necessary before commencing any work on it.

NORMAL OR AVERAGE This is a condition of hair which is neither porous nor resistant, dry nor oily, weak nor damaged.

Courtesy: Gillette Company Research Institute, Rockville, Maryland

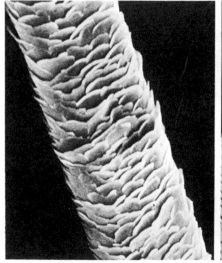 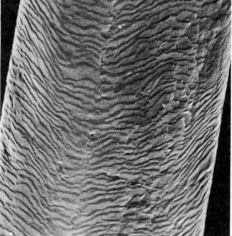 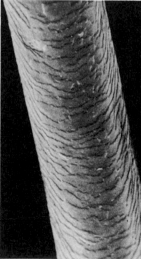

POROUS　　　　　　**NORMAL**　　　　　　**RESISTANT**

RESISTANT This is hair which, due to its physical condition, will resist penetration by permanent wave solutions, permanent tints, or any liquid and therefore is more difficult to process.

Most of the difficulty is due to the tough, compact, multi-layered cuticle that does not allow the solution to penetrate through into the cortex. Penetration is absolutely necessary, as the changes that create the wave or produce a new color can only occur within the cortex layer.

Hair with this tough, compact cuticle often has a coarse, wiry texture which usually gives additional problems.

CAUSES OF POROSITY VARIATIONS Not all cases of hard-to-wave hair are due to the resistant nature of the cuticle. Excess lacquer or film sprayed on the hair may duplicate the effect of a resistant cuticle.

POROUS HAIR has either a large, loose cuticle surface or excess space between the imbrications. This will allow rapid absorption of moisture or chemicals into the cortex.

HAIR DAMAGE

Natural

The porosity may be due to the natural development of the cuticle, which may range from very resistant to highly porous.

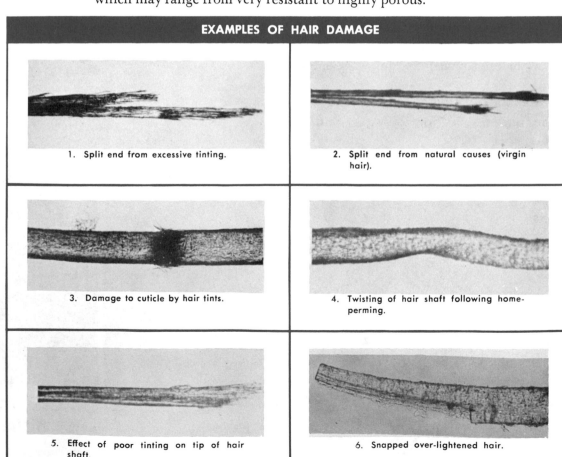

EXAMPLES OF HAIR DAMAGE

1. Split end from excessive tinting.

2. Split end from natural causes (virgin hair).

3. Damage to cuticle by hair tints.

4. Twisting of hair shaft following home-perming.

5. Effect of poor tinting on tip of hair shaft.

6. Snapped over-lightened hair.

Chemical damage

In addition, high porosity may be due to previous exposure to harsh chemicals such as strong bleaches or permanent wave solutions. These may have damaged, or entirely dissolved large areas of the cuticle, leaving certain areas of the cortex exposed. *At these points, excessive damage can be caused even through "normal" hair treatments.*

Difference in porosity

Even along the shaft of a normal hair, changes in porosity may be found. These differences make it difficult to regulate the affects of solutions in order to achieve uniform results. It is usual to find such areas at the ends of the hair and these ends have to be given special handling.

TREATMENT OF EXCESSIVE POROSITY

Hair with excessive porosity must receive treatments with special protective creams in order that other hair services may continue. Otherwise, the hair must be left without service until normal regrowth allows trimming of the affected section.

Tinting can present special problems due to such areas of greater porosity. These areas of the hair soak up the tint much more rapidly, giving rise to uneven coloring along the hair shaft.

COLOR FILLERS may be applied before the tint in order to even out porosity. The filler is a jelly-like substance (a mixture of proteins and keratin) which can be applied directly to the cuticle. This is done by rubbing and massaging the filler onto the hair and then combing and brushing it along the shaft.

The porous sections of the hair shaft take up the filler more rapidly than the less porous sections. Because the filler has similar chemical properties as the hair, it has the effect of evening-up the porosity of the hair along the entire shaft. This makes permanent waving, lightening and hair coloring easier to control and permits improved results with less damage.

MISCELLANEOUS HAIR PROBLEMS

DAMAGED HAIR Apart from excessive porosity, the hair may show other signs of damage, such as brittleness, split ends, rough, dry, harsh, lifeless look, tangling, knotting and matting when dry, and a spongy feel when wet. This hair type has a lack of gloss or sheen, shows lowered elasticity and has poor manageability. The hair will break under slight strain and thus has to be handled with extreme care.

OILY HAIR has a limp, lank look and may also present special problems. Shampooing is the necessary treatment to remove the excess oils which will hinder penetration of solutions into the cortex. Oily hair is hard-to-wave hair, but it is not necessarily resistant hair. Removal of the excessive oils usually returns the porosity to normal.

DRY HAIR has a dull appearance, a rough, harsh feel, has poor manageability and is difficult to brush, comb or style. It has a higher static electricity content and these charges give a repulsion effect (fly-away) to the ends of the hair fibers.

Cause

The dry condition may be due to a lack of natural oils or because these oils have been removed by harsh or strong shampoos. This allows the moisture in the cortex to evaporate, giving rise to the symptoms of excessively dry hair.

Treatment

Because of the lack of the oil coating protecting the cuticle, this type of hair is more porous than it would be otherwise. This dry hair requires conditioning treatment to replace missing oil and to restore it to a normal condition.

VIRGIN HAIR has not been given any previous chemical treatment at all. In this condition it is the best hair to manage, but use caution, there are fewer virgin heads entering shops today. The reason is that many patrons damage their hair with "home-kits," unskillfully used, before they seek professional care.

HAIR QUALITY

The quality of the hair is shown by some of the following characteristics:

BODY This is a loose term used to indicate how the hair stands up to or resists, various external influences. These influences are usually acting to ruin or disrupt the condition of the hair. Resistance of the hair to the pressure of hats, winds, pillows or the use of comb and brush indicates that the hair possesses "body."

TREATMENT "Body" is the spring, or "bounce" in the hair. This may be altered by damage to the structure of the hair. Lack of "body" is undesirable and creates many problems to the practitioner. However, an attempt may be made to restore the natural "body" of the hair by the following methods:

External

Hair lacquers, gums or resins, etc., may be sprayed on or applied to the cuticle of the hair, which causes it to stiffen, thus giving the illusion of body.

Internal

Special, mild acid rinses may shrink and harden the hair and thus partially restore its lost body. The damaging effect of alkaline lighteners may be decreased by these acid rinses which are applied as soon as the excess lightener is rinsed from the hair.

As an example, the use of a protein acid rinse not only coats the outside of the hair with proteins in order to form a stiffened coating, but also hardens the cortex due to its acid content.

ELASTICITY This is an outstanding quality of hair that allows it to withstand a great deal of stretching but still return to its original length when it is released. When we pull or drag on the hair, it usually results in the hair being stretched. The hair resists being stretched and this is indicated by the tension felt by the fingers as we pull on the hair. The tension is developed only within the cortex. The degree of tension caused by the amount of stress on the hair, depends on the nature of the hair and the amount of moisture in the cortex. Within certain limits, the hair may be stretched without damage and it will spring back to its original length after release. As long as you keep within these limits, this process may be repeated again and again without any noticeable damage to the hair.

ELASTIC LIMITS OF HAIR		
HAIR CONDITION	MOISTURE CONTENT	RESULTANT ELASTICITY
Normal hair (dry)	5–10%	20 – 30%
Wet hair	30%	50—60%
Hair (dampened with permanent wave solution)	30%	(damaged) 70%

Once the hair is dampened with permanent wave solution, it begins to soften so that no tension is felt when it is stretched. As a result of this softness, it is easy to overstretch by tight winding or by pulling. Overstretched hair will not return to its former length as it is now damaged and weakened. Other examples of stretching the hair occur during combing, brushing, winding, pinning and styling. However, little or no stretching damage is caused by these operations.

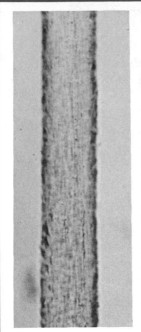

1. Hair before stretching.

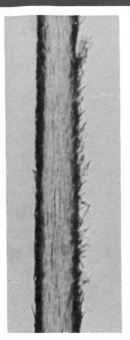

2. Slight stretching is loosening cuticle scales.

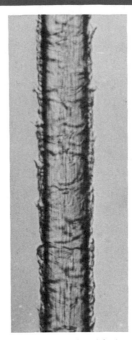

3. Separation of cuticle from cortex has begun.

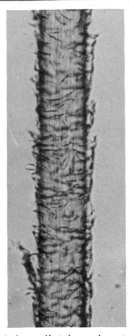

4. Immediately prior to breakage showing weakness due to excessive strain.

ELASTIC NATURE OF CORTEX Because of its elastic ability, hair is able to withstand relatively great forces, e.g., normal hair is stronger than copper wire of the same diameter.

In order to give this strength, pliability and elasticity to the hair, the cortex is built like a series of coil springs. These are wound around one another in a complicated fashion, but each is free to move backwards and forwards.

ACTION OF CUTICLE The freedom of movement is one reason for the outstanding properties of hair. These stretching movements are unrestricted by the scales of the cuticle, which can slide in and out, providing a continuous covering for the cortex even while the hair is in the stretched position. This arrangement is of the utmost importance in understanding the wide range of physical properties of hair.

CHAPTER 8

CHARACTERISTICS
OF HAIR

TEXTURE OF THE HAIR

The "hand" or feel of the hair is the manner in which we usually judge its texture. The texture of the hair can also be measured by its appearance, manageability and the way it reacts to trimming, brushing, combing, waving, and styling.

Because of its importance, it is vital for the success of his work that the practitioner take into account the wide variations of the texture of the hair.

Courtesy: Gillette Company Research Institute, Rockville, Maryland

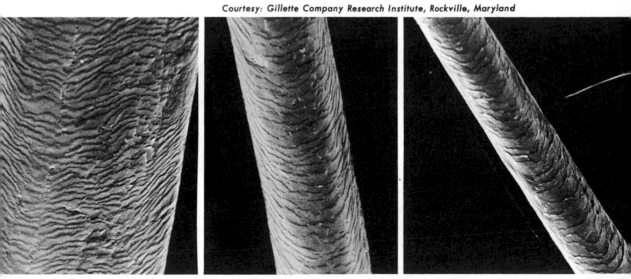

Illustrations of coarse, medium and fine hair, magnified 1200 times.

Although we speak of texture as if it were a single property of the hair, it is, in fact, produced by a number of separate and distinct properties. Each one of these may vary widely and give rise to changes in hair texture. As each one in turn may vary, it is not surprising to find that texture varies from person to person and even varies widely on the same head of hair. These factors are:

1. Size or diameter
2. Nature of cuticle
3. Density of hair
4. Natural characteristics
5. Length of hair
6. Direction of hair growth
7. Moisture level of cortex

SIZE OR DIAMETER In strand or fiber thickness, the hair is described as being from fine to coarse. Because the cortex is approximately 90% of its bulk, it is mainly variations in the cortex that give the hair its thickness.

NATURE OF CUTICLE We constantly squeeze the hairs, stretch or rub them together when we handle the hair and our sense of feel is in constant use. So the cuticle, being the outside layer of the hair, is very important when it comes to assessing the texture.

Size of imbrications

The imbrications may be loose with large free ends. As a result the hair becomes entangled easily as we try to squeeze, slide or compress the adjacent fibers of different hairs together. This gives an impression of coarseness and roughness to the touch.

On the other hand, a fine, smooth cuticle resists entanglement and thus gives the opposite impression.

Action of natural oils, etc.

The presence of oil on the cuticle may change our impressions of hair texture. A dry cuticle surface would feel different from the same hair coated with natural or artificial oils. Hair lacquers, sprays, protein conditioners, etc., may also give quite different impressions of texture from the true one.

DENSITY OF HAIR In the handling of the hair, quite a large number of individual hairs are involved. If the hair is thick and abundant on the scalp, it will feel quite different in texture from the same type of hair that happens to be thin and sparse. This is simply because our hand can take hold of more hairs when the density is thicker.

NATURAL CHARACTERISTICS   By its natural characteristics alone, hair can be wiry and tough or soft and silky. This factor is very important in designing a suitable hairstyle. If we do not take into account these natural tendencies and the manner of hair growth, many hairstyles will not hold and will loosen up in a very short time.

LENGTH OF HAIR   If the hair is cut very short, there always remains a feeling as if it were tough and unmanageable. A striking example of this is the stubble on the chin of males. If this stubble is allowed to grow, it eventually changes from the steel bristles on the unshaven chin to a silky, soft, flowing beard. If the legs are shaved you will feel the same effect until the hairs regain their former length.

DIRECTION OF HAIR GROWTH   The direction of each of the follicles plays an important part in the texture of the hair. Although the follicle usually emerges at an angle from the skin, this angle is not in the same direction for all follicles. Furthermore, the follicles are not evenly distributed all over the scalp, but they occur in groups of from 2 to 5.

These groups are arranged into definite orders or patterns. From these patterns we get natural partings, cowlicks, widows' peaks, whorls, crowns, fringes and other individualities of the hair.

Affect on hairstyling

The hair stylist must take into account the natural tendencies of the hair and their directional patterns. When we attempt to style or comb the hair, we must be careful to follow the natural lines and discover its real texture.

MOISTURE LEVEL OF CORTEX   The nature of the cortex and its relative moisture content also influences the apparent texture. Dry, unruly hair has different handling characteristics when it is dampened and softened by moisture or setting solutions. The humidity in the atmosphere plays a part (as does the oil film on the outside of the cuticle) in maintaining desirable moisture levels.

Application

Because moisture softens the texture of the hair, nearly all setting work is done in a dampened condition.

CONCLUSION

1. The immense and unending variety in texture of human scalp hair is at least one important factor to consider in determining why professional hair work is seldom routine and monotonous.
2. The successful practitioner is one who can adapt the natural differences in hair texture to give more pleasing and longer lasting styling effects.

HAIR TYPES AND LOCATIONS

RANGES OF TYPES Although we refer to "hair" commonly as being scalp hair, this is only one of the many types of hair that are well known. Hair, in some form, is found on the entire body except the palms of the hands, the soles of the feet, the lips, the backs of the end joints of the fingers and the eyelids. There are, in fact, at least 10 different types of hair found on separate and distinct areas of the body.

DIFFERENT RACIAL PATTERNS

Distribution of the types of hair on the body has been very useful in such studies as the migration of different races in the world, such as American Indians, Australian Aborigines, Africans, Japanese, Polynesians, among many others.

Beards, moustaches, and body hair show marked differences in density, distribution and pattern. Some races (Ainus of Japan) are extremely hairy over the body, while others are almost hairless (American Indians). A number of races, throughout the world, have hair with typical characteristics with relation to length, texture, color, curl or density.

MEDICAL AND CRIME DETECTION IMPORTANCE

Hair is of great interest to the plastic surgeon and to the doctor investigating physiological growth and the problems of aging. The police criminologist finds the endless varieties in the shape and form of hair to be unique with each individual. The experts claim that a person's hair is as easily identified as his fingerprints when it is observed under a microscope. The factors examined may be:

1. Thickness of hair shaft.
2. Type of cuticle scales.
3. Nature of pigment present.
4. Characteristics of the medulla.

The variation in each one of these factors is significant and may identify the suspect as to age, sex, habits and other individual characteristics.

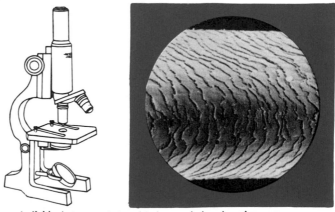

Individual characteristics of hair revealed under microscope.

MAIN TYPES OF HAIR

Hair exists in three main types, each of which has its own separate features. The distinction is usually based on the length of the hair.

However, it does not appear that different types of follicles are involved but rather that changes take place within the human body or in the papilla. In general, the soft, fine hair of the baby is gradually replaced by the stronger hair of the child. Then in turn the child's hair is changed to the adult type. The three main types of hair are:

1. Tertiary or terminal hair
2. Secondary hair
3. Primary hair.

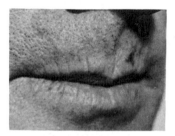 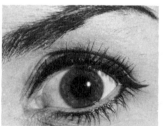 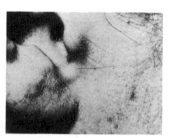

(a) Smooth hairless area of skin (lips), with the shaved hairy male skin.

(b) Secondary hair of the eyebrows and eyelashes together with fine primary hairs on face. — (Courtesy: "Structure and Function of Skin" — Academic Press)

(c) Cheek and part of the ear of a woman, showing fine vellus hair and tertiary hairs of scalp.

TERTIARY OR TERMINAL HAIR (long hair)

This is the long, soft hair found on the scalp. Because of its obvious importance it is the type usually referred to as "hair." It can be found on the beard and moustache of adult males and is also present on the legs, arms and body of both males and females. These hairs grow in groups of 2 to 5 (especially on the scalp). In these groups, the *hairs may be of different ages and consequently of different lengths*. A woman's scalp hair is usually longer and thicker than the hair of a man.

FEATURES The follicles of these long, soft hairs lie at an angle to the skin. This angle causes the hairs to grow in a sloping direction to the surface of the skin. The direction or grain of the hair fibers is readily felt by running the fingers or a comb through it. At particular points on the scalp there may exist a sudden change in the direction of the hairs, as in a natural parting.

Sometimes the follicles merge together at their openings on the skin surface. This gives rise to multiple hairs or what appears to be several hairs coming from one follicle.

Tertiary hair contains pigment and so it has a characteristic color (except in the case of an albino). On the scalp and beard (of a male) it frequently possesses a natural wave.

Each hair has at least one sebaceous gland associated with the follicle. The function of the gland is to produce a natural oil (sebum). This oil forms a film on the outside of the hair shaft and the outer layer of the epidermis. Each hair has an arrector pili muscle and so is able to demonstrate the characteristic "goose-pimples."

It is this hair that thins out with age in some individuals and so gives rise to areas completely devoid of hair (baldness). In other individuals it may slowly lose its pigment and become grey with age.

SECONDARY HAIR

The secondary type of hair is the stiff, short, bristly coarser hair found on the eyelashes, eyebrows and within the openings or passages of the nose and ears.

The follicles of these hairs usually lie at right angles to the surface of the skin and thus the hairs stand straight out away from the skin. They do not possess arrector pili muscles.

OTHER FEATURES

1. These secondary hairs usually increase in thickness and number with age, particularly on the eyebrows of the older male.
2. They are often curved (particularly in the case of eyelashes).
3. They usually also possess a large medulla.
4. The hairs range in length from ½″ to ¾″ but they sometimes grow to approximately an inch.
5. They are more sensitive to the touch than are scalp hairs and therefore act as protection devices for delicate organs such as eyes, ears and nose.
6. Because of their essential protective functions, it is very unusual to lose these hairs even in severe cases of baldness.
7. The eyelashes are particularly sensitive, and cause a reflex action of closing the eyelids whenever the eye is in danger of being contacted by a foreign object.
8. The purpose of the eyebrows is to prevent sweat, water, oils or chemicals running down from the scalp and entering the eyes. For this reason alone, it is not wise to completely remove or shave these hairs.

PRIMARY HAIR

This type of hair is also known as lanugo, vellus hair or "fuzz." It's the baby fine hair that is present over almost the entire smooth skin of the body.

OTHER FEATURES

1. These hairs have no medulla.
2. They are often unpigmented and so are difficult to see unless examined in strong light at the proper angle.

3. They have no arrector pili muscle but they do possess sebaceous glands.

4. These hairs are very short with a length of about ½″. Their function is to aid in the efficient evaporation of perspiration.

CONCLUSION

Recognition of the different types of hair is vital to plastic surgeons. Skin grafts must be taken from areas with the same hair pattern and type since the new grafts will continue to grow their own particular kind of hair. If this happens to be on the face, there will be a great deal of embarrassment and discomfort caused to the patient.

Although the three main types of hair are well recognized, it does not appear that there are also different types of follicles necessary to grow them. On the scalp of a baby, the first hairs are primary, and these gradually change until, in the older individual, the type found is terminal hair.

Now, in adult males, there often occurs a drop in activity of the follicles and they go back gradually to the early, downy type of hair. Later on even this type is slowly lost and all growth of hair ceases. This area of the scalp is then completely and permanently bald.

GROWTH OF THE HAIR

RATE OF GROWTH   The hair on the scalp grows at the average rate of ½″ per month or a total increase of 6″ to 7″ in length for each year.

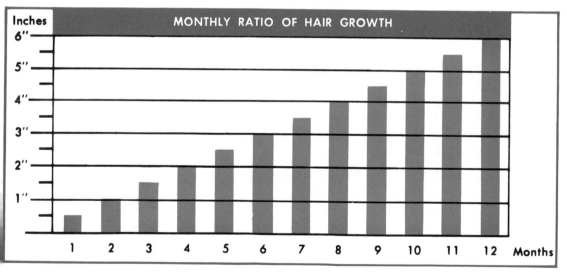

This normal average growth varies with the type and location of the hair. Hairs growing around the margin of the scalp (or hairline) grow very slowly. On the crown and on the back of the head the hairs grow at their best and are therefore the longest.

When very young, the follicle may produce as much as ¾″ to 1″ a month. As it gets older, it grows hair more slowly until at last it ceases to produce any growth at all.

LIFE OF FOLLICLE Each follicle produces hair for some definite period only. Then it has a short resting stage before again forming new hair growth. This active period of the scalp follicles varies from 2 to 4 years (which is typical). During the life of the follicle, new hair is formed at the bulb and this additional growth pushes the older part of the hair further and further away from the papilla.

LENGTH OF HAIR (Maximum) Hair may reach a total visible length of 22″ to 28″ if left untrimmed. Longer hair is sometimes seen in women, but it is rare to find hair exceeding 36″ in length. (World record is 6 feet 1 inch.)

EFFECT OF SEASONS It is reported that the maximum growth of the hair occurs in young women between 15 and 30 years of age. Growth appears to be faster in summer than in winter.

REASON FOR CONSTANT TRIMMING As each separate follicle has an individual cycle of growth, adjacent follicles can have maximum and minimum rates. This means that frequent trimming (other than that required to keep the hairstyle at a definite length) is necessary in order to avoid the uneven ends caused by this unequal growth.

NUMBER OF HAIRS ON SCALP The average number of hairs on the normal scalp have been estimated as:

Natural Blonde Hair — 140,000
Natural Red Hair   — 90,000
Natural Brown Hair — 110,000
Natural Black Hair   — 108,000

This is done by carefully counting the hairs on a definite known area of the scalp (e.g., 1 square inch). When this figure is known, the total area of the scalp is measured as best it can.

Therefore number of hairs in 1 square inch X Number of square inches of scalp hair = Total number of hairs on scalp.

It would take far too long to count all the hair on each scalp separately. Besides, what is wanted is only a rough estimate for use as a guide.

DIAMETER OF THE HAIR The diameter of the hair appears to vary within certain limits:

Natural Blonde Hair	— 1/1500 to 1/500 (of an inch)
Natural Black Hair	— 1/400 to 1/140 (of an inch)
Average Male Scalp Hair	— 1/525 to 1/300 (of an inch)
Average Female Scalp Hair	— 1/500 to 1/250 (of an inch)

HAIRS SHOWING RANGE OF THICKNESS
(When magnified to the same proportion)

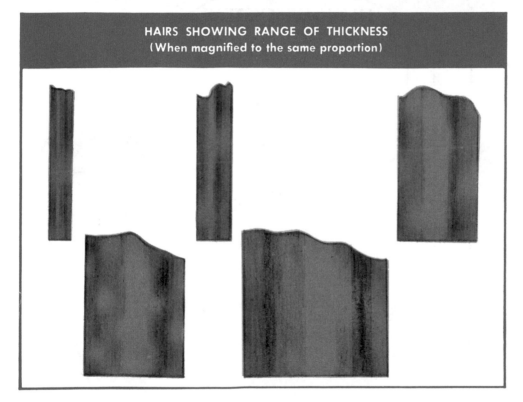

Thus a woman's hair is not only longer but is a little coarser on the average than a man's hair. However, the diameter of each hair is by no means uniform throughout its length. Depending on circumstances (e.g., ill-health) the variations in diameter can be very great indeed.

The hair of a child is soft and fine, but later it gradually develops into the stronger hair of the adult. *For this reason alone it is not advisable to give young children an adult permanent wave or other treatments involving strong chemicals.*

LOSS OF HAIR   Because our hair is not truly essential for life, any threat to or serious change in our state of health may be reflected by some corresponding change in our hair. However, we can very easily lose all of our hair without it in any way affecting our general health.

SOME CONTRIBUTING FACTORS IN HAIR GROWTH

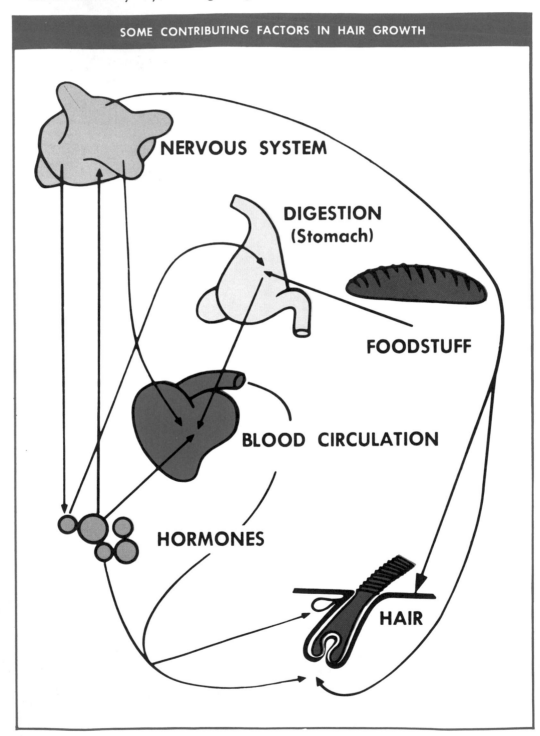

NERVOUS SYSTEM

DIGESTION
(Stomach)

FOODSTUFF

BLOOD CIRCULATION

HORMONES

HAIR

EFFECTS OF BLOOD AND LYMPH SUPPLY A growth of 6" to 7" of scalp hair per year is considered average or normal growth. Let us now examine what can influence this growth rate.

The growth of the hair depends mainly on the circulation of lymph and blood fluids through the papilla. This essential flow has two purposes:

1. To supply the hair with nourishment.
2. To remove cell wastes and other unwanted products from the region of growth.

(Accumulation of these by-products seem to poison or slow down the work of the papilla in producing hair.)

CONTROL OF THE BLOOD AND LYMPH SUPPLY The circulation of the blood and lymph is controlled by the following:

(a) General health
(b) Diet
(c) Age
(d) Hormones and glands
(e) Nervous system

AFFECTS ON HAIR GROWTH Good health is essential for strong hair that has a natural softness and lustre. In periods of ill-health both the hair growth and production of natural oils (sebum) may slow down or cease. The hair then becomes brittle, dry and harsh in appearance. Many drugs taken to combat illness may also adversely affect the hair and hinder the chance for successful hair services which involve chemical change.

Ill health caused by anemia of the blood, hepatitis, fever, bad teeth, diabetes and other long and severe illnesses affect hair growth markedly. Approaching motherhood can also impose a strain on the growth and nature of the hair.

The diameter of the hair becomes thinner during a period of illness although it later will return to normal thickness on regaining good health. However, there could remain a weak part of the hair shaft that can easily break under a strain caused by even slight stretching. This weak part remains in the hair until that section has grown long enough to be trimmed off.

OTHER CONTRIBUTING FACTORS IN HAIR GROWTH

DIET and nutrition have previously been mentioned, together with well balanced meals, as important factors in maintaining natural hair growth.

AGE Elderly people invariably show the affects of the passing years by a progressive thinning or loss of hair. On the other hand, youngsters tend to have a healthy, vigorous growth of hair.

HORMONES AND GLANDS Hormones are substances manufactured by glands. These hormones are circulated around the body by means of the blood and lymph systems. Hormones have some curious affects on the different types of hair:

1. During adolescence, hair begins to grow on the arms, legs, armpits, and other parts of the body.
2. The growth of beard and moustache hairs in males is under hormone control.
3. Effects of aging on the hair are due in part to the hormone changes, for example, change-of-life may cause weaker, drier hair in older females.
4. Thickening of eyebrow hairs (especially in adult males).
5. Common male baldness is considered to be a direct result of hormone influence.

EFFECTS OF WORRY A further major factor in hair growth is the freedom from long periods of emotional tension and excessive worry. Both real and imaginary problems very often combine to create a more or less constant state of hypertension, confusion and prolonged anxiety in the mind of the individual.

This anxiety state is recognized as one of the main factors in causing dull, lifeless hair. Even baldness can result from continued strain and from the lack of relaxation of the scalp muscles, which often takes place. Exactly how this happens is unknown, but experts think that some restriction is produced that interferes with the supply of nourishment or removal of cell wastes at the papilla.

Reducing Nervous Tension

The value of healthy exercise and outdoor activity, with its associated fresh air and sunshine, cannot be overstressed. Not only does activity of this kind build up your constitution, it also provides for healthy relaxation. This gives freedom from those daily cares and tensions that often combine to give the familiar "run-down" feeling.

The improvement in general health and well-being is reflected by a more desirable appearance and sheen of the hair (provided, of course, the hair is kept clean).

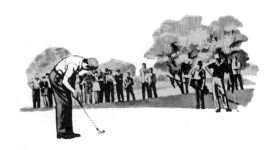 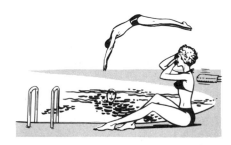

HAIR GROWTH CYCLE

REGULAR LOSS OF HAIRS   The shedding of hair is not exactly regular, being more noticeable in the morning and at certain other periods. No sensation of pain is felt when these hairs are pulled away from the scalp. The reason is that these hairs are dead even at the base or bulb of the hair. You may have noticed that when the scalp is brushed or combed there are invariably found a number of loose hairs. These have detached themselves from the scalp and may be seen on the brush, comb, coat or pillow.

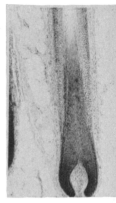

A normal hair and follicle also showing hardening of cortex and cuticle. (lighter areas).

LENGTH OF CYCLE   Each follicle has a definite age and when the hair reaches this natural limit, it falls out or is brushed or combed out. The follicle then has a brief period of rest (from 2 to 6 months) and then begins once more to produce a young new hair. On the scalp, this cycle of growth and replacement is from 2 to 4 years. The life span of the follicles of a woman's hair is about 25% longer than those of a man.

BED-HAIR   When the hair reaches its maximum age, an air space slowly develops between the medulla and the top of the papilla. Following which, the cuticle of the hair is no longer formed by the outer cells of the papilla and the cortex shrinks in thickness. A short period later the complete hair bulb loosens and separates from the papilla. At this stage the hair is known as a "bed-hair" and it lies loosely in the follicle. The papilla completely dies away and the follicle closes in over it. If the neck of the follicle is tight, it will continue to hold the "bed-hair" for a period of time.

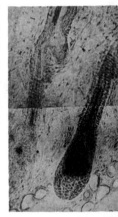

A young follicle just starting to produce a hair. Note bed-hairs of previous cycles which have not been brushed or combed out.

SHED-HAIR   The "bed-hair" may be pulled out by the daily brushing and combing, or it may be removed by shampooing or any other form of pulling or friction. Sometimes the "bed-hair" remains in the follicle long enough to be pushed out by the fresh, young hair itself. As the hair is now quite dead and has no attachment to the papilla, it results in a fallout of hair that is not painful and it comes away rather easily.

The hair fall is more noticeable in the morning since some 8 hours (sleep period) have passed from the last time the hair was disturbed. During the day the general care given to the hair removes those hairs ready to fall out and therefore no accumulation is present. The dead, detached hair is known as "shed-hair." Under the microscope the base of the "shed-hair" has a club-like, tattered appearance.

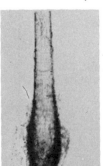

A typical "shed-hair" illustrating club end.

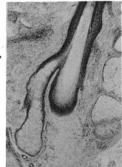

A "bed-hair" in an old follicle. The follicle has shortened past its sebaceous gland.

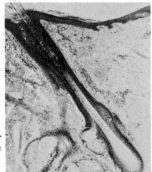

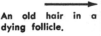

An old hair in a dying follicle.

EFFECTS OF CYCLE   Some 50 to 80 hairs are shed daily, from the scalp, in the normal cycle. This means that 50 to 80 new hairs must also appear each day in order to maintain a constant number of active scalp follicles.

In certain cases, patrons may suddenly realize that their hair is being excessively shed. To avoid this loss they may deliberately refrain from their usual brushing or combing. In the salon this patron may show an alarming loss of hair during a shampoo or in the preparations for a styling.

A greatly increased loss may be due to some definite disorder or upset of body health. If excessive loss of hair continues, it will result in a condition of thinning hair or ultimate baldness.

REPLACEMENT OF HAIRS

Normally, after the dead hair is shed there is a period of complete rest for the follicle. Then the cycle of growth is repeated. How this actually takes place is in debate even among the experts. There is some doubt as to whether:

1. An old papilla reforms and revives itself.
2. An entirely new papilla is formed in the old follicle.
3. The new growth of hair appears from other follicles that have remained dormant during the previous cycles.

In any case, the new young hair repeats the same cycle of growth as its predecessor (provided, of course, that there is no interference with the blood supply to the papilla and to the area of the germinal matrix, and no injury takes place to shorten its life span) .

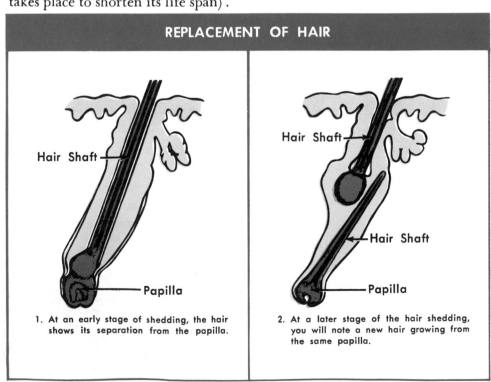

REPLACEMENT OF HAIR

Hair Shaft

Papilla

1. At an early stage of shedding, the hair shows its separation from the papilla.

Hair Shaft

Hair Shaft

Papilla

2. At a later stage of the hair shedding, you will note a new hair growing from the same papilla.

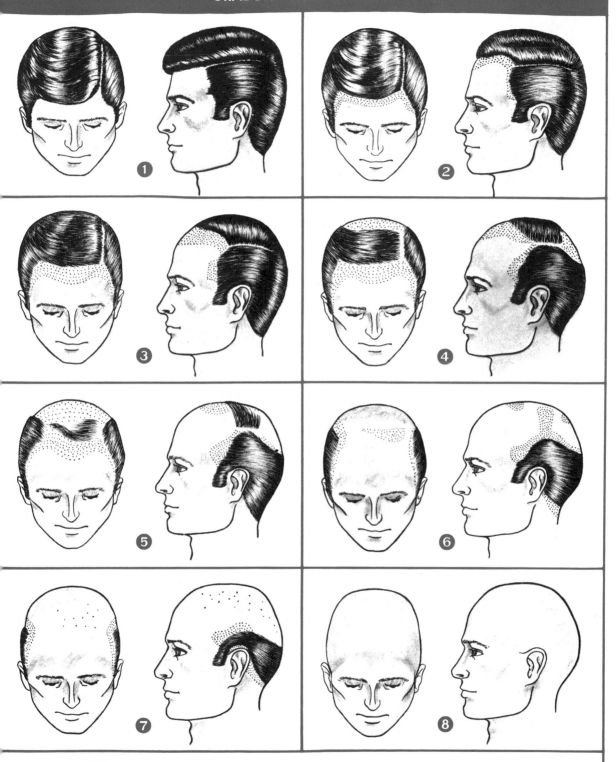

Unless it is caused by some severe illness or unusual phenomenon, scalp baldness does not occur overnight. It is rather a gradual process, usually caused by some form of alopecia, during which the hair growth cycle is slowed down, interrupted or discontinued entirely.

The above sketches illustrate the gradual loss of hair which occurs in the usual case of progressive baldness.

DIFFERENT THEORIES As a general rule, the longer the particular type of hair grows in length, the greater the period of time the follicle will continue to produce this hair.

Scalp hair has the longest cycle of growth. Hair on the eyelashes and eyebrows has a cycle of only from 4 to 5 months. The rate of growth of these hairs is only about half that of normal scalp hair. But, while the follicle rest period may be as long as 6 months on the scalp, the eyelashes and eyebrows require only 9 weeks for regeneration of the next cycle.

REASONS FOR HAIR GROWTH CYCLES

Although we know the details of these hair growth cycles, we are unable to pinpoint the real reasons for them.

DIFFERING THEORIES A number of theories have been put forward:
1. The cells in the papilla gradually accumulate a number of substances which retard and eventually stop hair growth.
2. The papilla is similar to all living cells and it cannot keep working indefinitely. It dies and another inactive follicle is then stimulated to produce a hair in its turn.
3. The papilla has a definite period of life and it then dies. This dead papilla is then replaced by a young active papilla (just as baby teeth are replaced by our adult teeth).
4. Hereditary factors play a very important part in the hair growth cycle.

CONCLUSION The question of hair growth cycles is tied up with facts we do not yet know. Evidence points to the rest period of the papilla as being a likely factor in creating the hair growth cycle. With abnormal changes in the physiology of the body, the papilla also shows that it may develop abnormal patterns in the regular cycle.

OTHER HAIR GROWTH CYCLES

ANIMALS Other creatures possessing hard keratin structures (wool, feathers, hair, fur, etc.) also show a loss or fall of these structures. However, moulting and shedding of hair in animals is seasonal and takes place at a definite period.

MAN In man, hair fall is continuous and there must be a continuous replacement of shed hairs. Therefore, a heavy shedding of hairs at a definite time is unusual and may indicate a disorder of the scalp. Some mild shedding of hairs does take place in autumn which is slightly in excess of the normal pattern. This indicates that even in man, there is still a tendency for seasonal loss of hair. But, of course, the loss of hairs still continues throughout the rest of the year in the regular growth cycle pattern.

VARIATIONS OF HAIR AND SKIN

TYPICAL FORMS OF THE HAIR

The form of the hair is due to its contour or shape. It can be readily seen on the scalp in three main forms:

1. Straight   2. Wavy   3. Curly

STRAIGHT HAIR

DISTRIBUTION   Unfortunately for the public, but fortunately for the professional, straight hair appears to be more common or general than naturally wavy hair. Some argument exists as to what is the true form of hair and it would appear that straight hair is the natural or original form.

Nevertheless, most people desire a form of hair which is not given to them by nature. Thus we see that hair waving and straightening are regular services demanded in civilized societies.

Whatever may be said about the psychological reasons for waving, *a wavy form of hair does provide the basis for versatile and professional styling.*

CAUSES OF STRAIGHT HAIR   Straight hair is formed naturally because of the pattern of cell growth at the papilla. Unless we can control this action of the papilla, no method of waving the external part of the hair can result in a truly permanent wave. According to some authorities, an examination of the cross-section of a straight hair typically shows a round, symmetrical structure. Other experts claim that this is not really true, since in their experience the cross-section may vary from round to oval without any change in the straightness of the hair.

Because of the structure of the hair cortex (from which hair derives its form), two posible methods of changing the form of hair are open to the practitioner.

WET SETTING

1. A hair set depends upon the alteration of the physical forces inside the hair.
2. Moistening the hair by means of water or setting lotions softens the hair so that it becomes pliable. Moisture, acting as a lubricant on the polypeptide chains of the cortex, permits a minor adjustment to its internal structure. Thorough drying after the hair is rearranged leads to the appearance of loose waves in the hair.
3. The changes that occur are not, however, permanent. If the hair is remoistened by rain or high humidity, it soon returns to its natural or straight form. If some means could be found to prevent the re-entry of moisture into the cortex, results would be permanent.

PERMANENT WAVING

1. More drastic changes are required if we want a more permanent change in the form of the hair. Chemicals, such as permanent wave solutions, must be used to alter the hair cortex sufficiently.
2. The winding or wrapping of the hair on rods provides the physical force necessary to effect a shift in the polypeptide chains. The hair is then hardened into the wave form by special neutralizers that chemically reverse the action of waving lotion.
3. This type of hair form change is more permanent than that produced by wet setting. But even in permanent waving the natural re-growth remains in the straight form, and so the change is not really a "permanent" wave.

WAVY HAIR

FEATURES OF WAVY HAIR This form of hair can vary from a loose wave, that has so shallow a curve that the wave is hardly noticeable, to over-curly hair.

CAUSE OF WAVY HAIR Naturally curly hair is believed to be due to an uneven growth pattern in the papilla. This effect is at a maximum in the adolescent but tends to diminish gradually as we get older.

The wave may also be affected by sickness, drugs, motherhood, diet, etc., which may cause the hair to return to the straight form for varying periods.

REACTION TO WAVING AND CURLING The loose, curly hair is readily combed and easily set into attractive styles. Most naturally wavy hair responds readily to waving and holds the wave fairly well, but short, tight, curly hair is difficult to handle because it usually tangles so readily. It forms "corkscrew curls" and extremely narrow waves and resists efforts to alter its natural texture and appearance.

OVER CURLY HAIR

FEATURES OF OVER-CURLY HAIR This form of hair is usually found on Africans and in some of the Pacific Islanders. It is relatively short and grows to approximately the same length all over the scalp.

CAUSES OF OVER-CURLY HAIR There is little doubt that over-curly hair is a special form of terminal hair. In cross-section it is said to be very flat. Experts can explain little about its origin but suggest it is caused by a difference in the nature of the papilla and germinal matrix in the follicles of the people concerned.

SPECIAL PROBLEMS Over-curly hair is difficult to handle and comb. It can be straightened with heated combs, caustics such as sodium hydroxide and special permanent wave solutions. Using chemical methods, the hair, converted to a softened condition, is combed straight and held there until ready for neutralizing. This action reverses the procedure which is found in the usual permanent wave method for waving straight hair.

PIGMENTATION OF THE HAIR

The natural color of the hair is due to the pigment (melanin) which is present mainly in the cortex. The natural shades or differences in hair color are caused by changes in the following:

1. Type of pigment
2. Difference in pigment granules.
3. Air spaces in the cortex.

TYPE OF PIGMENT

Scientific investigations of the many colors of the hair have discovered only four different natural types of pigment, which are:

(a) black
(b) brown
(c) yellow
(d) red

These four pigments invariably occur as mixtures, and this explains the unending variation in human hair colors.

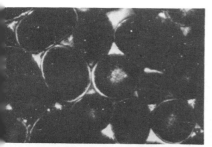

Natural black straight hair. (only black hairs) (These hairs absorb light intensely.)

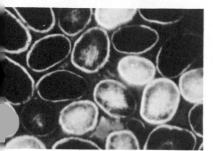

Natural brown straight hair. (contains black, brown, yellow hairs) (Note that there is no color in the cuticle.)

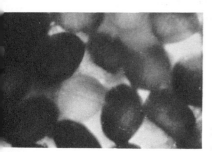

Natural blonde straight hair. (golden shade) (mostly dark hairs with lighter colored hairs)

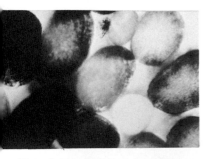

Natural red straight coarse hair (auburn shade) (contains yellow, red, brown, black hairs) (This hair has a large cortex with a thin cuticle layer.)

BLACK   Most black hair is really a combination of black and brown pigments. Oriental hair is claimed to be one example of pure black hair. Black is the dominant or most powerful of the hair pigments. If one parent, is dark haired then there is a strong tendency for the children of that marriage to also have dark hair.

BROWN   Of all the natural colors of the hair, the majority are found in the brownette range. Mixtures of brown with black pigment produce the darker brown to nearly black shades. On the other hand, if it is associated with the yellow or red types of melanin, we find the lighter shades of brown to blonde hair. Brown pigment is more powerful than the yellow or red.

YELLOW   Natural blonde hair contains yellow pigment in addition to various amounts of brown and red. It is the most changeable shade of hair coloring. Even in the same shaft there may be wide variations in pigment types. This is the weakest pigment and true natural blondes are very rare. Both parents must have light-colored hair, or at least carry the red or yellow pigments themselves in their cells.

Because of the mixture of pigments in blonde hair there is a tendency for the hair to darken as the person gets older.

Blonde hair is usually the finest texture of hair, suggesting that there is a link between the melanophores (pigment producing cells) and the hair growth control of the papilla. There are also more hairs on the scalp with this type of hair than with any other color.

RED   Red pigment is often found together with black pigment, giving attractive rust or copper shades. Brown or yellow sometimes occurs to give variations in the basic red coloring.

Red hair is peculiar in that it often has a stronger texture than other hair.

AIR SPACES

The presence of air spaces in the cortex can also vary the natural color of the hair greatly.

VARIATIONS IN HAIR COLOR

Not only are there variations in pigmentation between different individuals, there may be separate colors on the same scalp. For example, a single hair of a natural blonde might vary from almost grey to a medium brown. However, bleached blonde hair has an almost uniform coloring over the entire head.

OTHER FEATURES OF PIGMENTS

PIGMENT FORMATION The pigment in hair is produced by special cells of the hair bulb and as the hair grows upwards, the pigment is carried in the cortex with the new growth. As the melanocytes gradually die they form into granules (little grains).

PIGMENT FORMATION IN HAIR

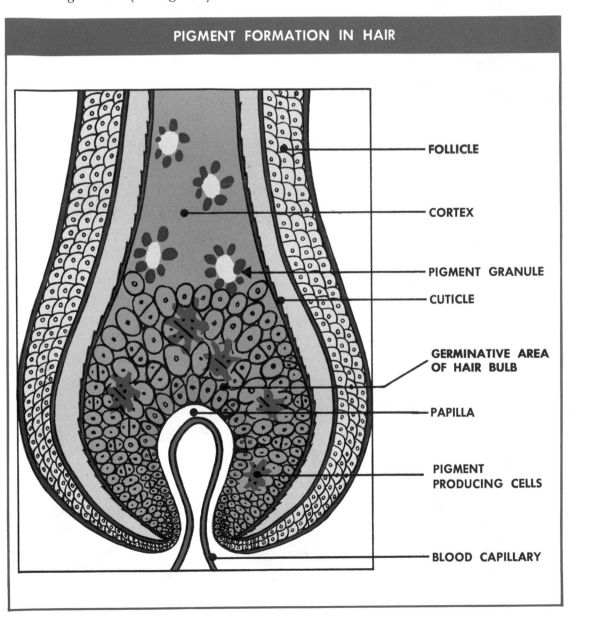

- FOLLICLE
- CORTEX
- PIGMENT GRANULE
- CUTICLE
- GERMINATIVE AREA OF HAIR BULB
- PAPILLA
- PIGMENT PRODUCING CELLS
- BLOOD CAPILLARY

SKIN PIGMENT Although the pigment of hair and the natural pigment in the skin are both melanin, there appears to be little relationship between them.

PIGMENT GRANULES

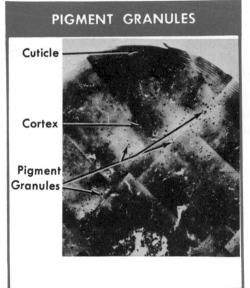

Cuticle

Cortex

Pigment
Granules

DIFFERENCES IN PIGMENT GRANULES

BACKGROUND PIGMENT This pigment can be found scattered throughout the cortex as diffuse or background pigment. It is only noticeable when the hair is almost white.

GRANULES The usual location of the pigment however, is in special cells inside the cortex called pigment granules. Pigment granules are very dense and, almost without exception, are composed of almost pure (well over 90%) melanin.

The pigment granules themselves vary:

1. They can be large or small in diameter.
2. They can contain a lot of pigment or very little.
3. They are gathered into clusters or are spread evenly throughout the cortex.

VARIOUS TYPES OF PIGMENT GRANULES

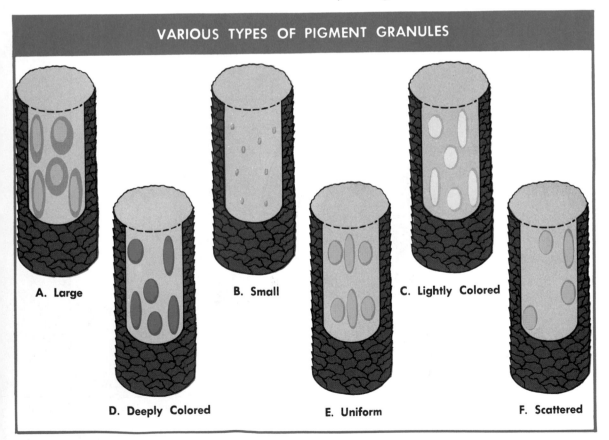

A. Large

B. Small

C. Lightly Colored

D. Deeply Colored

E. Uniform

F. Scattered

In bright sunshine the hair itself appears to be of a different color than it is at night, because sunlight is a more intense or stronger light. Because of the subtle influences of light and reflection on the pigments inside the cortex, the natural color of the hair is ever changing yet remains pleasing to the eye. The cuticle itself however, is completely colorless. With tinted or color rinsed hair, some color always remains on the cuticle. It must be noted that, the less that remains on the cuticle and the more color that can be introduced into the cortex, the more natural will the results appear.

FEATURES OF NATURAL HAIR COLOR Under the searching eye of the microscope, natural hair color may be seen as the result of:

1. Absence of color in the cuticle.
2. Presence of pigment granules in the cortex.
3. Patches of color in hair fibers, both from different areas of the scalp and within the hair fiber itself.
4. A pleasant, soft, deep color with no brassy quality.

GREY HAIR

Grey hair is due to the fact that some hairs lose their natural pigment, while others do not. This mixture of white and dark hair gives the outward appearance of being a dull grey color (pepper and salt).

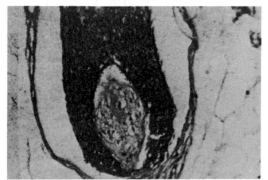

Ageing hair bulb with grey hair. Granules' are formed but lack pigment.

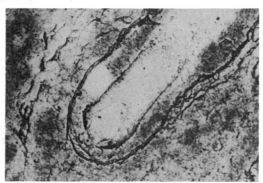

Albino hair showing no granules or pigment in bulb.—Courtesy: Biology of Hair Growth—Academic Press

Grey hair is usually just as strong as naturally colored hair. It is simply the result of some breakdown in the normal pigment production of the hair papilla.

ALBINO HAIR In some people there is a complete lack of hair pigment. This deficiency is known as albinism. Albinos have little or no pigment in their hair, skin and eyes, and because of the latter condition cannot stand bright sunlight.

It is a hereditary defect and so tends to appear in certain families, although there may also be normal children born in the same family.

DANDRUFF OF THE SCALP

DEFINITION   Dandruff is a condition of the scalp where an abnormal number of scales from the outer epidermis are constantly being shed. These thin, powdery scales lodge in the hair and fall out onto the shoulders where they look very unsightly.

The problem of dandruff is very widespread; indeed a recent survey of pharmacies, beauty salons and barber shops shows that dandruff occurs in at least 75% of the patrons coming to these centers for hair treatments or products. An odd fact that has emerged is that, in the case of people working in public relations (as in radio and T.V.) the level rises to 95%.

The rate of dandruff is higher in men than in women and is also more prevalent in winter than in summer.

TYPES OF DANDRUFF

COMMON DANDRUFF   Dandruff may vary widely in appearance, but the most common type is that of a simple loss of dry, flat, epithelial scales.

The scales are very difficult to remove by simple brushing or shampooing. They tend to detract from the appearance of a healthy head of hair and for this reason cause much upset and distress to the individual. However, if this type of dandruff is kept in check by proper scalp care, it may only present a minor psychological problem.

OILY TYPE   A more severe infestation is that of the oily type which has a patchy, crusting form. These scales are much larger and yellowish in color. If the crust is lifted from the scalp, the skin underneath is reddened and inflamed and accompanied by considerable itching.

This type of dandruff is found very often on the scalp of young babies and is then known as "cradle cap."

Courtesy: Gillette Company Research Institute,

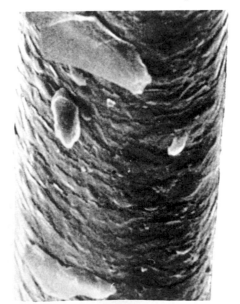

Normal hair with dandruff flakes adhering to hair fibers.

Unfortunately, in spite of its wide distribution and the long scientific investigation of dandruff, there still remains serious doubt about its exact cause. The theories that have been put forward include the following:

EXCESSIVE CELL PRODUCTION The most current theory concerning dandruff treats the condition as a speed-up in the shedding of skin scales on the scalp, combined with a high rate of skin cell production. The increased number of micro-organisms found on such scalps is due to the fact that they have more loose skin to grow on.

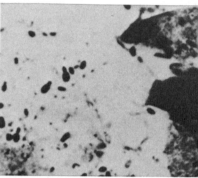

Bottle bacillus showing scales of epidermis or "dandruff" (magnified 600 times). — Courtesy: Hair & Scalp—Edward Arnold

Treatment would involve more frequent shampooing in order to remove excess scales. Special medications, designed to decrease the rate of cell multiplication in the basal layer of the epidermis, appear to give some relief.

NERVOUS ORIGIN Another theory suggests that dandruff is due to emotional upset of the body system, due to worry, strain or tension.

This theory stands up reasonably well when checked with statistics. It is true that nervous people suffer more from dandruff than placid persons. Country folk have less dandruff than their city cousins.

The higher rate in people working under pressure and strain (e.g., radio, T.V. executives) shows that there is some relationship between emotional stress and dandruff. It has been determined that excess worry, continued strain and hypertension affect the growth of the hair. It is not unreasonable to say that the normal and protective mechanisms of the skin system are interfered with in a similar manner.

COMBINATION OF INFECTION AND NERVOUS CAUSES This last theory combines the first two theories. It supposes that dandruff is caused by an infection by some germ (including the bottle bacillus) on the scalp of a person suffering from severe upset of his nervous system.

TREATMENT OF DANDRUFF

REGULAR CARE Some facts about dandruff are well known. The person with dandruff must treat his scalp with greater care than normally. Regular medicated shampoos are essential.

CHANGE OF MEDICATION In addition to a risk of dermatitis, another peculiarity of the medicated shampoos is that they must be changed regularly. The active ingredients used range from:

1. Coal tars
2. Hexachlorophenol
3. Flowers of sulphur
4. Metallic sulphides (selenium sulphide)

(This information is carried on the label of the container. *READ IT!*) These medicaments must be used in rotation, as resistance to the shampoo may build up. One particular product or brand may appear to be winning control of the dandruff, then, slowly, the dandruff returns until it is just as bad as before.

PROBLEM OF TREATMENT   Strong disinfectants cannot be used on the hair. The dandruff scales (SOFT KERATIN) must be dissolved from the hair (HARD KERATIN) without harming the scalp (SOFT KERATIN).

FUNCTION OF TREATMENT   The dandruff treatment must:

1. Remove the excess scales from the scalp and hair.
2. Not penetrate into or harm the healthy part of the epidermis.
3. Destroy causative microorganisms.
4. Slow down reproduction of epidermal cells in the scalp.

REMOVAL OF SCALES   If the dandruff is the simple, mild, dry type, good results may be obtained with the regular use of a hairbrush. This will help to loosen the scaly, powdery flakes that stick to the scalp and hair and remove the greater portion; thereby preventing an unsightly buildup.

Regular removal of the dandruff helps the scalp to stay healthy. Dust, debris and dandruff scales harbor the suspected bacteria and fungi that make the scalp unhealthy.

RISK OF TRANSFER   Practitioners may unwittingly help the spread of this condition if they do not do their part in the maintenance of high standards of salon or shop hygiene. Dandruff should be handled in the same manner as any other infectious disorder. Furthermore, if you suffer from dandruff, it is wise to keep your own brush, comb and anything else that comes in contact with the hair scrupulously clean by frequent washing and sanitizing.

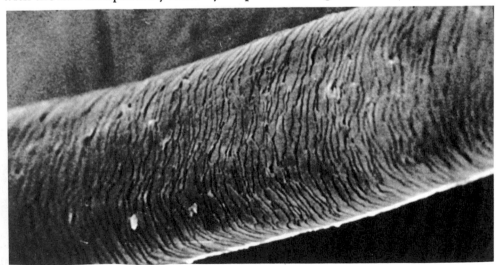

Normal clean hair fibers —Courtesy: L. Wolfram, Gittelle Research Institute, Rockville, Maryland

THE SEBACEOUS GLAND

IMPORTANCE   The value of this gland is emphasized when we discover that tertiary (terminal) hair follicles possess at least one sebaceous gland and in many cases, up to six are clustered around the follicle.

STRUCTURE

Under the microscope each gland appears as a bunch of grapes. The cells inside the gland break open continuously, sending their contents (sebum) into a special canal or duct leading up the side of the hair follicle.

Because of this special canal alongside the hair, the secretions of sebum are able to be transferred continuously over the whole area of skin. In addition, the oils are spread along to the tips of the hair.

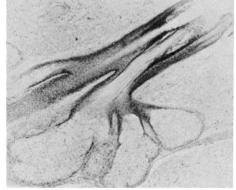

Sebaceous glands clustered around a single hair follicle. A special duct or passage ensures a constant flow of natural oils from the skin and hair shaft.

FUNCTIONS OF SEBUM

It is the function of this all important sebum which we will now investigate. Sebum possesses many properties that are beneficial to the skin and hair.

LUBRICATION

EXTERNAL   Because sebum is essentially a mixture of natural oils, it reduces friction on the skin and hair. Smoothness and slipperiness of normal skin are due to the oils which coat it. There is no need to be reminded of how rough our hands can feel when the sebum has been removed by constant washing in strong soaps and detergents. We can hardly say that having roughened hands is a life-or-death matter. However, the professional practitioner should be aware of the role that sebum plays in preserving natural attractiveness, as well as essential features of the skin.

INTERNAL   The natural oils supply this external lubrication, but the more important internal lubrication is supplied by the normal moisture content of hair and skin.

PROTECTION

MOISTURE LOSS   It has been frequently mentioned that this coating of natural oils protects against the loss of vital life-giving moisture from the skin and hair. More that half of our outer skin and about one tenth of the hair consists of water. There is a constant threat to the maintenance of this high level because of the dry atmosphere around us. If we did not have this coating of oils to stop evaporation, we would dry out as if we were laundry on the clothes line. Because of the high volume of water in the cells of the skin, when we do lose moisture (for various reasons) the skin shrinks and contracts. This contraction of drying skin can break small blood vessels and cause painful pressure on nerve endings. Skin conditioners are needed if there is any danger of the skin drying up.

SPECIAL PROPERTIES OF SEBUM

Sebum also possesses powerful bacteria and fungi inhibitors that prevent the mass invasion of the skin and hair by these destructive organisms. When we consider the fact that every object the skin contacts provides more chance of attack from hostile bacteria and fungi, we realize just how much we depend on sebum for our survival. The skin would otherwise provide an ideal "home" for these tiny intruders, as it is warm, moist and supplied with ample nourishment. Sebum is slightly acid, has a protein content, and in many ways will benefit the hair in a manner imitated by commercially prepared conditioners.

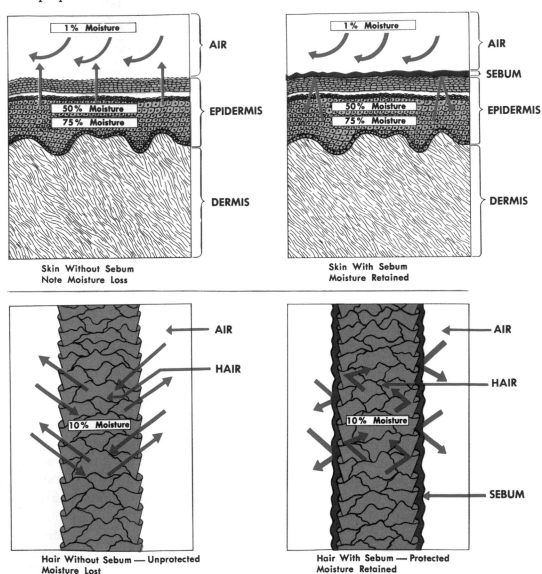

Skin Without Sebum
Note Moisture Loss

Skin With Sebum
Moisture Retained

Hair Without Sebum — Unprotected
Moisture Lost

Hair With Sebum — Protected
Moisture Retained

Skin diseases and scalp complaints are much more common in the child or the elderly person. For example, ringworm (a fungus which grows on the skin in a particular pattern) is not an uncommon complaint of the child, but is rarely, if ever, found on the adult.

A reduction in the protective properties of sebum takes place at adolescence, when the activity of the gland is often disturbed. In many teen-agers, the actual amount of oil secretion increases and causes a greasy skin, but the sebum frequently loses its bacterial action. The bacteria enter the hair follicle and begin to multiply and soon a thick colony of bacteria forms in the follicle.

Other skin troubles may follow, for example: boils, furuncles, car-buncles, pimples, acne, and blackheads.

TREATMENT OF SKIN PROBLEMS

Care must be exercised in the treatment of blackheads and acne. If simple hygiene is ignored, then the result will be to assist the spread and even aggravation of the trouble. Acne, as an example, can lead to scarring of the skin for life.

REMOVING BLACKHEADS Squeezing with the fingernails to remove a black-head, is temporary at best, and may even create more blackheads in the area. The skin must first be thoroughly cleaned by warm water and soap, then a cleansing lotion applied to remove the last traces of excess oils and to soften the skin. Special extractors may be used to remove the hard plug, or the skin may be gently squeezed by using a facial tissue. A suitable mild antiseptic skin cream should then be massaged gently into the affected area.

Caution:

Great care must be exercised in the removal of blackheads. If this is not performed carefully and correctly, it can cause infection and permanent scarring.

Antiseptic soaps (such as those containing hexachlorophene) should be used regularly on the skin. This counteracts the excessive greasy nature of the oils and helps to remove harmful skin bacteria.

CONTROL OF SEBACEOUS GLANDS

HEALTH As in all functions of the body, there is a close relationship between the activity of the glands and general health.

In ill health the secretions are slowed down or cease. As a result the skin and hair become dry so that they look dull and lifeless. Lustre or sheen of the hair, on the other hand, relies, to some extent, on the coating of sebum.

AGE We have already seen how the activity of the sebaceous gland depends on our age. Elderly people rarely have this normal activity and so their skin and hair become dry and dull.

DIET The type and amounts of food we eat also have an effect on the glands. Carbohydrates, in particular, cause more oils to be produced. Teen-agers often consume excessive amounts of sweets, chocolate, pastry, cakes, biscuits, etc., and these foods serve to maintain an over-oily, greasy skin.

HORMONES The hormones circulating in the bloodstream have a powerful effect on the sebaceous glands. Male hormones over-stimulate the glands, and young men tend to have oily skin as a result.

At adolescence or puberty, there is usually an upset in the type and rate of sebum production. At times the skin is dry, then, at another time, it is too oily. It may often be disfigured by pimples, blackheads and acne.

Disorders of the thyroid gland also affect the sebaceous glands, and as a result, people with simple goiter often have a dry, scaly skin.

SHAMPOO There is NO connection, however, between shampooing the hair or washing of the skin and increases in the natural level of oils. (This is similar to the misinformed statement that cutting or shaving the hairs causes them to grow faster.) Merely removing the oils at the skin or hair surface cannot stimulate the sebaceous gland which is deep inside the follicle.

Only those factors which work below skin level can cause any decrease or increase in the secretions of this essential gland. As a result, a person with an oily skin and hair has to shampoo the hair more frequently than others.

CHAPTER 10

EFFECTS OF HAIR SERVICE OPERATIONS

This area of the text will be devoted to a study of the effects of the following common professional operations upon the hair:

1. Brushing
2. Combing
3. Cutting
4. Shaving
5. Singeing
6. Plucking
7. Lightening (bleaching)
8. Shampooing
9. Permanent Waving
10. Coloring

BRUSHING

Brushing is very beneficial to the hair for the following reasons:

IT STIMULATES the circulation of the blood and lymph supply to the scalp. This helps to remove accumulated cell wastes more effectively, thus promoting healthy hair growth.

At times the scalp tends to lack its vital blood supply because of the bony framework of the skull. This necessary, hard, protective covering for the brain somewhat restricts the normal muscular activities that assist the circulation in other areas. As a result the blood supply to the scalp is reduced.

In some individuals this may also be aggravated by a very tight scalp. Any form of massage, which is carried out regularly, will assist the circulation and is therefore, beneficial. A pleasant tingling sensation is a sign that brushing has stimulated circulation and is assisting the health of the scalp and hair.

IT TRANSFERS SEBUM (natural oils) from the skin surface along the cuticle of the hair shaft. The coating of oils stabilizes the moisture content of the hair and maintains it at the correct level (approximately 10%). This moisture acts as an internal lubricant and the natural oils act as external lubricants. The oils thus lessen the tendency for the hairs to mesh together or form knots, as they would when too dry.

The oils on the outside of the cuticle also serve to emphasize the natural luster or sheen which is so pleasing to the eye. Dry hair is dull and unattractive.

BRUSHING REMOVES DEAD EPITHELIAL SCALES or dandruff from the hair. and scalp. Superficial dust, dirt and foreign matter may also be removed this way. This debris favors the growth of bacteria resulting in the unpleasant smell of dirty hair. Brushing the hair well before shampooing assists the shampoo to remove the smaller particles of grit and scales that the brush leaves behind on the hair and scalp.

STIMULATES RETURN OF NATURAL LUSTER The dull, dry, "flyaway," brittle appearance of some types of hair may be corrected by a program of regular brushing. Improvement will not take place immediately, but if the brushing is continued, a noticeable change will be seen and the hair will slowly regain its natural luster. (Conditioners applied to the hair will give immediate correction, but it is better to restore the natural activity of the sebaceous gland by brushing.)

EFFECT OF BRUSHING ON SEBACEOUS GLANDS

UNDER-ACTIVE GLANDS In the older patron, the changes that accompany old age will also cause a drop in the activity of the sebaceous glands. Brushing will help to offset some of these natural changes and stimulate the glands.

OVER-ACTIVE GLANDS With the over-active sebaceous glands giving rise to oily, limp hair, it is still advisable to give regular brushing to the hair and scalp. The over-activity of the glands, with resulting greasy hair, is not caused by any amount of brushing. Where this oily hair is present, the effects of the over-activity of the glands may be lessened by more frequent shampoos.

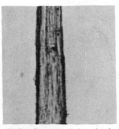

Hair damaged by faulty brushing.

PROBLEMS OF BRUSHING

Some styles of hair (particularly where back-combing techniques are used) do not lend themselves to regular brushing. The lack of necessary attention will cause irregularities to develop in the hair. Simpler styles are better for the purposes of daily brushing and general care.

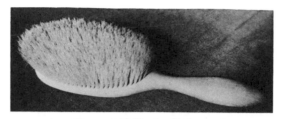

Stand-up Brush

There has been a great deal said about the brush itself. While many of these opinions are debatable, certain facts are known.

1. The professional is more skillful in the art of brushing the hair than the typical customer.
2. The spaced visits to the shop by the patron means that the harder brushes can only contact the hair at infrequent intervals.
3. Nylon brushes have been severely criticized because of their hardness. However, they are cheap and are easily cleaned and sanitized. This factor must be carefully considered with relation to the risk of cross-infection (from one patron to another).
4. Natural bristles are the best for a brush because they are softer than nylon and are made of natural keratin. This reduces the friction and wear between the hair and the brush.
5. The bristles of any brush should be set into tufts or rows. This allows the loose, "shed hair" to collect in the grooves without interfering with the action of the bristles.

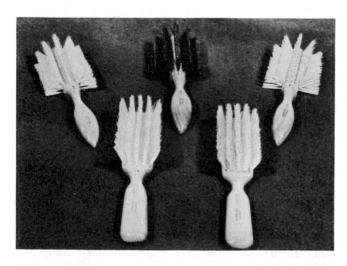

Various shapes of hair brushes used by professional hair-care practitioners.

CONCLUSION   The hair at the front of the scalp often shows the effects of brushing more than the other sections of the hair. The cuticle layer is more roughened and so the porosity of this area is greater, this fact must be considered in performing other professional hair services.

COMBING

Combing has physiological benefits on the hair similar to brushing.

NATURE OF THE COMB Because of the construction of the comb it must be handled with even more care than the brush. The teeth of the comb should never be allowed to scratch or injure the scalp. The teeth of a good comb should have rounded points, with a fine taper and space between them where they join at the base. *Avoid combs that pinch the hair at the base of the teeth,* causing pulling and tugging. Combs with broken or irregular teeth should be discarded.

CORRECT COMBING TECHNIQUES Injury to the hair and breakage may follow the incorrect combing of snarled or matted hair. The knots must be separated without undue effort or tugging on the shaft or scalp.

The skilled practitioner starts from the ends of the hair and gently works back towards the scalp. The unskilled person may try to force the comb through the hair, starting at the scalp. This causes great strain or breakage of the hair.

USES OF COMBING

1. Combing will remove attached scales and debris even more effectively than the brushing. Combing separates the hair into parallel strands which can then be gathered into convenient sized panels or sections.
2. Combing is very useful to remove excess water from the hair after shampooing or rinsing.
3. Tints, creams and fillers can also be spread along the shaft of the hair by the comb. This evens out the application quickly and simply.
4. Combing is helpful in distributing and sectioning hair for various shop techniques and operations.

In professional practice, the comb is used to perform many tasks and there is a wide variety of useful designs available.

Caution:

On virgin hair, combing would be the main initiator of damage. Careless action of the comb slowly abrades the cuticle to a point where the cortex splits longitudinally. The pressure of the comb is highest at the fiber tips and it is here that most damage appears as split ends.

SUMMARY OF COMBING AND BRUSHING Both combing and brushing have a psychological or emotional effect on one's personality. It is remarkable how quickly a patron will regain composure and confidence with a few strokes of the brush or comb through the hair.

Scientific discoveries have shown that in primitive and ancient societies, the brush and comb have been used on the hair for countless generations. This shows that early man realized their usefulness and modern man has verified this fact by continuing to employ them.

However, these simple but valuable tools, incorrectly used, can seriously damage the hair and scalp. If correctly used, however, they will help beautify and contribute greatly to the health of the hair.

CUTTING

AFFECTS ON HAIR GROWTH Cutting *has no affect* on the growth of the hair. Cutting does NOT stimulate hair growth. The action of cutting takes place some distance from the scalp, in the dead section of the hair shaft. In general, only those factors which affect the living part of the hair, its papilla and follicle, can alter the growth rate of the hair.

BENEFITS OF HAIRCUTTING AND SHAPING:

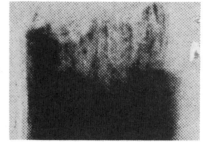

A fine hair the day after having been cut with good scissors. Note the sharp ragged edges.

1. The hair is kept shorter than the length it could really attain. Whatever may have been said about long hair in the past, modern living and the grooming industry demands a simple, shorter style. Short hair is easier to brush, comb, shampoo, wave, tint and style. On the other hand, long hair requires constant attention and it may even present a source of danger or risk of injury if the wearer is employed at work that involves close proximity to machinery.

2. Cutting off the distant ends of the hair shaft removes that worn, porous, unattractive outer portion that is often split and damaged.

3. Thinning may be used to reduce bulk, where the density of the hair is too great.

4. Cutting is necessary to even length, because of the unequal growth rate from adjacent follicles.

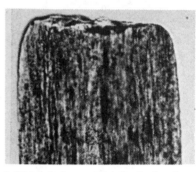

A thick hair four weeks after having been cut.

REASONS FOR FREQUENT TRIMMING

At the end of the individual life cycle of the follicle all further growth of hair ceases. But active, *young follicles* produce hair at a maximum rate of ¾″ to 1″ per month. Cutting or trimming is required to even up the ragged, untidy ends of the hairs. This trimming for correction of uneven growth is required more frequently than would be necessary if each individual hair were to grow at a uniform rate.

Cutting of the hair is also needed because of changes in trends and fashions that require new styling and shaping of the hair.

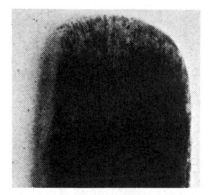

Hair six months after being cut. Note rounded-off end. — *Courtesy: Hair and Scalp, Edward Arnold*

CAUTION Thinning the hair with a razor involves a sliding, flat stroke which has a tendency to slice off strips of the cuticle which thus exposes the cortex of the hair. Subsequent harsh chemical treatment and combing will produce severe damage or breakage at these exposed points.

SHAVING

EFFECTS ON HAIR GROWTH Shaving is really a form of cutting by an instrument that cuts off the hair close to the skin.

As with the case of cutting, there is *NO* effect on the hair growth. This myth was exploded by Dr. Mildred Trotter at the Washington University School of Medicine.

Under her observation, 3 girls shaved their left legs from knee to ankle, twice a week for a period of 8 months. At the end of this time, microscopic examination revealed that there was absolutely no increase in the diameter of the hairs before or after the shaving period.

Another experiment was conducted to examine the hairs on the scalp and legs of 12 girls before the summer started. These girls continued to go swimming and sunbathing in the hot sun. After the season was over, the microscope revealed that the sun and wind had no effect on the growth, number or texture of the hairs.

REASONS FOR COMMON MISBELIEF After shaving there is, however, an illusion of growth that has given rise to the false idea that shaving really does affect the growth. Let us examine those points which appear to support the idea that shaving does cause an increased hair growth.

1. The shortness of the shaft of the shaved hair allows changes in its length to be noticed more easily. If the hair was shaved right to the skin and then allowed to grow only 1/16", we would readily notice this. However if the hair was already 6" long and it also grew 1/16" (in the same period as the shaved hair) no one could tell without some accurate way of measuring.

   Taking the example of the male with a full beard, it is impossible to detect the daily increase in beard growth. It is a different story with the clean shaven person and his "5 o'clock shadow" when the growth of the bristles can be seen on the very same day.

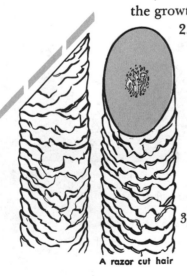

2. Because the follicles of terminal hair are not at right angles to the skin, shaving exposes more actual area of hair to the eye.

   Now, cutting the hair with scissors usually takes place at right angles to the direction of growth. But shaving gives an angled shape to the ends of the hair fibers due to the angle of the follicle to the skin. When the hairs grow out from the skin they keep their "thickened" appearance, especially as they are being compared with the white background of skin.

3. Apparent coarseness is caused by the short, shaved hairs being held more erect by the follicles clasped firmly around them.

A razor cut hair

SINGEING

EFFECTS ON HAIR GROWTH   Singeing is bad for the hair and it has no affect on growth.

DISADVANTAGES

Burning the tips of the hairs causes gases to be formed inside the hair shafts. These gases create great pressure and often cause the ends of the hairs to split.

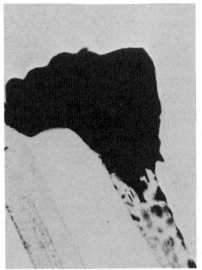

Singed hair twenty minutes after.

Courtesy: Hair and Scalp, Edward Arnold.

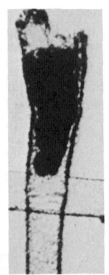

Singed hair fifteen days later. Note charring and swelling of cortex.

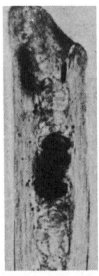

Singed hair after three months. Note extent of damage to the hair and rounding of end in the usual manner.

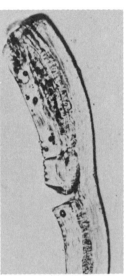

Singed hair after three and a half months showing complete breakdown of hair ends. This hair had not been treated with any chemicals after singeing.

A blackened knob is formed as a swollen cap at the ends of the hairs. This is not only unsightly and detrimental, but a complete waste of time. This knobby end is very soon broken off by the action of combing and brushing and so nothing is gained but split, damaged hair.

REASONS FOR PRACTICE   Singeing was based on the false theory that the medulla was actually a hollow tube in the middle of the hair. This tube was supposed to lead up from the papilla and was thought to be a canal out of which certain "juices" flowed and so were lost to the hair. The singeing was supposed to cap this tube and prevent this loss.

PRESENT KNOWLEDGE   In actual fact, the medulla is not just a hollow tube. It is made up of single cells in one or two rows or columns. In some cases the medulla may be broken up into sections, or even entirely missing from the hair. The drying of hair is really caused by the loss of cortex moisture through the cuticle and not from the medulla.

PLUCKING

DISADVANTAGES

1. Plucking the hairs can be a dangerous practice when carried to extremes or when performed under unsanitary conditions.

2. For the growth of an active hair to be prevented, the papilla itself must be destroyed. Merely plucking the hair out of the follicle is not enough. However, repeated plucking may achieve this purpose by the strain on the narrow neck of the papilla. When the papilla is broken off in this way the blood vessels attached to it are also damaged. Bleeding follows this and the open follicle fills up with blood from the ruptured capillaries. Bacteria can easily enter this open wound in the skin causing local inflammation.

3. If the eyebrows are plucked, chemicals used on the hair (especially tints and dyes) may run down from the scalp and enter the open follicles and the eyes. This has been known to cause a painful swelling or even temporary blindness. Eyebrow tints, if improperly used, may also cause this type of eye damage.

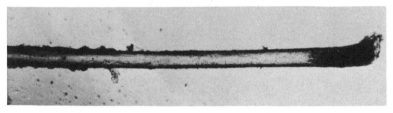

An old hair plucked from follicle. Hair is detached without pain.

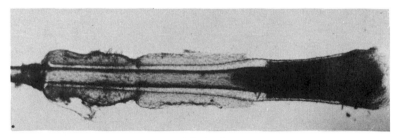

A normal active hair plucked from follicle. Part of follicle wall remains attached.

PRECAUTIONS Notwithstanding, tweezing or plucking the eyebrows continues to be practiced. The practitioner can reduce the risks following this treatment by these precautions:

1. Implements used should be kept clean and sanitized.
2. The skin should be kept free from oils and dirt by proper sanitary measures.
3. To protect the eyes, thinning of the eyebrows should take place from the lower hairline. This leaves the upper hairs to continue

their protective function of preventing liquids from running down from the brows and entering the eyes.

4. Complete plucking of all hairs from the eyebrows should never be practiced.

5. After plucking the hairs, the open follicles should be closed by a mild antiseptic skin ointment.

EFFECTS OF LIGHTENING (BLEACHING)

THE ACTION OF LIGHTENING Lightening the hair consists of treating the pigment in the hair with strong lighteners. These special chemicals (lighteners) serve to change the natural pigment into a colorless form.

DISADVANTAGES Lighteners must be strong chemicals in order to create the required change in the pigment. Extreme care must be taken to prevent damage to the structure of the hair. If precautions are not taken, the cuticle may be damaged or even removed. In the places where the cuticle has been removed, the lightener will damage the cortex itself.

Bleaching (lightening) damage is more likely to be caused by overlapping during a retouch. Lightening pastes or creams are easier to apply accurately and for this reason are safer to use than liquid lighteners.

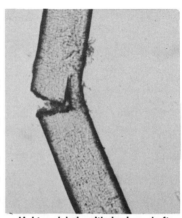

Lightened hair with broken shaft

Courtesy: Gillette Company Research Institute, Rockville, Maryland

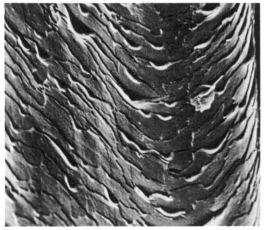

Damage to scales of the cuticle caused by lightening (bleaching) magnified 2100 times.

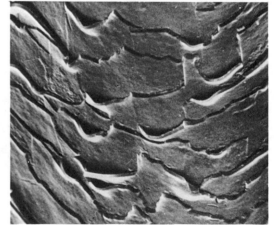

Damage to scales of the cuticle caused by lightening (bleaching) magnified 4200 times.

EXTRA PRECAUTIONS Research has shown that the bleach is not always thoroughly rinsed out of the hair after the lightening process. A weakening of the hair after the patron has left the salon often occurs.

This type of slow damage may be minimized by:

1. Giving the hair a thorough rinsing with warm water.
2. Applying a mild acid rinse.

USE OF CONDITIONERS Lightening causes the hair to appear dry and brittle. This is the result of chemical action on the natural oils of the hair. Conditioning (before or after) is often necessary to restore a more healthy appearance.

CONCLUSION

Lightening is a process that requires a great deal of knowledge and technical skill. If the practitioner is to achieve the desired change in hair color without excessive damage to the physical properties of the hair, a high level of understanding and ability must be attained.

SHAMPOOING

Proper shampooing with an appropriate shampoo is of great benefit to the hair.

IT CLEANSES THE SCALP of dirt, debris, dandruff scales, sweat and oils. These materials, if left on the hair, create very favorable grounds for the growth of harmful bacteria and fungi. The presence of such bacteria gives rise to unpleasant odors, in addition to the risk of actual hair damage.

Courtesy: Gillette Company Research Institute, Rockville, Maryland

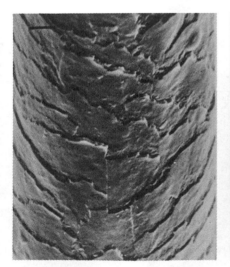 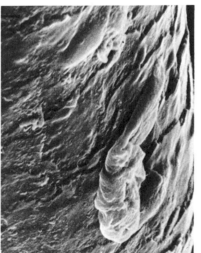 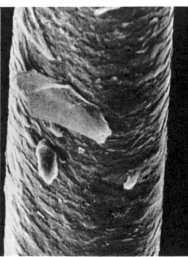

Normal clean hair, magnified 5000 times.　Normal hair with accumulated sebum and debris, magnified 7500 times.　Normal hair with dandruff flakes adhering to fiber, magnified 1260 times.

IT INCREASES ABSORPTION OF solutions such as rinses, waving and setting lotions through the cuticle into the cortex.

STIMULATION Massage of the scalp during the shampoo helps to improve the supply of blood and lymph to the scalp.

AFFECT ON SEBACEOUS GLANDS Shampooing has NO affect whatsoever on the activity of the sebaceous glands. Sebum does not have to be removed to keep these glands working, since the action of the glands depends on much deeper physiological reasons. Individuals with over-oily skin and hair need a shampoo more frequently than does the average person with normal activity of the sebaceous glands. The simple truth is that—the over-oiliness requires more frequent shampooing, NOT that frequent shampooing causes over-oiliness.

PROBLEMS IN SHAMPOOING The main problem with the modern shampoo is that the rinsing out of all traces of excess shampoo is vital. The work of the practitioner can be seriously affected by leaving a film of shampoo behind, in the hair. More failures in the shop can be traced to this one source (neglecting to completely rinse out the shampoo) than to any other single reason. This is especially true when highly alkaline shampoos are used.

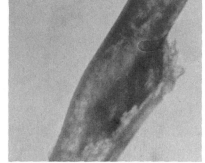

Hair after continued washing with highly alkaline soap. Note swelling and severe damage to shaft.

PERMANENT WAVING

NEED FOR PROFESSIONAL PERMANENT WAVING It should require no mentioning that the skillful use of waving solutions depends on the direct care and attention of the practitioner. Wavy hair is more attractive than straight hair and provides a wider choice for rearrangement in suitable, fashionable, longer lasting styles. Permanent waving is an accepted and indispensable professional service.

PROBLEMS IN PERMANENT WAVING

Notwithstanding these many advantages, permanent waving must be approached with caution. The solutions used do have strong chemical effects on the keratin of the hair, scalp and hands. Some damage to the hair usually results from any and every permanent wave.

The loss in strength of the hair may vary from 25% to 50%, even under expert control. However, this loss in physical property of the cortex can be tolerated. If carelessly applied, however, the solutions may cause an unacceptable amount of damage.

In extreme cases the hair may be almost dissolved. In others there may be damage to the cuticle resulting in weak, highly porous hair. The cortex damage can give rise to loss in quality and condition. Overprocessing can lead to excess frizziness, failure of curl to hold and hair breakage.

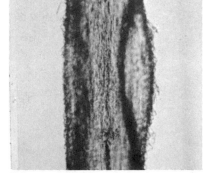

Hair showing area of greater porosity. When cold waving, this would require pre-conditioning treatment to avoid this type of damage from "thio."

As a protection, porosity and texture of the hair must be carefully assessed by testing before and during the processing of the wave.

The use of strong permanent wave solutions may remove the natural oils from the hair, giving rise to excessive dryness. To correct this, various materials are added to the waving solution (cream type).

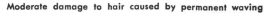

Moderate damage to hair caused by permanent waving

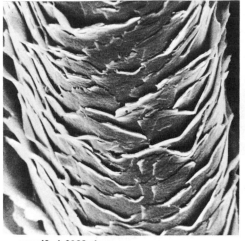

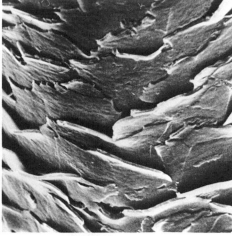

—magnified 2100 times.   —magnified 4200 times.

SPECIAL PERMANENT WAVE SOLUTIONS

The original *quality* and *condition* of the hair has a very great affect on results in permanent waving. For this reason the waving solution comes in various strengths.

1. Strong—for resistant hair.
2. Normal—for average hair.
3. Weak—for porous hair.

THE SPECIAL PROBLEM OF HOME PERMANENT WAVES

Many home permanent waves are sold and used indiscriminately by untrained and unqualified individuals. Most cases of damage to hair, through these practices, are the result of people with restricted budgets being forced to use materials of poor quality, which are applied unskillfully.

One type of home permanent wave that requires special caution is the non-neutralizer, non-rinsing, one-step waving solution. These solutions work because they contain metallic salts. However, these salts are left on the hair after the treatment because rinsing cannot be permitted when using them. These salts have a weakening, drying action on the hair and the trouble they cause is often complained about to the practitioner in the shop. The salts left in the hair continue to give trouble in tinting and in future permanents.

REPAIR OF DAMAGED HAIR There is little that can be done for badly damaged hair other than to cut that section completely off by trimming. Minor forms of hair damage may be repaired, to some degree, by acid rinses, special fillers or protein conditioners.

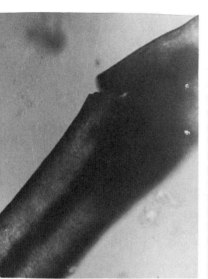 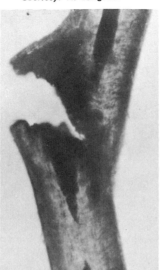 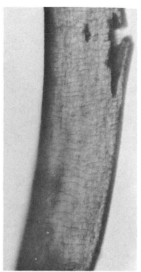 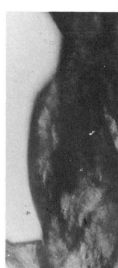

ECONOMIC IMPORTANCE OF PERMANENT WAVING

The affluence of our society and the rise in incomes have greatly stimulated professional permanent waving. The practitioner can assist this trend through an earnest effort to always give the maximum value to the patron. The patron should be able to clearly recognize the benefits of long training and experience in the application of a professional wave.

CONCLUSION   Finally, it can be stated that the possibility of some damage to the hair exists with any form of permanent waving. But, provided the practitioner realizes this and carries out the work carefully and correctly, hair waving can have vast decorative, psychological, economic and social values in our present society.

COLORING

TYPES OF HAIR COLORING   The use of color is of ever increasing importance in the shop and salon today. There are 3 main types:

1. Temporary rinses.
2. Semi-permanent tints.
3. Permanent tints.

MODERN TINTS   The old-fashioned methods of dyeing, merely coated the cuticle with some pigment which resulted in a harsh, unnatural, unattractive appearance. The natural color pigment of the hair is found only in the cortex and the medulla and NEVER in the cuticle. Modern tints are aimed at getting the maximum color into the cortex itself. They have a wide color range and are more simple to apply, being creams or pastes and not drippy liquids.

119

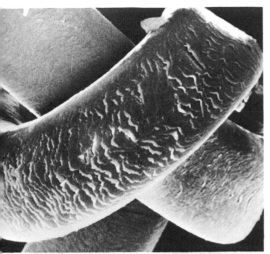
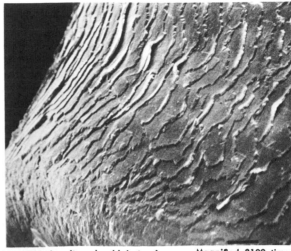

Magnified 630 times   Normal hair tied into a knot. Note: Putting it under high tension   Magnified 2100 times
causes small fractures and causes cuticle scales to begin to lift off.

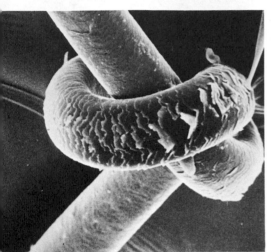
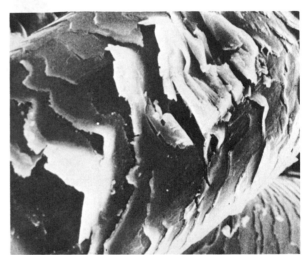

Magnified 630 times   Permanent waved hair tied into a knot emphasizes the cuticle damage   Magnified 1600 times
caused by permanent waving.

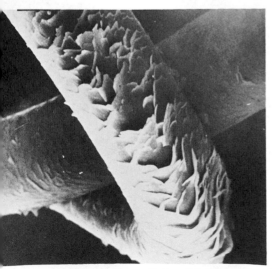
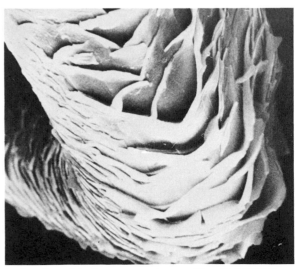

Magnified 630 times   Lightened hair tied into a knot emphasizes the cuticle damage caused   Magnified 2100 times
by lightening.

Courtesy: Gillette Company Research Institute, Rockville, Maryland

DISADVANTAGES:
1. Permanent tints (aniline derivative types) can cause skin reactions or dermatitis, and so have to be used with care.
2. The lighteners and developers or boosters used in the pre-lightening phase can cause dryness or brittleness of the hair.
3. A certain amount of hair damage is produced by most permanent tints.

CONCLUSION Tinting is a highly specialized branch of hair treatments. It is also very exacting, for one cannot tell with certainty what the final result will be, especially when color-matching previously tinted hair. Not everyone has the delicate color sense necessary for perfection in hair coloring; this work requires very high professional skill.

Photos of hair which has been subjected to various waving and coloring processes. To the naked eye this hair looks normal and quite nice. *Courtesy: Gillette Company Research Institute, Rockville, Maryland*

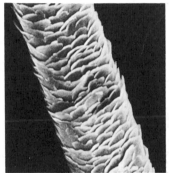 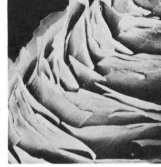 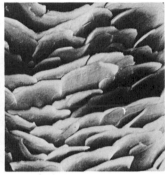

Magnified 1080 times   Magnified 2100 times   Magnified 2100 times

EFFECTS OF OTHER SPECIALIZED MATERIALS ON HAIR

We will now examine the effects of the following chemical materials commonly used on the hair, such as:

1. Conditioners
2. Lacquers
3. Hair foods
4. Hair removers.
5. Fillers

CONDITIONERS

Conditioners are used on the hair to restore (to a degree) a healthy condition to damaged hair. The need for conditioning is based mainly on the increase in the porosity of the cuticle layer of the hair.

REASONS FOR USE
1. Movement of substances through the natural protective barrier of the cuticle must be strictly controlled. If the natural oil layer is removed by careless treatment of the hair, the porosity is increased to a harmful level.

2. The cuticle itself may have been damaged or removed by harsh chemicals acting on the keratin of this important layer. A substitute protective layer must be applied.

SPECIAL FEATURES   In modern salons and shops conditioners may be applied to the hair as a routine measure. Chemists have given the practitioner a number of these hair treatments. Many are used as hair creams or so-called "nutritive" creams for regular treatment of dry hair. They usually contain a mild acid for the purpose of partially restoring body in the hair by shrinking and hardening the cortex and the imbrications of the cuticle.

TYPES OF CONDITIONERS   The modern artisan can now draw on a wide range of hair conditioners. ·

PRE-CONDITIONERS

These materials are applied to porous or dry hair before starting any work on it. The condition of this hair is such that its highly porous nature will expose it to serious damage if it is not protected beforehand.

The ingredients used often have several purposes:
   (a)   They contain *protein fillers* that coat the hair and even out the porosity.
   (b)   They also have *lanolin and cholesterol*. Lanolin is a soft natural oil (wool fat). Cholesterol is a waxy type of substance not easily removed by the chemicals used, and so protects the hair during any later work.

CONDITIONERS (additives)

These materials (usually lanolin), are added to the chemicals which are going to be used on the hair. They are found in shampoos, permanent wave solutions, tints, lighteners, creams, etc.

They are mostly emulsions formed by suspending the conditioning agent in the material. This gives these preparations a milky or creamy appearance. However, newer type lanolins are now available that remain clear or water-like in the emulsion form.

This type of conditioner is particularly useful for hair that is damaged or weakened and permits successful waving, lightening or tinting.

CONCLUSIONS

1. As the treatment of hair with strong chemical agents continues, we see an overall deterioration in the natural condition of the hair. It would be safe to say that at no other time in our history has the human hair been in such a poor state. As a result most patrons need conditioning treatments.

2. In the case of an older patron, the condition of hair always suffers as a result of age. It is up to the practitioner to tactfully suggest appropriate hair reconditioning to these patrons.

3. A patron should be able to regard the practitioner as a well informed guide to maintaining hair in a natural, healthy condition. So it is up to the practitioner to show interest and know-how in the rapidly changing science of these vitally important hair cosmetics.

CLEAR PROTEIN FILLERS

Protein fillers are made from cheap, waste protein materials—scrap leather, hooves of cattle or even turkey feathers. The protein is chopped up and then cooked under pressure, with caustic soda, for a definite period. After cooling, the mixture is neutralized by acid (hydrochloric or sulfuric) to pH 7.0–7.5. This contains soluble proteins, peptones, proteoses and free amino-acids. Peptones and proteoses are small chain polypeptides soluble in water. A part of the hair, when damaged, is converted to short chain polypeptides. The ends of these chains protrude from the hair shaft (if not already washed away). The protein, hydrolysate (so called because it is hydrolized or partially digested), contains many freed positive and negative groups. The damaged hair also contains these same groups. When in contact with each other, the groups in the hair, which are positive (*plus*), attract those solubilized short chain proteinizers which are (*negative*) and vice-versa.

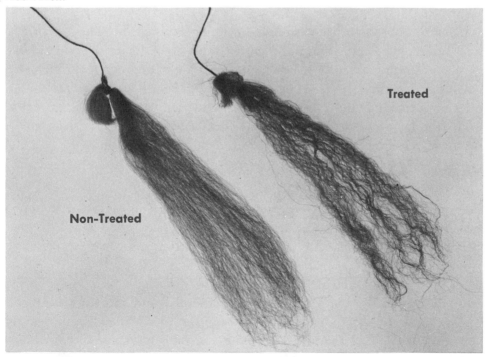

The above photo shows hair swatches (virgin black) bleached identically, with left swatch without substantive protein. Both swatches were bleached identically demonstrating the compatibility of substantive protein with bleach. You will note the differences in length, combability, brittleness, and strength. The non-protein-treated swatch is harder and rougher than the protein-treated swatch.

Hence the hair and the proteinizers form salt bonds between each other and this is basically why the protein substances join with the hair. For the same reason, hair coloring, especially water rinses and semi-permanent color rinses have a great affinity for these molecules. They also attach themselves to the hair by salt bonds.

COLOR FILLERS

In normal hair the salt bonds are evenly distributed. In damaged hair the new salt bonds formed may give a patchy hair coloring effect. Thus, a color filler in the form of a protein treatment or cationic rinse will even out the salt bonds which would have otherwise formed at the site of the chemical damage. The job of the protein color filler is to regulate the distribution of salt bonds or repair damaged hair (by joining onto it additional protein substances). The material usually contains certified colors and is adjusted to an acid pH to also restore H-bonds in the cortex. Fatty materials (lanolin, waxes, etc.) also help to condition the hair by reforming the usual water-inhibiting layer so that the porous cuticle cannot release excessive moisture.

OTHER TYPES

Not all clear gel hair fillers are protein types. Some of them are made from oil/water emulsions, especially thickened or gelled with a pH lower than 7, that is—mildly acid (3.5–4.0). They contain the usual conditioners, oils, waxes, higher fatty acids and also have as an active ingredient—cationic compounds.

CATIONIC COMPOUNDS have been known for many years. They form the basis of the old cream rinses. But the disadvantages of cream rinses—stinging of eyes and scalp, difficulty in uniformly applying the product through the hair, and low viscosity—have been overcome. By using higher molecular cationic compounds there is no stinging, and the gelled form is easier to comb through the hair. The material is applied after hair is shampooed and towel dried. It is combed through before setting.

REASONS Hair is normally charged negatively by static electricity accumulating on the cuticle. The excess electricity causes "fly-away" ends. Shampoos often make this condition worse. There are always some shampoo molecules (particularly soapless ones) left behind on the shaft. All commercial shampoos are themselves negatively charged, or at least increase the negative hair charges.

Cationic compounds are charged positively (at least their "tails" are). They are attracted by opposite charges on the hair and so neutralize them. The negative charges built up in the hair serve to attract the positively charged cationic compounds. The more the hair is exposed to weather, is lightened, is tinted or even waved, the more intense a negative charge will it possess, and thus the benefit derived from a treatment with a cationic compound will be more visible.

The gel is attracted to damaged cuticles, even more so after permanent waving, lightening and tinting. The adsorbed cationics restore the gloss and sheen to the hair. It gains a soft, silky feel and the acid restores "body" to the cortex. The treatment makes the hair more water repellent so the hair is less affected by humidity in the air.

The compounds are claimed to reduce the "crinkly" and dry feeling of the hair after permanent waving. They neutralize the excess shampoo residues and improve the flexibility of the hair. It is claimed that hair coloring takes better and more evenly if the hair is first treated with these rinses. Some foaming type hair tints contain positively charged or cationic agents. They clean the hair as well as color it.

HAIR SPRAYS

The development of the aerosol or pressure-pack can, has resulted in a vast increase in the use of hair lacquers and other sprays. In this form they are simply and easily applied on the hair and are invaluable for holding the hair in place and in controlling the loose ends.

DISADVANTAGES OF CHEAP LACQUERS The old-fashioned hair lacquers, using shellac and thinners, leave a hard, brittle film on the hair. This film is not only unattractive but is also very difficult to remove. Most cheaper brands of hair lacquers still rely on shellac to a large degree.

Some resistant conditions of hair may be due to this brittle, unnatural coating, and it must be removed from the cuticle prior to permanent waving.

NEWER TYPES OF SPRAYS More advanced hair sprays have a plastic base and are partly water soluble. This means that their removal from the cuticle can be more easily effected. The surface film that they leave on the hair is more natural looking and is resilient and elastic.

The increase in use of setting sprays continues and some supporters believe that their future development may be in the field of complete permanent waving, to replace the long chemical procedure now used. If the problems involved could be overcome, this would lead to vast changes in present day methods of permanent waving.

HAIR SPRAY DANGERS Warning must be given about the dangers in the use of certain lacquer hair sprays. Contact with the skin of some sensitive patrons may produce dermatitis. The vapors, when breathed in excessive amounts, may give rise to certain lung reactions. Doctors warn against this constant exposure in the salon or shop.

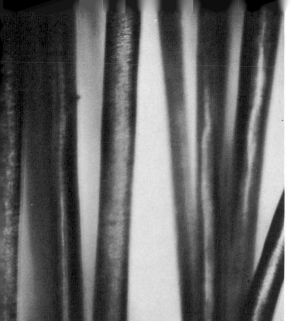

Hair before it is treated with hair spray.

Courtesy: Gillette Company Research Institute,

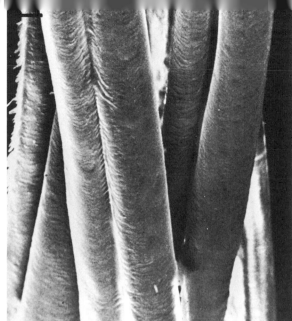

Hair sprayed with hair spray, magnified 600 times. Note two fibers in foreground bonded together.

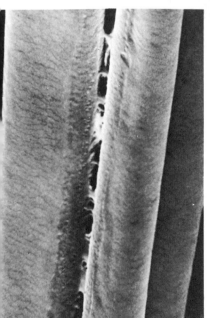

Hair sprayed with hair spray, magnified 750 times.

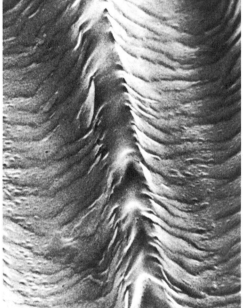

Hair sprayed with hair spray, magnified 2100 times. Note how fibers are bonded together with hair spray.

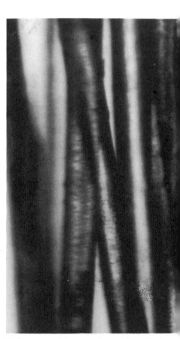

Hair set with good quality hair spray. Note even spread on hair cuticle.

Spray techniques

If you are using a pressurized can, press the valve release button down slowly and spray only enough to hold the hair lightly in place. Keep your head away from the spray stream and do this work in an open area. Of course, you must pay attention to safeguarding your patron, but the practitioner is more liable to be exposed to prolonged contact. However if the spray is used in an intelligent manner, there is no cause for alarm.

HAIR FOODS

CLAIMS VS. FACTS Constant public claims by some uninstructed advertisers try to tell us of the great "advantages" of their products in restoring the nutrition to "hungry" hair. But long and careful investigation by scientists has failed to produce any proof that the hair can be nourished by external means. Restoration of hair growth cannot be achieved by merely rubbing some patented, advertised product onto the scalp.

The hair growth is strictly controlled by the papilla and unless the treatment aims at this level, all attempts at restoration will be wasted. Because of a general refusal to recognize or accept this fundamental factor, many individuals squander their time and money on ineffective remedies.

NO hair tonic will directly cause the stimulation and growth of new hair once the papilla has died.

POSSIBLE BENEFITS *If there still remains a little life* (activity) in the papilla, *hair tonics* can be of some benefit in the following manner:

Alcohol Content

They usually contain alcohol, or spirits, as a solvent for their "active" ingredients. Alcohol can penetrate fairly readily through the skin and it has a dilating affect on the small scalp blood vessels, which causes more blood to pass through them.

Under the microscope the skin of an older person suffering from hair loss shows a reduction both in size and number of these essential blood vessels. In such a case, the increased size of blood vessels may assist growth of hair.

Regular Massage

The regular and religious massage with which hair tonic supporters rub the alcohol product into the scalp has a beneficial effect on the blood and lymph circulation to the follicle. In other words, methylated spirits or alcohol may be just as good on their own as in expensive hair tonics.

Conditioning Effect

Many hair tonics contain oils or waxes that are rubbed along the hair cuticle. These conditioning agents restore the natural appearance and moisture to the cortex. This removes the dry, brittle look which is often associated with poor hair.

Dandruff Ingredient

In the case of the "restorative" for balding or thinning hair, there is often an anti-dandruff agent added. These materials remove dandruff scales that harbor destructive fungi and bacteria. Any new growth of hair which may appear is then protected.

HAIR REMOVERS

DEFINITION   Hair removers or dipilatories, are creams or pastes used for the removal of unwanted hairs from the face, legs, armpits, and other parts of the body.

EFFECTS

1. Unlike shaving, the cream removes the hair right down to the mouth of the follicle. As a result this method is more effective and longer lasting.
2. The depilatories are closely related to permanent waving agents and act by first weakening the hair, then dissolving it.

PRECAUTIONS   Unfortunately, the hair shaft is similar in composition to the skin, both being varieties of keratin, and so skin damage is possible at the same time.

Providing the skin is reasonably healthy, and the time of application of the cream is not too long, little damage appears to be done. But on no account should they be used on an inflamed surface nor closely followed by the application of any chemical or deodorant.

After complete removal of the hairs, the area should be gently washed and carefully dried in order to prevent skin irritation resulting from continuing chemical action. Natural oils, removed in the process, can be supplemented by the application of cold cream or some other moisturizer.

CHAPTER 11

BASIC PRINCIPLES
OF COSMETIC CHEMISTRY

Introduction

The modern practitioner uses a number of techniques and scientific processes to achieve the objective of dressing and improving the hair. We cannot go very deeply into the science of chemistry but the more we know about the nature of chemical substances, the more likely we are to be confident and efficient in meeting problems in the shop.

The manufacturer and the scientist have cooperated as much as possible in an effort to simplify the work of the professional. However, this offers no guarantee, as the artisan still must accept final responsibility for the materials used and the effects produced on the patron's hair and scalp.

CHEMISTRY DEFINED Chemistry is the scientific study of the structure of things and the changes that take place in them. For example, a study of the changes that take place in the hair during permanent waving is part of the subject of chemistry.

THE STRUCTURE OF THINGS

MATTER is the material of which the world (including us) is made. Matter can have the form of a solid, liquid or gas. The change from one form to another can be brought about by heating or cooling, e.g., water (a liquid at ordinary temperatures) can be cooled to produce ice (a solid) or heated to form steam (gas). *These are physical changes.*

ATOMS AND MOLECULES

A close investigation shows that all matter is actually composed of countless billions and billions of extremely tiny particles called atoms. Most atoms are joined to form larger particles called molecules. *A molecule is formed whenever two or more atoms are joined together.* While atoms are very reactive, molecules are much more stable. Much of the study of cosmetic chemistry is concerned with how molecules of different substances behave. Molecules may have only 2 atoms or may have many atoms combined in various ways. The tendency for atoms to react to one another explains the endless number of substances which are already known and those which may be discovered in the future.

ELEMENTS

Closer study of atoms and some molecules (containing like atoms) show that large numbers of atoms are identical and so are the resulting substances. These similar atoms (about 100 different kinds) are known as *elements.* Some common elements are:

Hydrogen	Iron
Carbon	Sulphur
Nitrogen	Phosphorus
Oxygen	

Each one of these elements is made up of different atoms and therefore each element itself is different. *Only one kind of atom is present in an element.*

ELEMENTS ARE THE SIMPLEST FORM OF MATTER. Until recently, they were thought to be made from indivisible particles. However, it is now known that each element consists of individual atoms, the properties of that element being the properties of these minute particles. Every one of the countless numbers of atoms in the universe belonging to the same elements is an exact replica of each other one. The behavior of these extremely tiny particles forms the basis of modern scientific research and knowledge.

For each of the 100 or so different elements there are corresponding atoms. Using modern techniques, atoms can be split (fission) or joined together (fusion). However, they then no longer have the properties of the element to which they formerly belonged.

But these techniques do not involve the chemical reactions that professionals wish to take place within the hair. A practitioner employs changes of a relatively simple nature.

ELEMENTS & COMPOUNDS

TYPES	DEFINITION	SMALLEST PARTICLE	ELEMENTS FOUND IN HAIR
ELEMENTS	SIMPLEST FORM OF MATTER	ATOM *(Cannot be broken down by simple chemical reactions)* *About 100 different kinds*	CARBON NITROGEN OXYGEN SULFUR HYDROGEN PHOSPHORUS ETC.
COMPOUNDS	FORMED BY COMBINATION OF ELEMENTS	MOLECULE *(Consist of 2 or more atoms chemically combined)* *Unlimited kinds possible*	**COMPOUNDS USED ON HAIR** WATER HYROGEN PEROXIDE AMMONIUM THIOGLYCOLLATE PARA DYES (Tints) AMMONIA ALCOHOL ACIDS ALKALIS

MATTER

FORMS

GASES
LIQUIDS
SOLIDS

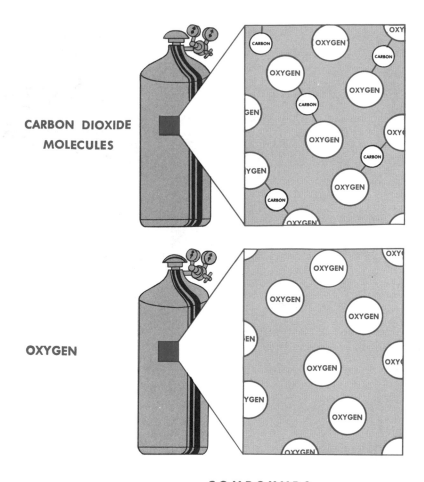

CARBON DIOXIDE
MOLECULES

OXYGEN

COMPOUNDS

There are far more examples of matter than the 100 elements alone. These additional substances consist of compounds or mixtures of compounds. Compounds are formed by the chemical combination of the atoms of one element and the atoms of another element or elements.

MOLECULES IN HAIR Hair is made of molecules which are arranged in a particular way to form KERATIN. This arrangement of molecules is not found in any other substance, so keratin is distinct and readily recognized as hair.

As different combinations of atoms are possible, an endless number of compounds can be made. Each compound has molecules with characteristic chemical properties.

On the hair these compounds may be harmless (no effect), harmful (damaging), or useful. Useful compounds have molecules that cause desirable effects when applied to the hair or skin in the proper manner.

Once the compound is made, it:

1. is *not* easily broken down again into its original elements.
2. does *not* resemble the original elements.

3. *is* similar to any compound formed in the same manner in any part of the world.

For example, water is a compound formed from the elements hydrogen and oxygen (H_2O).

CHEMICAL SHORTHAND (SYMBOLS)

To further clarify the meaning of the word "molecule," let us for a moment consider the compound water. You have all heard the term "H_2O." This bit of chemical shorthand clearly indicates the elements found in the compound, "Water," and also the number of atoms in the molecule. The letter "H" stands for hydrogen and since there is a little number 2 following the letter "H," it indicates that there are two atoms of hydrogen. The letter "O" stands alone, which means there is only one atom of oxygen.

Similarly, there are many atoms of various elements that can be joined together in numerous ways, each combination forming a different compound with its own unique formula (e.g., CO_2—Carbon Dioxide). This accounts for the almost unlimited kinds of compounds that can be formed.

Now, in rendering professional services we deal mainly in the use of compounds on the hair. Once a basic understanding of the differences that exist between elements and compounds has been established, as well as their composition, we can go on to the next area which deals with the solubility of compounds.

SOLUBILITY OF COMPOUNDS

Compounds are soluble or insoluble in different liquids. The liquid that dissolves a compound is called a *solvent*. The compound that is dissolved is called a *solute*. The resulting mixture of the compound and solvent is known as a *solution*.

SOLUBLE IN WATER

When a substance dissolves in a liquid, the result is known as a clear or "true" solution. The most common liquid used for making such solutions is water. Water is a liquid which acts as a solvent on many compounds. Its ability to dissolve compounds stems from the natural attraction between molecules of that compound and the molecules of water.

Dispersion of these dissolved molecules takes place within the solvent by stirring or the natural movement of molecules of the liquid. A characteristic of liquids and their solutions is that their molecules are in constant motion.

IMPORTANCE This complete separation of the molecules of the dissolved compound (solute) with the movement of water molecules allows the compound to pass through the imbrications (cuticle) of hair.

Water is the safest and best solvent to use for this purpose. It will not harm the hair or remove its natural oils. Afterwards, fresh water will safely rinse away the excess molecules of the solute when their purpose is complete.

SOLUBILITY OF COMPOUNDS

SOLUBLE IN WATER (SOLVENT)

COLD WAVING CHEMICALS
HYDROGEN PEROXIDE
SETTING LOTIONS

SOLVENT
COMPOUND

REQUIRED COMPOUND IS
ADDED TO CORRECT VOLUME
OF WATER (solvent).

MOLECULES

MOLECULES OF COMPOUND
ARE SEPARATED AND
COMPLETELY DISPERSED IN
SOLVENT. MOLECULES MOVE
EASILY WITH LIQUID.
(as a solution).

MEDULLA
CUTICLE
HAIR CORTEX

MOLECULES OF COMPOUND
ENTER CORTEX OF HAIR WITH
THE SOLVENT.
THE SOLUTION THEN CAUSES
CHEMICAL CHANGES
IN THE HAIR.

INSOLUBLE IN WATER (NON-SOLVENT)

(USE ORGANIC SOLVENT eg. ALCOHOL, ACETONE.)
SEMI-PERMANENT RINSES
PARA TINTS

NON-SOLVENT
COMPOUND

COMPOUND IS MIXED
WITH WATER
(in which it is not soluble).

MOLECULES OF COMPOUND
ARE NOT SEPARATED
BY WATER.

COMPOUND CANNOT ENTER
HAIR CORTEX BECAUSE
MOLECULES REMAIN CLUMPED
TOGETHER AND WILL NOT
PASS THROUGH
IMBRICATIONS.

134

Unfortunately, there are many substances that are not sufficiently soluble in water (*insoluble*). As water cannot separate their molecules, they remain joined together.

In this insoluble state, these compounds cannot be effectively used to make changes in the hair cortex. Their molecules remain clumped together on the cuticle and do not penetrate into the cortex.

ORGANIC SOLVENTS can be used because they may dissolve substances that are normally insoluble in water, e.g., hair colorings. Examples of organic solvents are benzene, ether, kerosene, alcohol (methylated spirits) and acetone.

Unfortunately, organic solvents present serious disadvantages when used in skin and hair preparations.

PROBLEMS WITH ORGANIC SOLVENTS

1. They remove excess oils from the hair, leaving it dry and lifeless.
2. As inflammable liquids, they are extremely dangerous.
3. Many are poisonous when breathed deeply.
4. They evaporate readily, leaving their dissolved substances behind in unsightly patches on the hair.
5. Their viscosity is usually very low. This means their solutions tend to run and drip easily, making their application on hair difficult to control fully.

EMULSIONS

DEFINITION   An emulsion is a mixture in which fine particles or globules of a liquid are suspended in another liquid with the aid of emulsifiers. An emulsion can be readily detected under a microscope, whereas dissolved molecules (in a true solution) are far too small to be visible.

REASONS FOR EMULSIONS   Water is best for use in the emulsion type of hair cosmetics since it helps carry chemicals more easily into the cuticle and/or through it into the cortex (for tinting, lightening, permanent waving, etc.). If, however, these products are mixed in water alone, the small drops so formed will, on standing, gradually separate into different layers (e.g., oil on water). Therefore, water cannot be used with these insoluble substances, which, nevertheless, are still required for proper hair care.

Emulsions are used to overcome the difficulties of applying substances to the hair which are insoluble in water. Emulsions are suspensions of small particles or droplets in an immiscible (incapable of being mixed) liquid. For example, oils are required to condition the cuticle of hair, either as special preparations (hair creams, conditioners) or with cosmetic treatments (permanent wave chemicals, hair tints, etc.). But these oils are not soluble

EMULSIONS

TYPES	EXAMPLES	IMPORTANT FEATURES
(O/W) OIL-IN-WATER THICKENER (0.5%) WATER (90%) (contains dissolved ingredients) EMULSIFIER OIL (10%)	COLD WAVE SOLUTIONS 1. Lanolized or milky types. 2. Creams or thickened types. CONDITIONERS NEUTRALIZERS TINTS (liquids or creams) LADIES' HAIRDRESSINGS BLEACHING EMULSIONS HAND LOTIONS	EMULSION "BREAKS" ON CONTACT TO RELEASE: 1. Moisture to enter hair and skin. (Softens, gives manageability, overcomes dryness.) 2. Oils remain on cuticle surface. (Reduces porosity and loss of moisture, increases sheen, lubricates skin and hair.) Can be thickened as creams for ease of application. (Gives appearance of "stronger" formulations.) Can be easily diluted by water.
(W/O) WATER-IN-OIL WATER (10%) EMULSIFIER OIL (90%)	CLEANSING CREAMS COLD CREAMS FOUNDATION CREAMS MENS' HAIRDRESSINGS	FORM STICKY GREASY PREPARATIONS. KEEPS HAIR STRANDS FIRMLY IN PLACE. USEFUL FOR REMOVING EXCESS GRIME FROM PORES OF SKIN. CANNOT BE DILUTED BY ADDED WATER. (Test for W/O emulsions.)

in water and would form a separate layer even after complete dispersion. If a mixture of oil and water is shaken vigorously, the oil will break into small droplets throughout the liquid. On standing, however, these dispersed oil droplets quickly rise to the surface, where they merge together as a separate layer.

If a special product, called an emulsifier (e.g., a soap) is present, it will coat the droplets of oil as they are formed. This stabilizes the oils and so forms an emulsion.

MODERN EMULSIONS The newer type of creams and milk lotions are popular forms of such emulsions. Emulsions are found in permanent wave solutions, shampoos, hair tints and creams, hand and body creams.

In commercial preparations, the droplets are made by homogenizers or blenders. The main requirements are that the droplets be very small and uniformly dispersed in the product. They must be stable in this condition for at least the average shelf-life of the preparation.

MAIN TYPES There are 2 types of emulsions used in cosmetic preparations. They are:

(a) Oil-in-water (O/W)
(b) Water-in-oil (W/O) Symbols

OIL-IN-WATER (O/W)

These emulsions are made of oil droplets dispersed in a watery base. This water base may, in addition, contain those dissolved substances required to carry out additional chemical reactions in the hair. Quite typical are neutralizers, permanent wave solutions and lighteners. The oil droplets may, in turn, contain water-insoluble chemicals such as oxidation tints.

However, the purpose of an emulsion is to apply a suitably dispersed conditioner easily and evenly to the hair. Once contact is made with the cuticle, the finely dispersed oil is adsorbed on the surface (the released oils, usually lanolin, spread over the imbrications).

This conditioning effect provides a pleasant sheen to the hair as it smooths the natural, rough surface of the cuticle. The oil layer also acts as an external lubricant.

Water molecules in the emulsion enter the cortex readily, carrying with them dissolved chemicals, such as:

1. Mild acids in hair conditioners and dressings.
2. Softening agents in permanent wave solutions.
3. Colored molecules in semi-permanent rinses.

Furthermore, the water molecules restore the natural moisture content (10%) of the cortex. This makes the hair soft and more manageable. Thus, the water content in the emulsion acts as an internal lubricant.

ONE ADVANTAGE OF O/W EMULSIONS is that they may be easily rinsed away by water. Thus, excess emulsion can be quickly removed when the desirable chemical action is complete.

Because they have a high water content (90%), O/W emulsions are milky, easy-flowing liquids. For special purposes, specific additives may be included as thickeners. These thickeners usually have extremely long, thread-like molecules which, by slowing down the movement of the emulsion molecules, make the emulsion thicker in both appearance and feel.

Tints, permanent wave solutions and bleaches may be formulated as creams and gels for special applications. *However, the strength of the active ingredient may remain independent of the viscosity or thickness of the emulsion. Thus it is impossible to compare the strength of the different brands or products solely on the basis of their visual appearance.*

TYPICAL FORMULA OF AN O/W EMULSION

In an emulsion, the following substances may be found:

oil type conditioner — usually a light mineral oil or lanolin.

emulsifier — a joining agent between the water and the conditioner, usually a form of soap.

thickener — to control the thickness of the emulsion or to make it look "stronger."

clouding agent — to give a pearly-white, attractive appearance.

active substance — insoluble chemical required for tinting, permanent waving, lightening.

perfume and water — to disguise unpleasant odors and impart a patron-pleasing odor to the hair.

WATER-IN-OIL (W/O)

These emulsions are made of water droplets scattered within an oily base. As such, W/O emulsions are much greasier than O/W emulsions. When formed with light mineral oils, they can be poured at normal temperature. Examples are baby cream and hair grooming creams.

W/O emulsions are used mainly as night preparations in skin cosmetics, or for the deep cleansing of skin tissues.

In men's toiletries they are limited to certain hairdressings. In general, men make less sophisticated demands on their hair cosmetics than women. Their personal habits include more frequent wetting of their hair, less concern if their hair is slightly oily, plus their normally shorter and closer hairstyles permit the use of water-in-oil emulsions.

TEST OF EMULSIONS W/O emulsions *do not mix with water* and are usually thicker creams.

O/W emulsions are easily diluted by water and as they already consist of approximately 90% water, are free-flowing, milky or creamy liquids. However, in special cases some O/W emulsions are thickened to form jellies or thick pastes.

BREAKDOWN OF O/W EMULSIONS Because of the complicated nature of the emulsion, the parts sometimes separate, on standing, into the water (the major part of the emulsion) and the active ingredients. Once this occurs the product should be considered useless and discarded.

ACIDS

FEATURES OF ACIDS A large and useful group of compounds are known as acids. The acids have a number of similar properties. Skin and hair are mildly acid in nature and are able to resist the effects of further acid contacts (providing it is not too strong). Acids have a sour taste, as shown by the taste of vinegar.

Acids can be neutralized by alkalies and so acid burns should be treated by a solution of sodium bicarbonate (mild alkali).

ACIDS USED IN HAIR TREATMENTS Mild acids are frequently used in hair cosmetics to obtain a wide variety of effects:

1. To remove soap scum left in the hair after a soap shampoo.
2. To strengthen weak hair or damaged hair. This adds "body" to the hair by shrinking and hardening the cuticle and cortex.
3. In neutralizers, to remove the alkali of any permanent wave solution remaining in the hair.
4. To stabilize hydrogen peroxide solutions. Stabilized hydrogen peroxide maintains its strength much better during storage.
5. In hair creams and dandruff treatments to maintain the sheen or luster of the hair. (By shrinking and hardening the cuticle.)

EXAMPLES OF ACIDS USED Acids used in hair treatments are weak acids, which cause no damage to the hair itself. Common items that are acid in nature are:

White vinegar — (acetic acid)

and

Lemon juice — (citric acid)

In hair treaments, acids are often used in neutralizers, cream rinses and conditioners.

ALKALIES

FEATURES Another large and useful group of compounds are called alkalies. These are much more liable to cause damage to the hair if applied carelessly or too strongly.

Alkalies have a flat "earthy" taste, as shown by the taste of bicarbonate of soda or baking powder.

Alkalies can be neutralized by acids and if the skin is accidentally splashed with a strong alkali, bathing with vinegar (weak acid) will help correct the condition and minimize damage.

ALKALIES USED IN HAIR TREATMENTS These are employed to:

1. Swell the hair, which permits better penetration of products such as permanent wave solutions, hair straighteners, setting lotions, rinses, lighteners and colorizers into the cortex of the hair.
2. Unstabilize (activate) hydrogen peroxide lighteners, thus preparing them for immediate use.
3. Remove oils from the cuticle in order to increase the porosity of the hair. (Alkalies tend to have a dulling effect on the hair because they open the imbrications.)

More care must be taken when using alkalies on the hair and skin than with the acids. Only mild alkalies can be used, such as ammonia, borax and soda. It is important that the practitioner be familiar with the pH values of products in order to avoid damage to the hair by ignorance of the effects of too much alkali or acid.

pH SCALE

Acids are neutralized by alkalies to form neutral solutions and alkalies are neutralized by acids to form neutral solutions. Furthermore, the properties of these acids or alkalies may be used in other solutions or emulsions which are otherwise neutral.

For example, if certain changes are needed in the cortex of the hair, it is desirable that the product be alkaline, e.g., permanent tints.

However, if the cuticle is the only part of the hair to be affected, it is advisable that the product be acid, e.g., a temporary rinse.

It is necessary to use *only* mild acid or alkaline solutions on the hair. Therefore, the chemist must know in advance the exact amounts of acid or alkali present in every product before it is released for use on the public. But using terms such as "mild," "strong," "weaker," gives only a very rough guide and therefore is unsatisfactory.

For greater accuracy a pH scale has been devised. The pH of a solution is the degree of acidity or alkalinity found in that solution.

THE pH SCALE

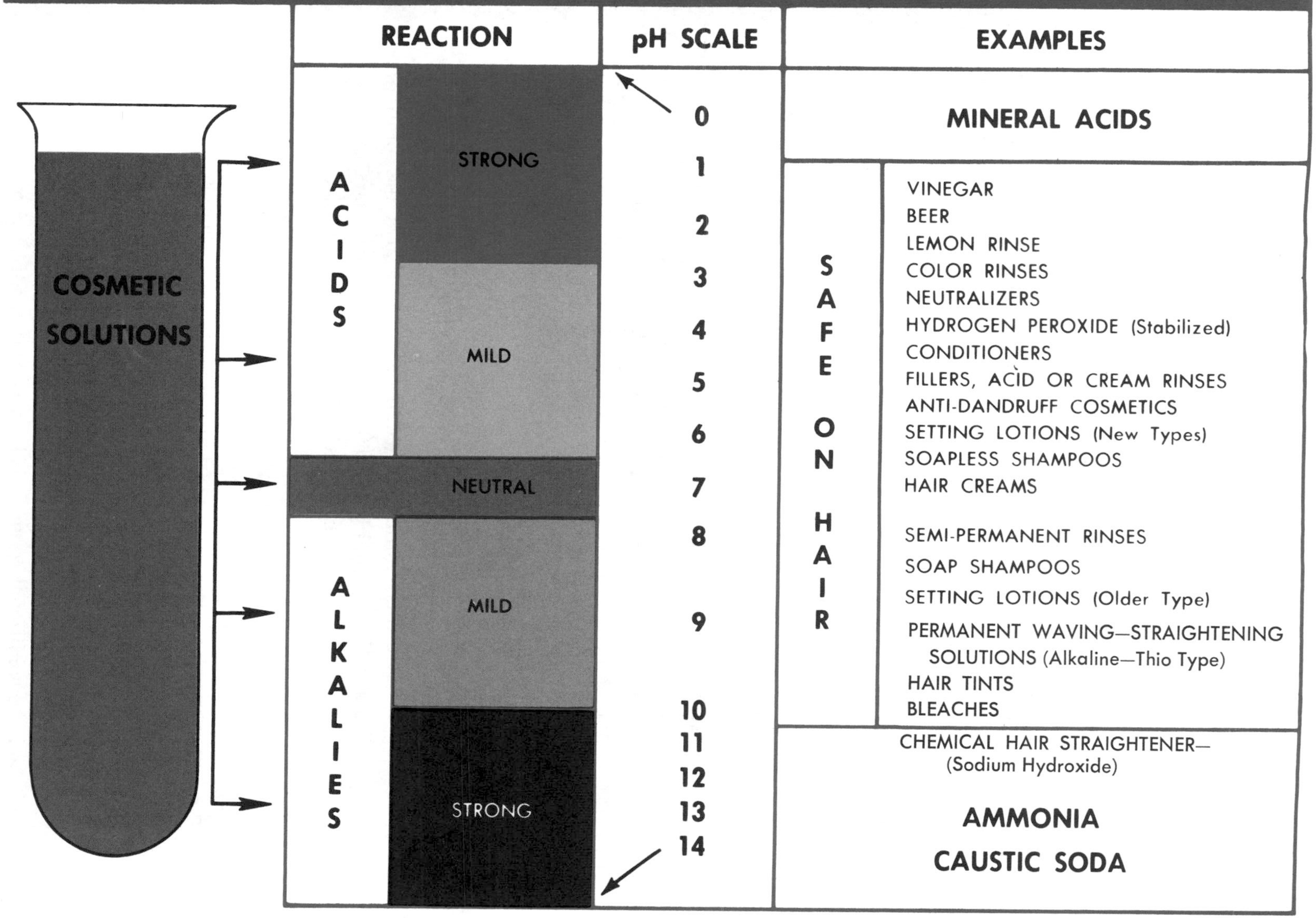

REACTION	pH SCALE	EXAMPLES
		MINERAL ACIDS
STRONG (ACIDS)	0	
	1	
	2	VINEGAR
MILD	3	BEER
	4	LEMON RINSE
	5	COLOR RINSES
	6	NEUTRALIZERS
		HYDROGEN PEROXIDE (Stabilized)
		CONDITIONERS
		FILLERS, ACID OR CREAM RINSES
		ANTI-DANDRUFF COSMETICS
		SETTING LOTIONS (New Types)
		SOAPLESS SHAMPOOS
		HAIR CREAMS
NEUTRAL	7	
MILD (ALKALIES)	8	SEMI-PERMANENT RINSES
		SOAP SHAMPOOS
		SETTING LOTIONS (Older Type)
	9	PERMANENT WAVING—STRAIGHTENING
		SOLUTIONS (Alkaline—Thio Type)
		HAIR TINTS
		BLEACHES
STRONG	10	
	11	CHEMICAL HAIR STRAIGHTENER—
	12	(Sodium Hydroxide)
	13	**AMMONIA**
	14	**CAUSTIC SODA**

SAFE ZONE HAIR

COSMETIC SOLUTIONS

141

NEUTRAL POINT A pH figure of less than 7.0 indicates an *acid solution*. Pure water would be found to have a pH of 7.0 as water is neutral (neither acid nor alkali). A pH figure above 7.0 would be alkaline.

ACIDS ON THE HAIR A pH figure of less than 7.0 indicates an *acid solution*. The smaller the figure becomes, the stronger is that acid solution. From pH 1.0 to pH 6.0 the hair is in a good condition and the cuticle scales press down tightly on the hair shaft, making the surface smooth and glossy. However, below pH 3.0, depending on the acid involved, the hair can become liable to damage or destruction.

ALKALIES ON THE HAIR A pH greater than 7.0 indicates an alkaline condition. As the pH increases, the hair swells. A mild degree of alkalinity, pH (7.0 to 10.0), is not considered "good," but is regarded as "safe" on the hair and permits the cuticle to have greater porosity. This increased porosity is useful in order to get certain solutions into the cortex more easily for treatments such as in waving, lightening, tinting and others. Above pH 10.0, the excessive swelling produced causes a marked degree of loosening of the hair cortex structure. This can lead to lasting damage or total destruction of the hair.

TESTING FOR pH The exact pH figure may be accurately determined by a sensitive electrical device called a pH meter. As a pH meter is an expensive instrument, other methods for testing the pH of a product may be used by practitioners.

Indicator solutions or pH papers show an appropriate color after contact with the test substance. By comparison with the color code supplied, the pH figure is found.

pH INFLUENCE ON HAIR PRODUCTS

With this information it can be shown that if the solution to be used has a pH between 1.0 to 10.0 it will probably be safe to use on the hair. However, it depends upon the type of acid or alkali used.

THE pH OF TYPICAL PRODUCTS For example, on the acid scale we find that a pH range of 3.0 to 1.0 indicates a safe but strong acid condition. Thus, organic acid rinses (vinegar or lemon juice) are used to strip hair of soap curds and add "body" as well. Color rinses also have a low pH figure.

From pH 3.0 to 6.0 covers the "mild" acid range. Thus *neutralizers* and *hydrogen peroxide stock solutions* are mildly acid. In general, solutions or emulsions with a mild pH figure are the best for damaged hair. *Conditioners, fillers, acid and cream rinses* treat damaged hair and help prepare it for additional services. Likewise, anti-dandruff cosmetics are mainly surface treatments for scalp and hair, and have a lower pH figure.

Setting lotions (new type) use wetting agents for better softening of the hair fibers. Thus, the need for alkaline setting agents has decreased. In addition, lightened hair needs milder setting conditions which the newer solutions can give in their mild acid state.

Next there are the *soapless shampoos* within the mild acid range of 5.5 to 7.0 pH. Thus the cuticle is cleaned without excess swelling and with little solution entering the cortex. Hair also handles better when shampooed in mild acids.

Hair creams or hairdressings are emulsions which contain mild acids. They condition the cuticle with their oils, and add body with their acid content. Although the precise neutral point on the pH scale is 7.0, the neutral range is considered to extend from pH 6.5 to 7.5.

In the alkaline pH range, hair has much more sensitivity than in the acid state. Only mild alkalies can be used, so all hair treatment products should, when possible, be kept below a figure of pH 10.0 unless they are to perform as depilatories.

For example, *semi-permanent rinses* are alkaline so that they can enter the cortex by swelling the hair. Alkalies have a softening effect on the hair as well. So lotions, which are alkaline, will soften and swell the hair. Unfortunately, the hair remains in this softened condition longer, so humidity can undo the set more quickly.

Soap shampoos are shown as alkaline (pH range 8.0 to 10.0). This is necessary because the cleaning action of soap is destroyed at lower pH's. Thus soap shampoos not only clean hair, but they soften and swell the hair as well. For lightened hair this is particularly undesirable.

Alkaline waving solutions must be kept above pH 9.0, otherwise the waving action slows down markedly. Higher pH figures give few problems on resistant hair. But for tinted and damaged hair this high alkalinity may be disastrous. One feature of permanent waving products is that *all neutralizers are acid*. So the hair is brought back to its normal, mild acid state (pH 6.5).

THE NEED TO NEUTRALIZE When using soap shampoos, chemical hair straighteners, hair tints and lighteners, all strongly alkaline products, if corrective treatment (neutralization) is neglected; these treatments will result in damage to the hair.

OUTSIDE THE SAFE RANGE of hair cosmetics (pH 1.0 to 10.0) we find first the mineral acids (pH 1.0 to zero). These acids are far too strong for use in the salon or shop.

Similarly ammonia and caustic soda are very strong alkalies. Ammonia is a chemical found in many shops. But practitioners must be extremely careful when using 28% ammonia water in liquid bleaches or lighteners. Cheap supplies often prove dangerous and costly in the long run, because they have not been properly tested or developed for results in the pH range that is best for the patron. Thus a knowledge of the pH figure of hair products gives extremely useful data.

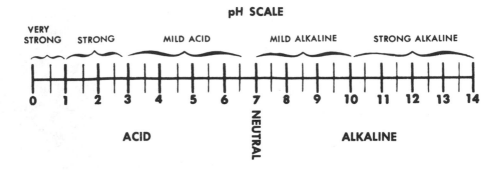

EFFECT OF pH ON HAIR

Very Strong Acid (pH 1.0–0.0)

These acids will dissolve hair completely, breaking it down to form soluble components. Strong acids also have a corrosive effect on the hands and scalp. So mineral acids such as nitric, hydrochloric and sulfuric *cannot* safely be used in the shop.

Strong to Mild Acid (pH 1.0–6.5)

Mild acids have an astringent effect on the hair. This means that they shrink the cortex in diameter, close the imbrications and give the hair more "body."

The cuticle scales press down more firmly, increasing the sheen or luster of the hair. Where hair has a history of damage, this astringent action is very important in restoring its physical condition and appearance. Mild acids also reduce the tendency to tangle and mat when handling wet or dry hair. Thus it is easier to shampoo, comb or brush out into a desired style.

Mild organic acids are also sold as acid rinses. Or, they may be included in neutralizers, cream rinses or fillers to overcome excess porosity of hair following alkaline treatments such as tinting, chemical straightening and permanent waving.

Color rinses in the mild acid range may have a remedial effect on hair fibers, as well as giving pleasing colors to hair.

Neutral (pH 6.5–7.5)

Solutions in the neutral pH range do not affect the hair very much. This is an advantage when requiring milder changes with already damaged hair. Thus, neutral waving solutions and some soapless shampoos have a neutral pH.

EFFECT OF pH ON HAIR

SOLUTION		EFFECT ON HAIR	IMPORTANT FEATURES
VERY STRONG ACID (pH 1.0–0.0)		DISSOLVES HAIR COMPLETELY	MUST NOT BE APPLIED TO HAIR OR SCALP.
STRONG TO MILD ACID (pH 1.0–6.5)		HAIR SHRINKS AND HARDENS BODY IS INCREASED CUTICLE IMBRICATIONS CLOSE UP POROSITY IS REDUCED SHEEN OF HAIR IS IMPROVED SOAP RESIDUES ARE REMOVED NEUTRALIZES TRACES OF ALKALIES	Acid or cream rinses restore body to bleached, porous hair. Conditioners and fillers overcome the excess porosity of damaged hair. Special shampoos reduce tangling and matting of hair and prevent color loss. Hair creams increase sheen. Color rinses provide temporary effect. Neutralizers remove residual waving lotion.
NEUTRAL (pH 6.5–7.5)		HAIR IS NORMAL DIAMETER TEXTURE AND LUSTER STANDARD	NEUTRAL WAVING SOLUTIONS ARE DESIGNED TO PREVENT EXCESS SWELLING OF NORMAL AND DAMAGED HAIR. MILD SHAMPOOS FOR NORMAL CLEANING AND MANAGEABILITY OF HAIR.
MILD ALKALI (pH 7.5–10.0)		HAIR SWELLS GREATLY. POROSITY INCREASES AS IMBRICATIONS OPEN. HAIR HAS A DRY, DRAB APPEARANCE.	TINTS AND BLEACHES PENETRATE EASIER AND CHEMICAL ACTION INCREASES. COLD WAVE SOLUTIONS FOR RESISTANT HAIR. SOAP SHAMPOOS TO OVERCOME ACIDITY OF TAP WATER. ACTIVATORS FOR HYDROGEN PEROXIDE.
STRONGER ALKALI (pH 10.0–14.0)		DISSOLVES HAIR COMPLETELY	MUST NOT BE APPLIED TO HAIR OR SCALP UNLESS USED AS DEPILATORIES.

Mild Alkali (pH 7.5–10.00)

Hair swells and softens markedly as the pH of hairdressing products increases. Hair becomes more porous as the imbrications open. Normally, resistant hair must be treated with mildly alkaline preparations to facilitate entry of compounds into the cortex.

But if any hair is left in a mild alkaline pH it will be softer and have little body. It will appear drab and dull because the imbrications protrude too much.

Mild alkalies tend to strip natural oils from the cuticle as well. This makes the hair dry and lifeless, as the natural moisture level in the cortex drops through evaporation.

Because soaps break down rapidly in acids, all soap shampoos must contain mild alkalies. Although this alkali maintains the cleaning action of the soap, its subsequent dulling of the hair fibers is well known.

Hydrogen peroxide solutions are stabilized by mild acids. So, if weaker hydrogen peroxide lighteners are needed, these acids must first be neutralized by mild alkalies. This forms the basis of liquid or cream bleaching mixtures.

Strong Alkali (pH 10.0–14.0)

Hair continues to swell in progressively stronger alkaline solutions and may reach a diameter of ten times the original size, even in mild alkalies.

Hair depilatories or hair removers have a higher pH range. Some hair straighteners have a pH from 10.0 to 12.0, which explains why these materials are so severe in their effect upon the hair.

When the hair is being destroyed in a strong alkaline solution, such as a depilatory, it first becomes gummy to the touch as the cuticle breaks down. Then the cortex turns to a soft jelly-like substance. Then the hair proteins are converted into water soluble products. The hair loses all its strength and finally passes into complete solution by swelling enormously.

CONCLUSION

Needless to say, the pH factor of hair cosmetics is of vital importance. The professional should be alert to the disastrous effects of excessive pH conditions on the hair.

For example: In the area of permanent waving there is a trend to use neutral or even acid permanent waving solutions, especially when the hair has a history of damage. Regular permanent wave solution will only work at a pH of 9.5 (approx.) which is too high for damaged hair. Merely reducing the strength of the permanent wave solution will not correct its excessive pH content. However, special permanent wave solutions pH 3.0 to 8.0 do not have this tendency. These solutions are mostly intended for porous hair

EFFECTS OF pH ON LIGHTENED (BLEACHED) HAIR

The numbered specimens show the effects of acids and alkalies on the diameter and imbrications of bleached hair.

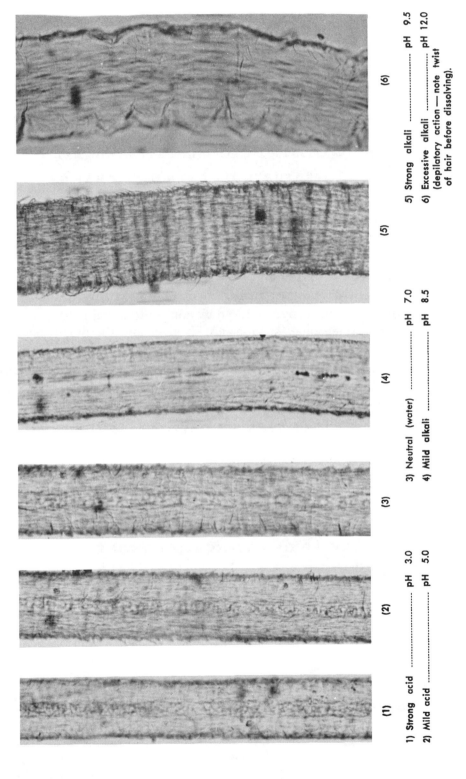

1) Strong acid .... pH 3.0
2) Mild acid .... pH 5.0

3) Neutral (water) .... pH 7.0
4) Mild alkali .... pH 8.5

5) Strong alkali .... pH 9.5
6) Excessive alkali .... pH 12.0
   (depilatory action — note twist
   of hair before dissolving).

for which the strongly alkaline solutions are unsuited. As they are very effective on porous, damaged hair, it is possible that in the near future we will see them used more extensively.

CHEMICAL CHANGES

DEFINITION Complicated changes which take place between the atoms of the elements are called "chemical changes." A chemical change signifies a permanent change and the formation of new substances or compounds. In many cases it is not possible to reverse the chemical action that has taken place. Therefore, a chemical change means that there is a more or less permanent change in the original matter and heat is generally involved.

FEATURES OF CHEMICAL CHANGES

SPEED OF CHANGES A rise in temperature always results in a speed up of this chemical change. An increase in the concentration of the chemicals used will also speed the reaction.

CONTROL OF CHANGES IN HAIR Chemical changes resulting from the use of a professional product (which involves some change to the hair) are usually quicker than changes induced by non-professional products.

The professional solutions are stronger and the practitioner often uses heat (steamers, hood processing machines) to further increase the speed of the change. Some manufacturers claim that quick results can be obtained from their materials, but the practitioners should remember not to sacrifice the safety of the patron in order to speed up the work.

DANGERS OF CHEMICAL CHANGES

ALL chemical changes require expert attention at *ALL* times. Even a minute of neglect may cause a great deal of damage to the hair. The hair has no power of self repair and so the unfortunate patron must wait for regrowth to restore the hair to its normal healthy condition.

EXAMPLES OF CHEMICAL CHANGES IN THE HAIR

PROCESS	CHEMICAL USED	CHEMICAL CHANGES
Permanent waving	1. Permanent wave solution . .	Hair is softened (Cystine is converted to Cysteine)
	2. Neutralizer	Hair is hardened (Cysteine is reconverted to cystine)
Lightening (bleaching)	Lighteners	Natural pigments are destroyed in cortex. (melanins are converted to oxymelanins)
Tinting	1. Para tints + 2. Developer	Artificial pigments are formed in cortex

PHYSICAL AND CHEMICAL CHANGES

TYPES	EXAMPLES	DEFINITION	USE IN COSMETOLOGY
PHYSICAL	STEAM WATER ICE HEATING AND COOLING OF WATER WATER IS FORMED BY PHYSICAL CHANGES	CHANGES OF A SUBSTANCE IN FORM FROM SOLID-LIQUID-GAS STATE NO NEW SUBSTANCE IS FORMED ACTION IS EASILY REVERSIBLE RATE OF CHANGES IS SIMPLY CONTROLLED	SETTING, FINGER WAVING, ETC. HAIR IS SOFTENED BY SETTING AGENTS — THEN HARDENED INTO WAVES BY DRYING.
CHEMICAL	ALKALI HEAT ACID REACTION OF ACIDS WITH ALKALIES (neutralization) WATER IS FORMED BY CHEMICAL CHANGE	PERMANENT CHANGES WITH FORMATION OF NEW SUBSTANCES ACTION IS <u>NOT</u> EASILY REVERSIBLE RATE OF CHANGE MUST BE CONTROLLED BY: a. TEMPERATURE b. CONCENTRATION c. TIME d. pH OF SOLUTION IN CONTACT WITH THE HAIR	<u>COLD WAVING</u> Keratin in cortex is chemically changed by waving solutions. Waves made permanent by reaction of neutralizers on changed keratin. <u>BLEACHING</u> Bleaches react with hair pigments to reduce color. <u>TINTING</u> Reaction of developer with tint bases forms tint pigments.

149

PHYSICAL CHANGES

DEFINITION Not all changes that occur in matter are severe or nonreversible, such as those found in a chemical change. Sometimes there is only a mild form of change known as a physical change. *In a physical change, no new substances are formed and the action is readily reversible.*

FEATURES OF PHYSICAL CHANGES

When a substance goes from the liquid to the solid or gas form it undergoes a physical change only. Example:

Ice — solid   Water — liquid   Steam — gas

Heating or cooling will change any form of water. This can be repeated as many times as you like without causing a permanent change. In other words, water remains water whether it be ice or steam. No new substance is formed.

EXAMPLES OF PHYSICAL CHANGES IN THE HAIR In the study of the hair we find that physical changes are used in setting, pin curling, roller curling or finger waving. Moisture can influence the hair by softening it and thus making it more pliable. A curl can be introduced in the hair and the hair carefully dried in the fixed position of the curl. The curl formed is an example of a physical change.

Unfortunately, as physical changes are simple and reversible, the curl will not hold. It gradually relaxes because the hair has a marked tendency to absorb moisture from the atmosphere and the hair reverts to its former condition.

Because of the tendency of humidity to relax the curl it is now customary to treat the hair with a setting spray. This forms a flexible coating on the hair cuticle and reduces the natural porosity of the hair. Less water vapor can now enter the hair and so the set will last much longer.

Setting is a valuable example of a physical change. It may be repeated as often as you like on normal hair, with very little risk of damage.

OXIDATION

DEFINITION Oxidation is a special example of a chemical change, but of a moderate kind. Basically, it means to combine or add oxygen to or with some other chemical.

FEATURES It was at first thought that only oxygen was involved in this type of chemical change, but we now find that other substances can act as oxidizing agents. Oxidation usually indicates that the substance is altered but not too severely, if the reaction is properly controlled.

In cosmetology, minor chemical changes in the hair caused by oxidation are very useful in the process of neutralizing, lightening, tinting and stripping.

OXIDIZING AGENTS

Oxidizing agents are materials which will cause oxidation of other substances. They are very active, sensitive materials. The most common one found in hair treatment is *hydrogen peroxide,* one reason being that it breaks down to form water and oxygen. Other oxiding agents are available for special purposes such as the neutralizer used in acid type permanent wave methods.

CONCLUSION

1. Oxidation brings about important chemical changes which are used by the practitioner to achieve certain effects in the hair. The purpose of these chemical changes is to cause mild alteration in the hair without affecting its properties.
2. Severe damage can be caused by sudden chemical changes in the hair and must always be avoided.
3. Excessively strong chemicals (such as lighteners, permanent wave solutions, chemical straighteners), must be used with great caution.

GENERAL PRECAUTIONS

The professional treatment of hair is becoming more scientific and so more chemicals are being used than ever before. Apart from reactions to the skin and hair (which have been briefly mentioned) there are a number of precautions needed in handling such chemicals in the shop.

1. All bottles, packets and containers must be accurately labeled. If a label cannot be read clearly it should be removed and replaced by a new one.
2. It is not wise to return parts of the contents of bottles back into the bulk container. All unused chemicals should be thrown away as it is false economy to try and save a few ounces at the risk of destroying a gallon of fresh material.
3. Materials should be removed from storage only when required and only in the estimated amounts needed.
4. All solutions should be checked and double-checked to see that they are the right ones and of the correct strength for the job at hand.
5. There is a real saving in buying products in bulk but only if the staff members are properly trained in handling these materials.
6. If there is any doubt about the contents of a bottle, it should be thrown away. All unlabeled bottles should be treated in this way automatically.
7. All materials should be kept in a cool, dry place. No bottles should be exposed to strong sunlight. On a hot day it may be necessary to put stocks of hydrogen peroxide into the refrigerator.

8. Plastic containers are very good for handling most materials (except strong lighteners) as they are very rugged. Glass should not be handled if your hands are wet or slippery.

9. Liquid should be poured carefully from the container, as it has a tendency to splash. If it happens to be ammonia or a strong lightener, it may cause severe burns. In cases of accidental spillage, these materials should be immediately diluted with plenty of warm water.

10. In carefully measuring amounts of solutions, the container or measure should be held at eye level. This ensures accuracy of amount and prevents fumes from entering your nose or eyes.

11. Mixing of ingredients (such as tints and developers) or breaking down of bulk solutions (such as shampoos) should be done thoroughly.

12. ALL manufacturers' directions should be read before starting to use the contents. It is surprising, the number of qualified artisans who admit to NOT having read the directions.

PRODUCT TESTING AND RESEARCH

No manufacturer would release a product unless it had been exhaustively tested and the proper recommendations and instructions given on the label (or given in appropriate literature).

If directions are disregarded, it is useless for practitioners to blame someone else for their ignorance. The public requires protection and expects the professional to act in its best interests. The chemistry of hairdressing products is changing very rapidly, and practitioners must keep in constant touch with new developments.

Because "such and such" a product has been used for some time does not mean that it will stay the same or always react on the hair in exactly the same way.

In the case of hair damage, when label directions were ignored, it will be impossible to get the support of the manufacturer. In certain cases, this could lead to serious medical and legal problems.

CHAPTER

12

SHAMPOO AND ITS CHEMISTRY

Introduction

The most fundamental operation performed in the salon or shop is shampooing. Shampoo is a Hindu word, which means "to clean." A recent survey found that professionals want a shampoo not only to clean but also to rinse out easily; produce a gloss on the hair without leaving a dry feeling, and at the same time leave the hair more manageable. In the light of these requirements, some of the best known shampoos are not very satisfactory, since they cause hair to become difficult to comb and produce a "flyaway" look. In addition, the hair feels rough to the hand and lacks natural luster and sheen.

AIM OF SHAMPOO

IMPORTANCE From the standpoint of cleanliness, attractiveness and personal hygiene, the care of the hair has become an important factor in our daily lives. Because of its structure, the hair must be treated carefully and not only the hair but the scalp also, must be kept scrupulously clean. Efficient shampooing is essential in order to maintain the hair and scalp in a clean and healthy condition.

PREPARATION   To effectively carry out the professional operations of shaping, waving, straightening, lightening and coloring, the hair must be properly cleansed and prepared.

Practitioners must remember that often this cleaning is done without considering the possible need for *special shampoos*. This fact is frequently overlooked or is not clearly understood. Selection of a shampoo should be based on hair and scalp variations such as:

1. Presence of dandruff.
2. An oily condition.
3. A dry condition.
4. Damage from previous treatments.
5. Kind of artificial hair coloring used.
6. Kinds of treatments that are to follow the shampoo.

RESPONSIBILITY   Although we are trying to look at matters of physiology and chemistry in the shop, there are economic complications to consider. For example, shampooing the hair is an operation that takes time, and time is money. Various firms wishing to sell their products use price and ease of application as selling points.

Despite the claims of salesmen, practitioners must remember that it is the overall picture that must be taken into consideration. Buying a brand of shampoo simply because it appears that it will save either money or work can be very misleading and costly. Low priced shampoos are not only cheap but they are often damaging to the hair and as a result may cause loss of goodwill and patrons. And, therefore, in the overall effect, they are very expensive.

COMMON PITFALL   Sometimes salesmen will advise that their products do not require a preparatory shampoo. But they neglect to advise that a shampoo *is* required for normal or oily hair, and that his no-shampoo method only works on dry, damaged or very porous hair.

The products not requiring a shampoo often have a creamy appearance because they are emulsions. Their action of cleansing the hair is identical to the function of the ordinary shampoo since they contain non-foaming detergents. Consequently, they have some cleansing action and will successfully prepare hair (normal, dry or damaged) for additional services.

CONCLUSION   Shampooing the hair should NEVER be thought of as something that can be done "any old way," for it must be done properly and in a conscientious manner. Success of later work on the hair depends greatly on proper preparation.

ACTION OF SHAMPOOS

A

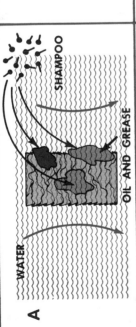

WATER

SHAMPOO

OIL AND GREASE

Sticky greasy surface attracts and holds dust and other particles of foreign matter to hair cuticle. Water alone is unable to clean hair because water molecules are unable to pull particles free from cuticle. Shampoo molecules have a strong attraction for hair, grease and dirt, etc.

B

DIRT

OIL AND GREASE

Proper massage during a shampoo insures that shampoo molecules are brought into direct contact with these substances.

Each tail of a molecule is attracted to grease and dirt.

Action of shampoo causes grease and oils to roll up into small globules reducing contact with hair cuticle.

EXCESS shampoo molecules are attracted to imbrications. Alkaline shampoos open imbrications causing tangling and matting during massage movements as fibers rub together.

C

WARM WATER RINSE

Currents of warm rinsing water remove dirt and grease because heads of shampoo molecules are attracted to passing water molecules. Tails of shampoo molecules plus attached dirt and foreign matter are bound to heads of shampoo following the rinsing currents of water. Thus foreign matter is removed ONLY during rinsing stages of shampooing.

D

CONTINUED RINSING

Excess shampoo molecules are less easily removed from hair shaft. Continued rinsing is essential to cleanse hair of shampoo. Time of rinsing is reduced by restricting amounts of shampoo. Excess swelling of imbrications is prevented by acid, soapless shampoos.

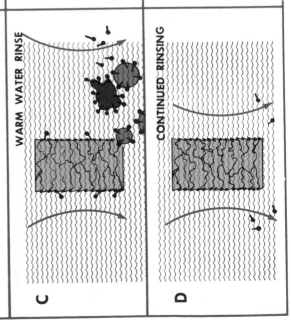

OBJECTIVES IN SHAMPOOING

OILY HAIR AND SCALP   There is no clear idea of what the general public, and/or the practitioner expects from a shampoo. The people with oily hair want a shampoo that really cleans. A stronger shampoo is required for the oily scalp because any excess removal of oils is quickly counteracted by the over activity of their sebaceous glands.

NORMAL OR DRY SCALPS   All patrons want a shampoo that carries the implication that the hair will still be left in a good condition after shampooing. A plain or cream shampoo may be used on patrons with normal or dry scalps. In every case the objective is to cleanse the hair and leave it feeling soft and silky.

Accordingly, we have the following main types of shampoos:

Clear shampoos—for greasy hair.

Conditioning shampoos—for normal or dry hair (cream or lotion type) .

FAULTY TECHNIQUES   The shampoo, itself, is of the utmost importance in cleansing the hair. Not all of the trouble, however, is entirely due to the shampoo product. Much of the cause of dry hair is the misuse of the shampoo by the practitioner.

Because of the apparent "simple" nature of a shampoo, it is usually given by the least experienced employee in the shop. Not that anything is wrong with this, but there is often very little supervision.

Manufacturers frequently complain about the resistance of the professionals and the general public to attempts made to educate them as to the merits of new products. These people buy a shampoo and then use it without even reading the directions or gaining the correct information about its use. After the gross misuse of the shampoo there are bitter complaints that the modern shampoo is far too drying and unsatisfactory.

EXCESSIVE SHAMPOO   A common error in shampooing is the use of excessive amounts of shampoo to clean the hair. Instead of just removing the *excess* oils, dirt and debris, the *surplus* shampoo leaves the hair very dry and hard to manage. Excessive shampoo is particularly damaging to lightened hair.

The stripping of ALL of the natural oils from the hair is a direct result of the excessive amounts of shampoo used. Only a small amount of the modern shampoo is required to clean the normal scalp because it is surprisingly efficient.

CONDITIONING SHAMPOOS

One attempt to help the practitioner has led to the cream or lotion type shampoo (containing lanolin or conditioner). But even here the product is misused, for "conditioner type" shampoos are usually intended to be employed in a two-stage application:

1st Stage
Normal strength of shampoo is used to clean the hair.

2nd Stage
Diluted strength shampoo should follow the first rinse. (This weaker shampoo allows the conditioner to be deposited on the hair shaft.)

PROPER RINSING

GUIDES TO PROPER RINSING Rinsing of the shampoo is a further step that is often improperly carried out. Rinsing must be complete and accurately timed. Absence of foam in the rinsing water is one indication that the rinsing has been adequate. The feel of the hair (squeaking or softness) is also used to tell us that this essential technique is completed.

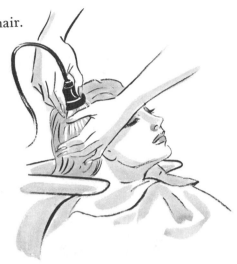

Every trace of shampoo must be rinsed off by a forceful jet of comfortably hot water.

RINSING PROCEDURE It is better to err on the safe side and make sure all excess shampoo is completely rinsed from the hair. Time this operation correctly, use strong jets of warm water and manipulate the hair so that no part of the scalp is missed.

FUNCTION OF FOAM (Lather) As regards to the "foam" itself, there is no evidence to show that foaming actually assists the cleansing of the hair and, in fact, it is thought to actually interfere with the cleansing process.

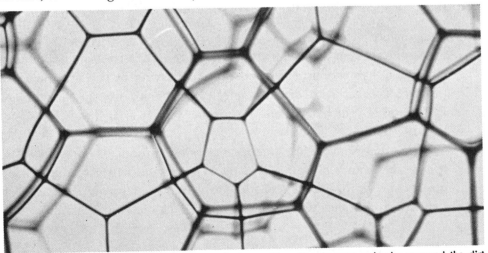

The action of a shampoo on dirt particles attached to a fiber. The shampoo molecules surround the dirt and help to lever it off with the aid of proper rinsing.—Courtesy: British Launderers Research Association.

A magnified view of foam bubbles. Courtesy: Dr. J. A. Kichener, Royal College of Science.

It is true that foam or lather is taken as a sign by the user that a shampoo is effective. However, many substances will clean the hair as well or better without foaming at all. These non-foaming cleansers are used in tints, permanent wave solutions and scalp treatments. These detergents are also used as wetting or softening agents for normal or porous hair.

EFFECTS OF SHAMPOOING

Not only is cleansing required, but shampooing contributes a great deal to the health and appearance of the hair.

1. Health

Healthy hair is good looking hair. The shampoo must remove dirt, debris, dandruff scales and excess natural oils; all of which can harbor bacteria. The strong smell of unwashed hair is primarily due to the presence of these bacteria.

Unlike most other structures in the body, hair has no power of self-repair. Fulfilling the life span of each hair strand depends on the removal of the bacteria, for if they are left on the hair various scalp disorders could result.

2. Luster

Luster or sheen of the hair is due to the interplay of light on the hair cuticle. The amount of natural oils on the cuticle influences this feature of the hair. Excessive removal of the oils by the shampoo will result in an unattractive, dull, dry appearance. However, the replacement of the oils by a conditioner or the use of a conditioner type shampoo will help maintain the desirable luster.

3. Color

The natural colors and shades in the hair are emphasized and heightened by a good shampoo. The removal of the dulling film of dirt on the cuticle allows the natural colors and highlights to be properly seen.

4. Manageability

The natural colors and shades in the hair are emphasized and heightened by proper shampooing. However, excessive drying by the shampoo may produce a great deal of static electrical charges on the hair fibers. Each strand of the hair repels one another to give a "flyaway" or "wind-blown" effect.

On the other hand, if the shampoo does not produce some static electricity, the strands of hair will cling together and will give the hair an unpleasant, limp, lifeless look. Excessively oily or greasy hair also has a similar appearance due to the complete lack of static electricity.

5. Odor

Clean, shampooed hair has an attractive fragrance of its own. This natural odor may be enhanced by the addition of a suitable perfume to the shampoo. As a result a patron may judge a shampoo largely on the desirable odor it leaves in the hair. For this reason, selection of shampoos must satisfy this basic appeal for a suitable fragrance, as well as its cleansing ability. Therefore, if a pleasant perfume is used, it may sharply influence the judgment of the patron. So, regardless of how well a shampoo cleans the hair, the patron will not be satisfied if the shampoo leaves an undesirable odor on the hair.

RESULTS OF POOR SHAMPOOING

Many of the problems in permanent waving can be traced back to poor rinsing of the shampoo. The shampoo still remaining in the hair prevents the entry of chemicals into the hair cortex and in some cases, reduces their potency. The shampoo is too often treated as unimportant and too little time is allowed for it. If the schedule is running late the time is often made up by "skimping" on the next shampoo.

Leaving the hair not properly cleansed can lead to losses in time, money and goodwill. This careless preparation of the hair can give rise to failure of the permanent wave, streakiness and uneven coloring or tinting, gumminess, stubbornness and dull appearance of a hairstyle.

HAIR CLEANSING PROBLEMS

CUTICLE SURFACE The nature of hair is the real cause of the difficulties in the cleansing and beautifying action of the shampoo. Since the hair is covered by the rough, hard, scaly surface of the cuticle, the ragged edges of the imbrications are well suited to catching and holding dirt and debris. If the hair is not properly cleansed this dirt and debris will leave the hair in an unattractive condition.

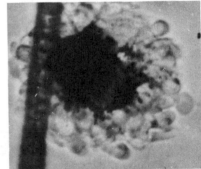

The action of a shampoo on dirt particles attached to a fiber. The shampoo molecules surround the dirt and help to lever it off with the aid of proper rinsing. — Courtesy: British Launderers Research Association.

LACK OF ATTENTION The skin is cleansed frequently because of the obvious implications of unwashed skin, but the need for frequent shampooing is often overlooked. Despite the fact that the total area of the scalp hair is nearly twice that of the skin area, this part of the body often receives the least attention.

HAIRSTYLE You often hear stories of people who go along for weeks without a single shampoo; the excuse being that they do not want to disturb their hairstyle. They apparently feel that their hairstyle is more important than a clean head.

ATTITUDES Many elderly patrons believe that shampooing the hair is unhealthy or unnecessary. People who work in dusty, dirty occupations need more frequent shampoos but they may not have the time to wash their hair every few days.

NATURAL OILS The film of natural oils on the outside of the hair helps to trap dust from the air. The slightly sticky surface then holds the dirt until it is washed off.

CUTICLE SCALES The cuticle scales, themselves, break off and fragments stick to the hair shaft. In addition, dandruff scales lodge in the hair and can be removed only by shampooing.

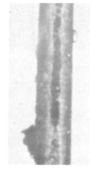 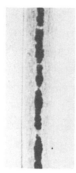

POSITION Being uppermost means that grit, dust and other foreign matter will more often fall onto the rough, sticky surface of the hair. Exposure to wind and other elements results in dirt being deposited in the hair.

THE DIAMETER OF THE HAIR Thick, coarse hair takes longer to clean than fine hair. The coarser hair has larger scales on the cuticle and so their rougher nature holds more particles of dirt on the hair.

Hair with attached dirt particles, dandruff scales and sebum coating.

Same hair after cleaning with a mildly acid soapless shampoo.

TYPE OF HAIR Certain types of wiry hair can be lathered and cleaned only with difficulty. Soft, pliable hair on the other hand, is easier to shampoo.

SUBSTANCES ON THE HAIR

There is a very wide range of foreign materials, which accumulate on the hair, that contribute to the need for regular shampooing:

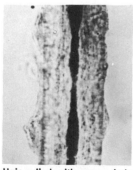

1. Lotions and lacquers leave a gummy residue that is difficult to remove.
2. Hair creams and conditioners contain various oils and a host of other substances.
3. Soap curds are found in the hair if hard water and soap are used to wash the hair at home. Soap films will also be left on the hair when it has only been rinsed in the bathroom basin without running water.

Hair soiled with excess hair cream which must be removed by shampoo.

NATURAL OILS There are many variations in natural oils found on the scalp and hair. In general, the hair of the teen-ager is at its oiliest. As a person gets older, the amount of oils decreases and the hair becomes drier.

ACTION OF SHAMPOO

The action of the shampoo occurs in two separate stages:

1. Wetting
2. Removal of dirt (rinsing)

WETTING

WETTING AND SURFACE TENSION   Most people would say that putting water on the hair "wets" it but, scientists have shown that this is not in itself correct.

The difficulty of wetting hair is due to the water, which has an important property known as surface tension. Actually, there always appears to be a film present on the surface of water. The surface seems to be under tension, hence "surface tension" is the name used to describe this property. As a result, water will not easily spread out on the oily cuticle of the hair, but forms as droplets along the outside of each shaft. Because the water drops will not spread out, the hair is not as "wet" as it should be.

EXAMPLE OF SURFACE TENSION   If the windshield of your car is slightly greasy or dusty and light rain begins to fall, what we notice is this:

The water refuses to form a thin, even layer over the windshield, but instead forms hundreds of droplets on the glass. These droplets scatter the light and you cannot see through the car windows properly.

But if the service station attendant sprays a detergent cleaner on the windshield, this treatment removes the oils and dirt. The rain then spreads evenly and you can see the road clearly.

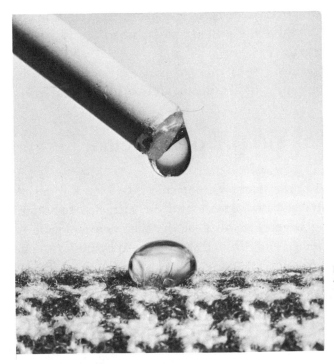

Drops of water showing the effects of surface tension and the lack of "wetting."—*Courtesy: Unilever Ltd.*

EFFECTS ON THE HAIR   The surface tension of water and the oily surface of the cuticle prevent the hair from being wetted. The water forms droplets along the shaft but in between them the hair is perfectly dry.

Furthermore, even where we find the water droplets, the hair is not properly wet. Air bubbles trapped within the imbrications prevent the water droplets from wetting the cuticle thoroughly, even at the positions where the hair is apparently "wet."

FUNCTION OF SHAMPOO   One of the functions of the shampoo is to lower the surface tension and allow the water to spread evenly along and between the imbrications.

THE NEED FOR SHAMPOO

SALTS   Water, alone is capable of removing those materials from the hair which are soluble in it. Salts, perspiration and certain chemicals may be rinsed from the hair quite effectively by the use of water alone.

GREASE AND DIRT   But, water alone will not remove grease, oils or dirt. The water molecules slide past these substances since they cannot get a grip on their greasy surface and pull them free from the cuticle.

A shampoo is required so that the water is sufficiently attracted to the foreign matter and can sweep it off the hair by a stream of rinse water afterwards.

EFFECT OF SHAMPOO   A shampoo carries out its function because the shampoo molecule is made of two parts, each of which has a separate task. In addition, the molecule cannot be easily pulled apart and so the two parts of the molecule must work together.

We will stylize the shape and size of the two parts of the molecule in order to clearly explain the nature of shampoos and to understand their properties.

FUNCTION OF SHAMPOO MOLECULE

HEAD —
(Water-
Loving.
Grease,
Oil-
Hating.)

SHAPE
OF
SHAMPOO
MOLECULE

TAIL — (Water-Hating.
Grease, Oil-Loving.)

HEAD   The task of the head of the shampoo molecule is to keep the tail of the molecule, along with attached dirt, grease and oil, attracted to water, especially during the rinsing stage. The head of the shampoo molecule is pushed aside by grease, oils, debris and dirt and shows no attraction for them.

TAIL   It is the tail of the shampoo molecule that has a special attraction for dirt, grease, debris and oils. The tail is called the "water-hating" part of the molecule as it has no attraction for water molecules.

NEED FOR USING WATER Many organic solvents (kerosene, alcohol, gasoline) can dissolve grease and dirt readily from the hair. However, these solvents are not very soluble or attracted to water. This means that they cannot be rinsed from hair by the use of water alone. Although the grease, etc., is removed, these materials are now replaced by a harsh, inflammable solvent which is left in the hair. Therefore, they are not suitable for general shop practice and hair is best cleansed with shampoo and water.

ACTION OF THE HEAD AND TAIL

PURPOSE OF SHAMPOO STRUCTURE Shampoo molecules are relatively large molecules which have been specially treated. The effect of this treatment is to give the shampoo a strong attraction for both grease and dirt and also for water. Therefore, it is the combined action of these two parts (head and tail) that allows the shampoo to clean the hair with the help of water.

This equal attraction for these mutually repelling substances (oil and water) produces a "tug of war" effect. The water molecules, instead of sliding past the grease and dirt on the hair, are able to sweep or pull these materials away from the cuticle.

Since the water-loving heads of the shampoo want to stay with the molecules of the rinsing water, and since the link between the head and the tail of the shampoo is extremely strong, the tail (with dirt, grease, oil and debris attached) is levered or lifted off the hair.

By stripping the hair free of these substances, the hair is left clean and saturated only with a harmless substance, water.

REMOVAL OF OIL

FIRST STAGE In the case of oils on the hair, the first action of the shampoo is to cause the oils to form into rounded droplets. This reduces the area of the oils in direct contact with the hair and weakens the hold that it has on the cuticle. The oil droplets have the "oil-loving tails" of the shampoo sticking inside them with the "heads" (oil-haters) projecting outward.

The heads act as "hooks" to grab hold of the streams of rinsing water and the oil is pulled completely free from the hair by this process.

FINAL STAGE Once the oils are lifted free from the cuticle and are in the rinsing solution itself, the rounded oil droplets become fully surrounded (emulsified) by the shampoo molecules. This prevents the oils from being re-deposited on the hair shaft and they are washed from the hair.

HOW DETERGENTS REMOVE OIL FROM HAIR

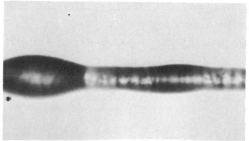

(No. 1 — Oil coated hair.)

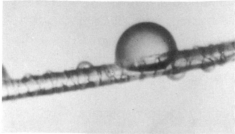

(No. 2 — Globule starting to form.)

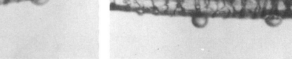

(No. 3 — Note the decreasing surface contact.)

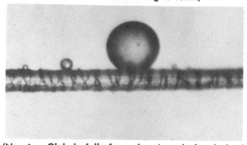

(No. 4 — Globule fully formed and ready for rinsing.)

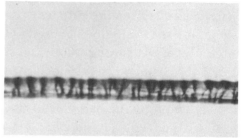

(No. 5 — Clean hair.)

REMOVAL OF DIRT AND GREASE

MECHANICAL REMOVAL Dirt, grease and other solid objects are more difficult to remove from the hair. The larger particles can be simply brushed or combed out, however, since hair has an attraction for dirt, most of the particles of dust will remain.

ACTION OF SHAMPOO When dirty hair is washed with a shampoo, the tails of the shampoo are attracted to the dirt and grease. As soon as contact is made between the dirt and the dirt-loving shampoo it develops an extreme reluctance to part company. This force or attraction is even stronger than the force that attracts the dirt to the hair in the first place.

VALUE OF MASSAGE Thorough mechanical agitation and massage of the scalp and hair are very important factors aiding the work of the shampoo molecules. These molecules have to be worked into and around *ALL* of the hair fibers. This is necessary to bring the tails of the shampoo molecules into touch with all the foreign material on the hair in preparation for the rinsing stage which follows.

FUNCTION OF RINSING

TIMING Removing all of the shampoo, oils, dirt and debris from the hair is the prime objective of the rinsing process. This technique is truly of critical importance and must be carried out properly and timed accurately.

RINSING ACTION Complete removal of all shampoo molecules from the hair is achieved by the agitating, surging action of the warm jets of water rushing past the hair fibers. To be effective, each jet of water must be directed along each strand of hair in order to achieve complete rinsing.

EXCESSIVE SHAMPOO Rinsing of ALL shampoo molecules is made much more difficult if an excess of shampoo is used. This excessive shampoo works its way deep into the imbrications of the cuticle and there it is almost impossible to remove by rinsing. Never use more shampoo than is really necessary to clean the surface of the cuticle. Excess shampoo is not only wasteful, it interferes with shampooing, is harmful to the hair, and will detract from its appearance.

FOLLOW MANUFACTURER'S DIRECTIONS

To avoid some of the problems caused by faulty shampooing, it is advisable to take note of the following:

1. Measure out the shampoo carefully
2. DON'T rely on guesswork for the correct amount
3. READ the directions carefully
4. The supplier knows his product far better than a practitioner thinks he or she does and his instructions should be followed implicitly.

SOAP SHAMPOOS

INTRODUCTION AND HISTORY The earliest known shampoos were those made by boiling laundry soap and water until a clear jelly was formed.

SOURCE Soap comes from natural sources (coconut oil or animal fats) and through treatment with alkalies can be made into a limited number of types. There are three main alkalies used for this purpose (caustic soda, caustic potash and ammonia).

TYPES OF SOAPS Although depending as well on the fat used, caustic soda usually forms a hard soap. Hard soaps are found as laundry soaps (as bars, cakes, chips, flakes, beads, etc.).

Dirty clothes are nearly always soiled by perspiration and body grease (both acid in nature). To counteract this acid so that the soap can continue cleaning, excess alkali is added by the manufacturer.

As the pH of laundry soaps are higher than 9.0 the alkali content has a bad effect on hair. With bleached hair, all soaps have a particularly severe action and are really too harsh to be used at all.

Toilet soaps are usually made from better quality animal or plant fats treated with caustic potash. This forms a soft, bland soap. However, these soaps are made into cakes and as such are not in a convenient form for a shampoo.

LIQUID SOAP SHAMPOOS

Soap shampoos are usually made with an ammonia "head" and a fatty "tail." As is common with soaps, these shampoos must also be made alkaline.

The pH of a good quality soap shampoo should be about 8.0–9.0. However, cheap soap shampoos are often in excess of pH 10.0. Although highly alkaline conditions favor the cleansing action of the soap shampoo itself, the alkaline content is not good for the hair.

ADVANTAGES OF SOAP SHAMPOOS   They do not remove too much sebum from the skin and hair and so these surfaces still retain some of their natural oils. Excess shampoo can be rinsed out of the hair without much difficulty.

DISADVANTAGES OF SOAP SHAMPOOS   They react with hard water in rinsing. This results in a soap scum which is left firmly attached to the cuticle causing a loss of the luster or sheen of the hair. In addition the wetting and dirt-removal properties of the soap shampoo are very poor by comparison with newer types.

FORMATION OF SOAP SCUM

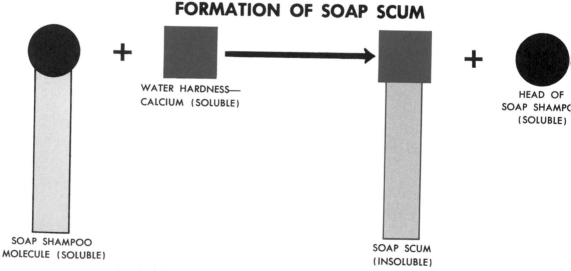

WATER HARDNESS—
CALCIUM (SOLUBLE)

HEAD OF
SOAP SHAMP(
(SOLUBLE)

SOAP SHAMPOO
MOLECULE (SOLUBLE)

SOAP SCUM
(INSOLUBLE)

HOW TO OVERCOME THESE DISADVANTAGES   More shampoo can be added to make up for that lost by the water hardness, or by using specially treated or soft water for the shampoo. (Distilled or rain water is excellent.) Water softeners can be installed to meet the great water requirements of the typical salon or shop, but they are somewhat expensive.

The wetting and dirt-removal properties of the soap shampoo may be improved by using water as warm as possible during shampooing.

The soap scum can be removed from the cuticle by a final mild acid rinse. Certain firms have special powders which are intended to be used in the rinse to remove soap scum and these are usually more suitable for professional use.

All of these acid rinses neutralize the excess alkalinity of the soap shampoo and cause shrinking and hardening of the cuticle. Acid cream rinses further restore the sheen to the hair because they cause the cuticle scales to press down on the hair shaft more tightly.

REMOVAL OF SOAP SCUM

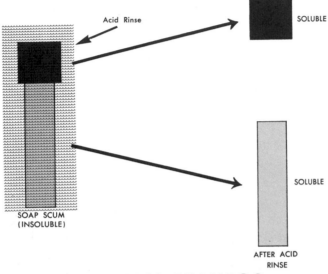

Acid Rinse

SOLUBLE

SOLUBLE

SOAP SCUM
(INSOLUBLE)

AFTER ACID
RINSE

SOAPLESS SHAMPOO

SOURCE Soapless shampoos are made from synthetic detergents (mainly derived from petroleum industry by-products) or from natural fats that have been chemically treated. These detergents were originally developed to overcome the serious disadvantages of soap in industry. The use of soap creates problems, as we have seen, and because they solve many of these problems, soapless shampoos have become very popular for professional hair service.

RANGE Over 200 different detergents are now available and more are being developed each year. Since we can "tailor-make" the molecules according to the purpose desired, synthetic shampoos have a tremendous advantage.

These new "tails" must be chemically or synthetically manufactured. One method is to take a natural fat and convert it to its fatty acids. These fatty acids are then treated in special chemical processes.

This changes the mixture of natural fatty acids into other compounds having a desirable molecular size and shape. In other words, the "tails" are preformed in exactly the length required for improved shampooing.

These selected fatty acids are neutralized with alkali (more often a mixture, with caustic soda predominant). The alkali forms the necessary "head" which is chemically joined to the "tail."

SOAPLESS SHAMPOO MOLECULES

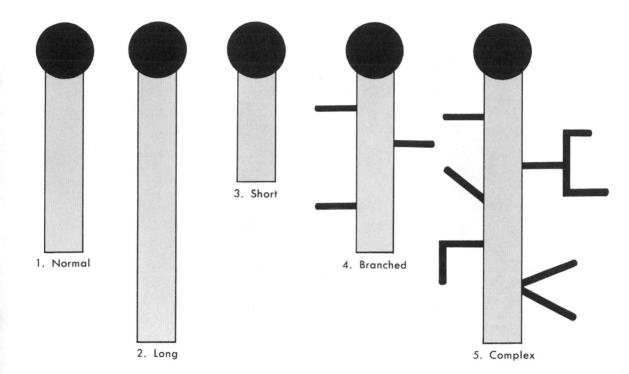

1. Normal

2. Long

3. Short

4. Branched

5. Complex

NEW TYPES Although the present soapless shampoos have a strong command of the market it does not mean that these shampoos are perfect and, therefore, they are being constantly improved. This results in better products continually becoming available for professional use.

ADVANTAGES OF SOAPLESS SHAMPOOS The wetting and dirt removal properties of soapless shampoos are excellent. They are not affected by hard water (they can clean hair readily in hard or salt water) as long as fresh water is used as a final rinse.

They do not depend on natural sources and this means their range and scope are almost inexhaustible. Furthermore, a steady decrease in price has put them within the reach of everyone.

They can be made acid without reducing the cleaning action. This allows them to be used on lightened and damaged hair without causing swelling or matting of the hair.

They can be highly concentrated to form thick liquids, creams or pastes. Then, by simply mixing with tap water they can be made ready for use in the shop. This is economical because it reduces shipping costs (transportation and containers) which would be extremely high if water were included. Water is very heavy and in a ready-to-use shampoo, there is approximately 80% water.

DISADVANTAGES OF SOAPLESS SHAMPOOS They are very difficult to rinse from the hair. They are excellent removers of oils and grease and therefore are inclined to strip the cuticle of all the natural sebum as well. This excessive removal of natural oils may result in dry, chaffed skin and dull, unmanageable hair. As a result, they may give an unpleasant sticky feeling to the hands when wet. These shampoos also present a danger in the fact that they may cause dermatitis by contact with sensitive skins.

HOW TO OVERCOME THESE DISADVANTAGES

1. *Reduce the amount of shampoo used.* Because of the stronger action of the soapless shampoo, very little is actually needed to thoroughly cleanse the hair.
2. A vitalizer, hand cream or hair conditioner after the shampoo will overcome the excess dryness of the hair, skin and scalp.
3. Additives or conditioning agents may be included within the shampoo itself. These agents act by:
   a) Reducing the cleansing efficiency of the shampoo.
   b) Depositing some of the conditioner on the hair shaft.

However, this technique of conditioning the hair by the shampoo itself can only be done effectively if the concentration of the second stage shampoo solution is reduced. Rubber gloves may be worn by the practitioner if sensitive to certain types of the soapless shampoos. Sometimes the brand of the shampoo should be changed to reduce the danger of dermatitis, since not all soapless shampoos will produce skin sensitivity.

USE OF SHAMPOOS

PURPOSE OF SHAMPOO The purpose of a shampoo is to:

1. Cleanse the hair and leave it in a normal, healthy, attractive condition.
2. Prepare the hair for some further operation, such as, permanent waving, hair coloring, etc.

If the hair is greasy or oily, then a preparatory shampoo is a necessity.

In some cases, for particular formulations, manufacturer's directions often state that shampooing "may" be omitted. Various wetting and shampoo materials (non-foaming) are already present in the solution in such cases. But they are only intended for use on dry or porous hair. In any case, a shampoo beforehand will give an idea of the porosity, from the feel of the wet hair; for example, a rubbery feel indicates cuticle damage.

WHEN PERMANENT WAVING, the shampoo may dilute the waving solution because of the presence of excess rinse water. If properly controlled, this will give greater control of the processing, especially for highly porous hair. The shampoo also acts as a swelling agent, for the hair swells up to 14% extra in diameter. The swelling allows easier and faster penetration of the permanent wave solutions.

PROPER TECHNIQUE The shampoo must be evenly and thoroughly distributed through the hair by finger and hand movements. This complete distribution is important in order to bring the shampoo in contact with all of the dirt and grime in the hair and permit the shampoo molecules to perform their special functions. The foreign matter on the cuticle is then removed by strong jets of warm water directed in such a way as to create surging currents over each strand of hair.

No shampoo, however, is completely satisfactory to the artisan since the required properties are numerous and demanding.

FEATURES OF A GOOD SHAMPOO
1. It should not form soap curds in ordinary tap water.
2. It should be neutral (or at least not highly alkaline) so as to prevent undue swelling or damage to the hair.
3. It should clean the hair completely and gently, without damage, and leave it soft and lustrous.
4. It should produce a thick, rich, creamy lather (so that we can recognize that rinsing is completed when there is an absence of foam).
5. It should not interefere with any other operation that might follow the shampoo.
6. It should rinse easily and completely from the hair.

SPECIAL SHAMPOOS

Certain shampoos can be simply called "gimmick" shampoos, which do nothing "extra" for the cleansing of the hair not already done by ordinary shampoo. They include "pearlescent" shampoos that contain pearly flakes that reflect the light (the flakes are a type of plastic that is often difficult to remove from the hair after the shampoo).

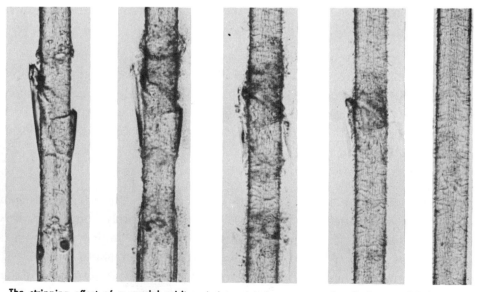

The stripping effect of a special spirit and detergent shampoo on a heavily lacquered hair strand.

JELLY SHAMPOOS (in clear sachets or collapsible tubes) are usually simply ordinary clear liquid shampoos that have been thickened by adding common salt.

OIL SHAMPOOS and powder, dry shampoos have all but disappeared. Their limited use has been taken over by newer improved types.

NUTRITIVE SHAMPOOS The practical value of "nutritive" shampoos and medicated (dandruff) shampoos remain as yet unknown. There are, however, possibilities of major developments in the future. Nevertheless, most "nutritive" shampoos now sold are only lanolin cream or oil type conditioning shampoos. Their action is to control the porosity of the hair by forming a protective coating over the cuticle.

OTHER BIOCHEMICAL PRODUCTS (such as, fish, eggs and various forms of protein), have been patented in special shampoos. These products function as moisturizers to control the moisture level in the cortex and, as a result, the manageability of the hair is much improved.

The combination of shampoo and colored rinses, shampoo and neutralizer, shampoo and alcohol for removing lacquer films, shampoo and lightener, are examples of the versatility of the modern shampoo.

TESTING OF SHAMPOOS

The chemist in the laboratory can make all sorts of tests with the shampoo, but there is still no substitute for the practical tests that the professional applies in the shop. To obtain reliable comparisons between different shampoos, conditions must be exactly the same. They include method of shampooing, temperature of water, amount of rinsing, uniformity of massaging the scalp, hardness of water, the hair texture, type and materials that have to be shampooed from the hair; all must be carefully controlled.

POINTS TO BE TESTED

The following points must be considered in order to decide if a particular shampoo is satisfactory or is better than the brand already in use in the salon or shop:

EASE OF DISTRIBUTION Some shampoos do not cover the head and seem to "sink into" the hair. It is rather difficult to spread them evenly or to raise a good lather. For effective shampooing the entire head must be thoroughly covered.

RINSING   Some shampoos rinse away fairly quickly while others continue to foam after what seems endless rinsing. While a 5 minute rinsing is about right for most shampoos, this period may not be long enough if the suds (or foam) persist. All suds, foam and shampoo must be removed for hair cleanliness.

COMBING   The combing of wet hair gives some indication of the roughness of the hair. Poor shampoos leave the hair rough to the touch because they raise and damage the cuticle. This makes combing difficult and care must be used to avoid breakage when matting and snarls are encountered.

LUSTER OF THE HAIR   The removal of the dulling dirt and film should produce a desirable sheen in the hair. This sheen is assisted by the cuticle scales remaining hard and firm and by a thin film of natural oils remaining after the shampoo.

Soap shampoos (alkaline) invariably leave a dingy soap scum on the hair which must be removed by special rinses since it detracts from the appearances of lustrous, healthy hair.

SPEED OF DRYING   Drying the hair is the most tedious step in the normal shampoo. It is also the most costly because of the time and equipment (hair dryers) involved. Some shampoos leave the hair saturated with water and, therefore, are slow to dry. This moisture is found in two places:

On the outside of the hair

As much as 50% extra water may be on the outside of the hair. The actual amount found depends on the shampoo used.

Inside the hair

Ordinarily, the hair will soak up about 30% of its weight in water during the shampoo. To set the hair, two-thirds of this moisture must be dried out again since the normal moisture content of the cortex is approximately 10%.

Dryers with well designed hoods are essential to improve the rate of drying. The temperature and volume of air directed onto the hair are limited. The use of excessive heat may create a distinct danger of damage to the hair and scalp. Patron comfort must also be considered and if the time of drying can be reduced by a better shampoo, this is a great advantage.

MANAGEABILITY   The ease of combing and setting the dry hair after the shampoo is a very important consideration. When the hair is dry there may be a tendency for excess static electricity to be produced within the hair. This causes "flyaway" or "scarecrow" effect as the hair fibers repel one another. Furthermore, the more the hair is combed or brushed, trying to achieve the desired style, the more it flies about and defeats these attempts.

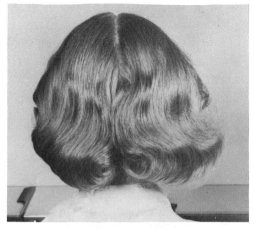

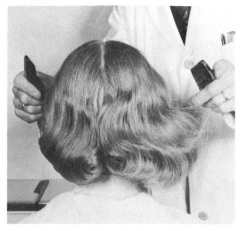

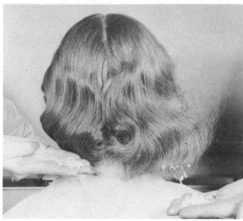

(Above left). Model with left and right hand sides of hair shampooed with "good" and "bad" shampoos respectively. (So called "half-head" tests are necessary to give a reliable comparison.)

(Above). Hair after vigorous combing and brushing. Note "fly-away" strands on right hand side. Further brushing will only increase the problem.

(Left). The hair cleaned with "bad" shampoo has an excess of static electricity. Attraction of pieces of paper to the hair indicates this state on the right hand side (poor shampoo) but not on the left (good shampoo).

Courtesy: Lever Brothers

On the other hand, some shampoos leave the hair flat and limp. Not enough static electricity is left in the hair and it appears to lack natural "body."

PRACTICAL WORK

SHAMPOO IDENTIFICATION A soapless shampoo can be identified in the following manner:

1. Shake the ready-to-use shampoo solution until a good foam is formed. Then add a small quantity of a mild acid, such as vinegar. Immediate collapse of the foam indicates a soap shampoo, whereas soapless shampoos remain unaffected.
2. Repeat the above test using hard water. Collapse of foam, with curds floating on the surface, indicates soap.
3. Test the pH of the shampoo with indicator papers.
   Acid—soapless shampoo only.
   Alkaline (or neutral) —can be soap or soapless shampoo.

SAFETY

Finally, the shampoo must be completely safe to use. Solvent shampoos such as kerosene or gasoline, are extremely dangerous. Some give off poisonous fumes, and there is an ever-present risk of fire, therefore, they are rarely used today. The shampoo should not affect the scalp or hair of the patron nor harm the hands of the practitioner while being used.

Shampooing often results in some of the shampoo trickling down the brows into the eyes. While the diluted shampoo (during rinsing) is harmless, there is always the risk that undiluted shampoo could enter and cause severe stinging of the eyes. Proper placement of towels and careful protective measures by the practitioner should prevent this problem. Some shampoos can cause severe irritation to the eyes while others seem to have little effect.

CONCLUSION

Shampooing of the hair is an essential part of hair care and should receive more attention. It is often overlooked as a possible cause of later difficulties. Because of this shortsighted attitude, practitioners fail to realize that the choice of the correct shampoo and proper application are vitally important. Even if the proper choice is made, the product cannot be expected to do its job satisfactorily if not used according to the specific directions. These directions are based on the research and "know-how" of a highly organized technical industry. Notwithstanding, the real potential of the modern shampoos, the actual performance and final responsibility for them must rest with the professional skill and application by the artisan.

CURLING AND WAVING OF HAIR

NATURAL WAVES IN THE HAIR

Before an investigation can be made of the changes that take place in the cortex of the hair during temporary or permanent waving, a brief look at natural waves in the hair should be profitable.

A few fortunate people possess naturally wavy or curly hair and in certain races tight, over-curly hair is typical. Although several theories exist, unfortunately, science has not been able to determine the exact cause of this natural feature of the hair.

CONTROLLING FACTORS

But, the type of wave and the characteristics of the wave are controlled by several factors such as:

HEREDITY   Before a person can have naturally curly hair there must be present certain factors that control the growth of this hair. The nature of these factors are not fully understood but they are handed down from the parents. If the parents have wavy hair then an offspring will be more likely (but not certain) to have the same type of wavy hair.

DIET   Although naturally wavy hair cannot be produced by eating some special food, the food eaten does affect the hair in some ways. A well balanced diet is essential for healthy hair whether it is straight or wavy.

When the diet is lacking in certain amino-acids (containing sulphur) the natural waves will flatten. Young mothers often complain of straightened hair and in the older person any natural waves have a tendency to become shallower partly due to changes in their diet.

HEALTH   As hair growth is bound up with all the body processes, any upset to the system will alter and change the tendency for waves. People convalescing from a severe illness can notice a slow return of the natural waves that they had lost during their period of poor health.

THEORY OF NATURAL WAVES

Certain theories have been advanced to explain exactly how the hair gets a natural wave. These theories include the following:

SHAPE OF HAIR SHAFT   Some claim that waves are due to the shape of the cross-section of the hair.

> If it is round—then the hair is straight.
> If oval—then the hair is curly.
> If flattened—then that hair is over-curly.

Although it is a fact that hair does have these shapes, there does not seem to be any clear cut proof of the facts that this theory would suggest. E.g., straight hair can be either round or oval and vice versa. Even if this theory is believed, it still does not explain why a round hair would only be straight, or that an over-curly hair must be flattened.

SHAPE OF FOLLICLE   Others claim that it is the follicle that is responsible for the wave and that the shape of the follicle determines that the hair will take a certain form. This theory is based on the fact that hair cells are soft when first produced and become completely keratinized or hardened before reaching the surface of the skin. If these cells harden in a straight follicle, the hair will be straight. If they harden in a curved follicle, the hair will be wavy or curly.

This theory could also be possible, but it still does not satisfy all conditions known about the hair. For instance, changes in diet, health, age, taking of drugs, motherhood, etc., will all change the wave in the hair without a corresponding change in the shape of the follicle. Whether or not the arrector pili muscle can act to change the shape of the follicle is also a matter of debate.

ACTION OF GERMINAL MATRIX   This theory claims it is the action of the germinal area near the papilla that decides whether the hair is to grow straight or otherwise. It is the function of the "germ" area to produce the cells which form the cortex which will grow out of the follicle as hair.

Straight Hair

Now if cells are being produced at an even rate all around, there is no reason why the hair should curl. If there is an even growth of cells, it follows that the hair would grow straight.

FORMATION OF NATURAL WAVES IN HAIR

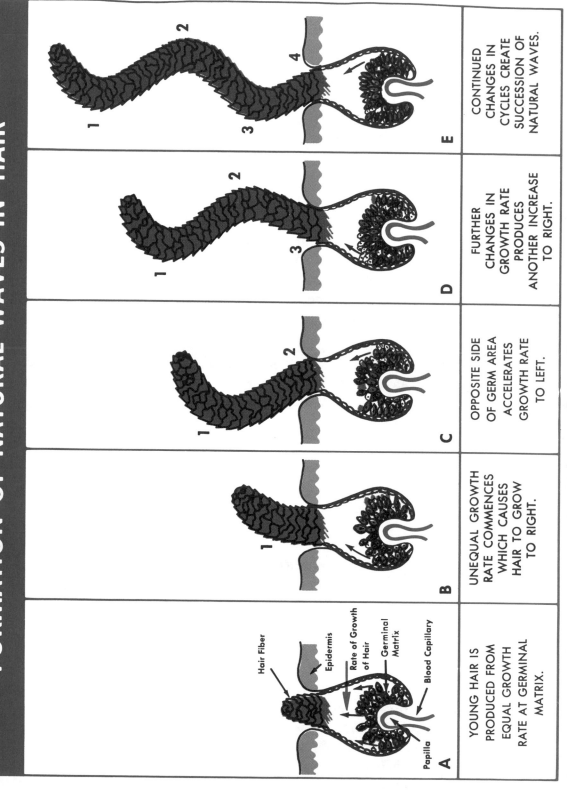

A — YOUNG HAIR IS PRODUCED FROM EQUAL GROWTH RATE AT GERMINAL MATRIX.

Hair Fiber

Epidermis

Rate of Growth of Hair

Germinal Matrix

Blood Capillary

Papilla

B — UNEQUAL GROWTH RATE COMMENCES WHICH CAUSES HAIR TO GROW TO RIGHT.

C — OPPOSITE SIDE OF GERM AREA ACCELERATES GROWTH RATE TO LEFT.

D — FURTHER CHANGES IN GROWTH RATE PRODUCES ANOTHER INCREASE TO RIGHT.

E — CONTINUED CHANGES IN CYCLES CREATE SUCCESSION OF NATURAL WAVES.

Curly Hair

But if at any time one side of the germinal matrix is producing more cells that the opposite side, the hair will grow in a curve. Obviously, if this extra growth of hair cortex on one side continues, the hair will grow in a circle. However, after acting in this way for a time the germinal area ceases this abnormal activity and produces less growth than before.

Then the alternate side of the papilla accelerates its rate of growth. This continues for a period of time and shifts the hair back to its original position. However, before it slows down it has produced curved growth in the opposite direction.

Changes in Cycle

This cycle is repeated over and over and the changes in the cycle take place at various rates. Over-curly hair is the result of a rapid rate of cell overproduction and change. If the change is slower, the hair grows in soft, loose curls. If the changes slow down further, then the growth rates would be the same and the hair would emerge straight or with a very slight wave.

ROLE OF AMINO-ACIDS Thus, the reasons why hair changes its natural shape can easily be due to the changes in the amino-acid chains in the cortex. More amino-acids are found on the outside of the waves than on the inside of the waves. But, because the hair does not grow into a circle, then the sum total of the left and right sides are the same when taken along the whole length of each hair fiber.

Therefore, the number of amino-acids in a strand of curly hair are the same as in straight hair, but at certain places (on the outside and inside of each curl) there appear to be differences in numbers.

UNIFORM WAVE FORMATION To form waves in the hair, these changes in growth rates must take place within many follicles in the same area and at exactly the same rate and direction. Otherwise there would be just a tangle of uneven and unruly curls in the hair.

EXTERNAL EFFECTS Although the actual growth changes take place deep within the follicle, the effects of the wave are not confined within the skin. The actual time taken to grow one complete wave in the hair would be at least one month, and by this time the changing hair fiber would have left the follicle. (The follicle itself is only $\frac{1}{8}''$ deep and the rate of growth is approximately $\frac{1}{2}''$ to $1''$ per month.) Therefore, a complete wave would take from one month to two months or more to form, depending on the rate of hair growth and the tightness of the wave.

CONCLUSION

Due to the period of time that it takes to form each natural wave in the hair, it is difficult to explain natural waves by means of the shape of the follicle or cross-section of the hair alone. Because of the present knowledge science has of the structure of the cortex, it is thought that the real cause of natural waves in the hair are changes in the hard keratin chains as they are formed. While no detailed studies have been done on wave formation in human hair, much work has been done on wave formation in wool, which illustrates the theory of uneven hair growth rate.

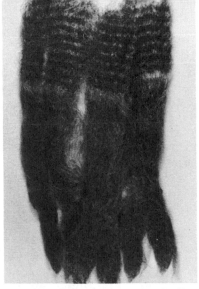

Photograph of wool (a hard keratin fiber similar to human hair) showing straight and waved sections. The straight section was caused by a lack of copper in the diet. Waves returned when diet was made sufficient for normal wool growth.—Courtesy: Wool Ind. Res. Association.

ARTIFICIAL WAVES IN THE HAIR

REASONS FOR ARTIFICIAL WAVES Depending on circumstances and the demands of fashion, most individuals seek to be different. In our society, most members have straight hair. However, fashion and style indicate an accent on wavy hair. Apart from a few lucky people who naturally have the exact hair formation they desire, the remainder spend their lives trying to get those waves which nature denied them.

STYLING Another point is that wavy hair offers much greater opportunities for the creation of different styles than does straight hair. But, as the aim in artificial waves is to copy nature, methods of nature must be imitated as closely as possible.

BASIC PROBLEMS IN ACHIEVING PERMANENT ARTIFICIAL WAVES

Natural waves in hair are formed because the outside of the wave contains more amino-acids than the inside of the wave. There are several ways for altering the position of the polypeptide chains present in straight hair and thereby create a wave or curl. These methods include the following:

STRETCHING If the hair (without previous treatment of any sort) is pulled around rollers or the fingers, then a kink or a wave can be formed in it. To do this the cortex has to be stretched on the outside of the shaft. Because tension is developed in the cortex as a result of this stretching, this tension slowly returns the hair to its original, unstretched, straight form. (Similarly, over-curly hair will spring back again on release.)) Thus, it is not possible to put permanent waves in the hair simply by arranging the hair into a wave without treating it in some way.

SPRAYING   The hair can be wound, as described previously, and before releasing it, sprayed with some fixative or lacquer. Although very large curls may be treated in this manner, the method usually fails. In order to hold, the spray has to be applied in so thick a film that the hair has a brassy, unnatural appearance. In addition, the lacquer or spray tends to crack and to flake and combing and shampooing the hair become very difficult tasks following this treatment.

CHEMICAL REARRANGEMENT   To be successful, the hair must be chemically softened so that the amino-acid chains will rearrange themselves into a "permanent" waved form. This is only possible if the cross-bonds holding the chains in their natural position are first broken. The cross-bonds must then be reformed and the hair hardened, with the new wave form becoming its stable or normal state.

If recently permanently waved hair is stretched, the waves should spring back upon release, indicating that the rearrangement of the amino-acid chains has chemically changed the basic nature or form of the straight hair.

THE FOUR MAJOR STEPS
USED IN ALL HAIR WAVING

There are four main steps by which the hair is altered in form. These same steps are found in setting, finger waving, permanent waving and thermal waving. These are only different techniques of waving hair, but the basic steps remain the same.

These basic steps are the following:

1. WINDING

METHODS   The hair to be curled is wound around some circular object (rod, roller) or is fashioned by the fingers and then pinned. The flexible nature of hair allows us to do this without previous treatment. In practice, the hair is often softened by water or pre-dampened with special solutions, beforehand, to make it easier to shape or wind on the rods or rollers.

DETERMINING WAVE SIZE   The size of the circular object decides the final size of the resultant wave or curl. A small rod gives a tight curl and the large curls or "jumbo" size rollers give the loosest curl.

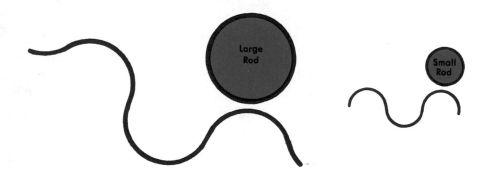

2. SOFTENING

METHODS   After the winding has been completed, the hair must be properly softened and the cross-bonds broken by special solutions. Sometimes softening is achieved by a shampoo before winding, particularly if the hair is not to be fully softened, as in setting. When stronger chemicals are used, it is usual to allow some time for the bonds to be broken and to assume their new positions, especially in permanent waving, and this is known as the *processing time.*

BONDS IN CORTEX

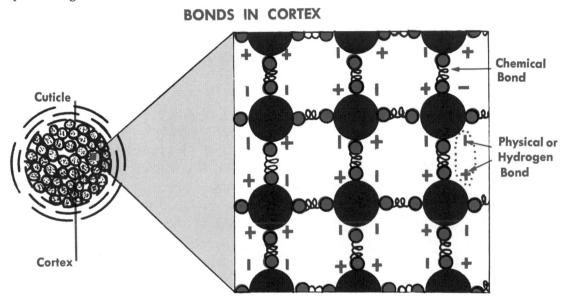

Hard keratin chains of cortex shown end-on. This arrangement of the cross-bonds in all directions gives great strength of flexibility to the hair. They also hold the hair in its natural form (straight, wavy or curly) and this form cannot be altered without first breaking one or both types of bonds.

3. HARDENING

METHODS   Before the hair can be unwrapped or released, the cross-bonds must be reformed*(while in the new position). If the hair is unwound before the completion of this step, the wave will be a complete failure.

Furthermore, in permanent waving, if the softening of the hair is too extensive, this hardening stage may not create a wave either. (The reason is that chains of keratin themselves may be broken and the hair damaged.)

4. UNWINDING, COMBING AND BRUSHING OUT

After the formation of the new bonds, the hair is removed from the rods or rollers or released from being pinned. The curls introduced into the hair are always slightly tighter than actually desired, so they can be brushed out into the planned style.

The positioning of the wound curls and the combing or brushing out after the hair is released are the final factors in the creation of soft, natural-looking waves.

*This is achieved by drying in the case of temporary waving, and by special chemicals and drying in the case of permanent waves.

WET WAVING AND CURLING

FEATURES A temporary hair set is produced by *physical changes* which occur within the hair cortex. Because of the nature of these physical changes hair can be set as frequently as desired. This is the basis of finger-waving, pin curling, roller curling and all wet setting.

For many years the artificial waving of hair by setting has been practiced. Originally, it was carried out by dampening or softening the hair with water or lotion. In this more pliable state the hair is carefully wound in curls, or on rollers and left to dry to its normal state (approximately 10% moisture in the cortex) .

SOFTENING

FUNCTION OF WETTING Water alone can be used because *it has the ability to break down the hydrogen bonds in the cortex.* These bonds, which occur on adjacent polypeptide chains, prevent them from moving. But, slipping or movement of the chains must take place before a proper wave can be formed.

Stretching that part of each hair strand which is on the outside of the roller or curl must cause a temporary rearrangement of the chains. Water lubricates the chains so that they can move relative to one another. However, even though hydrogen bonds are broken, the total amount of movement is very small because the strong sulphur bonds are completely unaffected by the water and continue to restrict slippage of the polypeptide chains.

PURPOSE OF SHAMPOO As the hair must be thoroughly saturated with water, a good shampoo will see that the hair is properly cleansed as well as wetted. Nevertheless, thorough rinsing of excess shampoo is essential to prevent such problems as gumminess, poor manageability and dull appearance of the hair.

PROPER METHODS OF SHAMPOOING Because of the importance of shampooing as it affects hairstyling, it is essential to shampoo the hair in a professional manner. Some patrons claim to have just "washed" their hair, but it is advisable also for the professional to give them a proper shampoo beforehand. (See chapter on shampooing.)

A recent survey revealed that only about 8 out of 10 people use a proper shampoo. The remainder use either hand or laundry soap. Furthermore, there are about 5 out of every 10 who rinsed their hair afterwards in the bathroom basin, wthout using running water.

These practices are completely contrary to present knowledge of shampooing. Modern science has clearly shown there is no substitute for the surging, agitating action of warm jets of water to effectively clean the hair and leave it free from excess shampoo.

ACTION OF SOFTENING

WATER Although, in principle, water will break H-bonds in the hair, in practice we have to assist the process. The more H-bonds broken, the longer lasting will be the wave. To help this softening function, the water should be made as warm as possible.

SETTING LOTION A better method is to use cool, diluted, setting lotions which contain alkalies such as borax or ammonia, together with wetting agents. These wetting agents will help the alkalies penetrate into the cortex. There, the setting lotion breaks the H-bonds and enables the hair to be softened and to take up a new, waved position. Some of the newer setting lotions (with a pH close to 7.0) accomplish the bond-breaking task without the swelling associated with alkaline lotions.

HARDENING

DRYING Various circular or round objects (rods or rollers) and also pins, clamps or clips, can be used to hold the hair in the waved or curled position until drying takes place and the H-bonds have been reformed. Body heat and evaporation by sun and wind can be used to help this drying and hardening process. But in the shop it is quicker and more convenient to use well designed hairdryers.

FIXATIVES The setting lotion usually contains various hair mucilages (such as, resins, gums, pectins). These substances dry out and act as fixatives. They also function as a moisture repellent layer on the hair cuticle to prevent humidity in the air from weakening the set too quickly.

The materials in setting lotions help to hold the hair in place, although a final, high quality hair spray helps to give a better and longer lasting combout. The term "fixative" is also used by some manufacturers to denote a neutralizer used following the application of permanent wave lotion or chemical relaxer.

CONCLUSION

POSITION OF CROSS-BONDS The hair is wet waved or set in a slightly stretched state, because the softening agents will not affect the S-bonds. Therefore, these unbroken chemical bonds must be stretched in order to conform to the curl or wave. The S-bonds are held away from their normal position by the combined holding power of the many altered H-bonds.

Although a single physical or H-bond is extremely weak, there are millions of them. Therefore, they can exert an overwhelming power over the S-bonds that are attempting to restore the hair to its normal straight form. The effect, however, is temporary and the hair style is also temporary.

CHANGES IN HAIR CORTEX DURING WET SETTING

S-BOND ⦵⦵⦵

H-BOND ➕ ➖

1. STRAIGHT HAIR
(Showing position of H and S Bonds.)

S-BOND
H-BOND

2. HAIR SOFTENED BY SETTING LOTION.
(H Bonds are broken.)

3. HAIR WOUND ON ROLLERS.
(S Bonds Stretched into Waved Positions.)

4. HAIR AFTER PROPER DRYING.
(H Bonds Reformed into Waved Positions.)

5. HAIR AFTER BRUSHING OUT INTO SET.
(Waves held only by H Bonds.) Hair Is Sprayed with Moisture-Repellent Barrier.

184

LOSS OF SET As soon as the hair absorbs moisture from the atmosphere (or if it is dampened by water or rain), it quickly returns to its normal, straight form. The set is lost because the holding of the hair in the new waves is normally maintained only by the strength of the countless number of altered H-bonds.

Consequently, when the hair is moistened by any means (intentionally or otherwise) these H-bonds are broken. At this point, the unchanged, stretched S-bonds are left free to straighten the hair with the result that the new waves relax.

A TEMPORARY WAVE

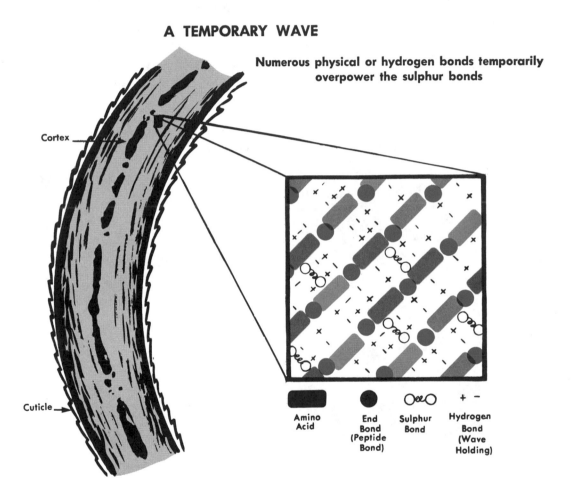

Numerous physical or hydrogen bonds temporarily overpower the sulphur bonds

Cortex

Cuticle

Amino Acid

End Bond (Peptide Bond)

Sulphur Bond

Hydrogen Bond (Wave Holding)

LOSS OF PERMANENT WAVES The same thing takes place, but for the opposite reasons. Hair, normally curly when wet (naturally or recently waved), can be held straightened or flattened until dry.

An example of this is seen as a result of the pressure of a hat or a pillow, or even wind, applied while the dampened hair is drying. Here the H-bonds are maintaining the hair in a straight form. Their greater number once again overcomes the power of the S-bonds, which, in this case, want to hold the "permanent" or natural waves in the hair.

REGAINING WAVES   Those who have a permanent wave know that however unruly their hair looks first thing in the morning, they can get it back into shape by slightly dampening and then combing it. The natural or artificial waves fall more easily into place after the hair has been slightly softened by the moisture on the comb. If, as a result of this treatment, a frizz develops in the hair, it shows that the permanent wave has been slightly overprocessed.

If the hair has only a set, such moistening will only cause a more rapid collapse of the waves and little can be done other than brushing and combing. When this fails to arrange the hair into an orderly appearance, then it must be reset in the usual manner.

ADVANTAGES   Despite the obvious drawbacks in relying only on the H-bond changes in the cortex, setting has a number of distinct advantages:

1. It is easy and relatively simple to do.
2. No chemical changes take place and so there is no risk of hair damage.
3. It may be repeated as often as necessary.

The popularity of hair setting and styling remains very high and it will continue to play a very important role in professional hair work.

CHAPTER 14

PERMANENT WAVING

Introduction

The development of permanent waving was a direct result of scientific investigation into the structure of the hair. Professors Ashbury and Speakman, doing research into keratin, discovered the chemical bonds within the cortex. Their prime concern was the cystine cross-bonds (links), connecting hair fibrils. Their importance in hair modification lead to practical permanent waving.

Using this information, a patent was taken out in 1936 for the first practical method of waving the hair into permanent waves. (Until this period, all advances in waving had been made by practitioners using hit-and-miss methods.) After 1945 permanent waving was gradually adopted as the prime method for permanently waving the hair.

Several unsuccessful permanent wave chemicals were used between 1936 and 1941 and discarded. They were rejected because of foul odors, poor softening, and the risk of poisoning or severe damage to the skin or hair. Recent research has produced a number of useful waving chemicals, such as, the neutral and acid waving solutions, which seem to be solving many of the problems encountered in professional hair work.

BASIS OF PERMANENT WAVING The modern permanent wave solution was prepared for commercial use because:

1. It was possible to break the S-bonds by using a permanent waving solution (processing), and that—
2. New S-bonds could be deliberately reformed in a waved position by using an oxidizer (neutralizing).

TECHNIQUE OF PERMANENT WAVING

The method can be conveniently divided into these main steps:

1. Shampooing (preparing the hair)
2. Wrapping hair
3. Processing
4. Rinsing
5. Neutralizing
6. Conditioning (when necessary)
7. Setting, drying and styling.

SHAMPOOING

All methods of waving or styling hair depend, to a large extent, upon proper preparation of the hair, and this is especially true in the case of permanent waving. It is essential that permanent waving solutions penetrate into the cortex before they can begin to soften the hair for a successful permanent wave.

CHOICE OF SHAMPOO   The shampoo itself must be carefully chosen and should be an efficient soapless type which will leave the hair in a good condition. In addition, the shampoo should not interfere with the chemical action of the permanent wave.

PURPOSE FOR SHAMPOO   Shampooing in permanent waving has a number of functions to perform. Dirt, dandruff scales, foreign matter, hair spray films, lacquers and gums must be removed because they make the hair cuticle resistant and will slow the entry of solutions into the cortex.

SOFTENS H-BONDS   The water and the mild alkaline conditions of the shampoo softens and breaks many of the H-bonds in the cortex. This makes the hair more pliable and easier to section and wind on the rods.

POROSITY AND PROCESSING TIME   Furthermore, the shampoo gives very valuable information regarding the porosity of the hair. If the hair soaks up the shampoo easily, then that hair is porous. If it prevents easy penetration then the hair is resistant.

Porous hair requires a much shorter processing time; resistant hair requires a longer processing time. The length of time the permanent wave solution must remain on the hair can thus be estimated.

UNEVENNESS OF HAIR POROSITY   Another problem of porosity is unevenness, for along the same shaft may be found areas of widely differing rates of absorption of the solution. This situation usually occurs at the ends of the hairs, but all along the hair shaft processing of the wave will be quicker in porous areas and slower in resistant areas.

PROTECTIVE ACTION OF RINSING The evenness of penetration of permanent wave solution can be aided by the shampooing stage, as the more porous areas will soak up extra water. This water, used for rinsing, tends to dilute the strength of the permanent wave solution which enters those porous sections and helps to even out its action. This weaker solution will give slower processing at the exact points where this is required.

PRECONDITIONING Over-porous hair may require a preconditioning treatment before applying the solution. Special fillers are now available to help correct over-porous hair, retard the process, and thus permit test curls to be taken.

CONCLUSION

It is wise to dampen the hair with warm water, even if shampooing or pre-dampening the hair with permanent wave solution is not carried out. This procedure helps the hair to take the solution more evenly.

There seems to be no reason for drying the hair (other than towel drying), after the shampoo. Drying the hair under a dryer is a time consuming process and, furthermore, by leaving the hair slightly damp the permanent wave solution will be absorbed more quickly and evenly.

AMMONIUM THIOGLYCOLATE

The discovery of solutions which will cause the S-bonds of the cortex to be more effectively broken was a major advance in permanent waving. Without going too deeply into their chemistry, a group of substances has been found which are suitable for this purpose.

PREPARATION The most commonly used waving solution is based on ammonium thioglycolate ("thio"). This compound is prepared from thioglycollic acid with the careful addition of ammonia until the pH is about 9.4 to 9.6 (i.e., alkaline). Thioglycolic acid is a fairly stable substance, so this chemical is better to store, ship or transport. However, used alone, it has only a little waving action on the hair and may be dangerous to the skin. It must be mixed with ammonia to be effective.

Formula

Thioglycolic acid plus ammonia = Ammonium Thioglycolate + Ammonia
(excess)   ("thio")   (pH 9.6)

PROBLEM OF SELF-OXIDATION

When combined with ammonia, the "thio" thus formed is very active on the hair and so powerful that it will extract oxygen from the air, thus weakening its power gradually.

PREVENTION To prevent this from taking place, the "thio" is usually packed in small bottles suitable for one application only.

Another method of handling bulk solutions is to add a waxy material to them. This material simply floats on the top, serving as a barrier, and thus prevents self-oxidation from the air space above the level of liquid in the bottle, especially as the level drops.

Yet another method employed is to use a solid or powder type "thio" permanent wave chemical. This comes in a capsule form (to prevent weakening in storage) ; it is dissolved just prior to application.

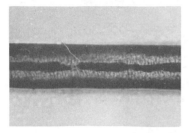

Virgin dry greasy hair before shampooing.

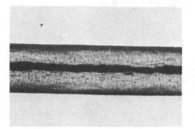

Same hair after shampooing and rinsing.

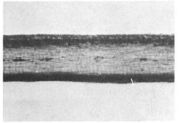

Hair (as before) in ammonium thioglycolate solution (pH 9.4) for 5 minutes. Slight swelling of imbrications.

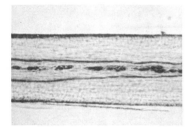

That hair in ammonium thioglycolate (pH 12.5) for 5 minutes. Severe swelling of cortex.

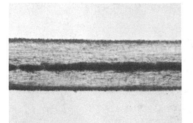

Hair from same strand in neutral waving solution (pH 7.5) for 5 minutes.

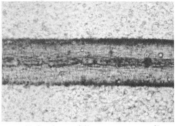

Hair in cold wave neutralizer (pH 3.0). Note droplets of conditioner in o/w type.

STRENGTH OF PERMANENT WAVING SOLUTION

The concentration of ready-to-use "thio" solutions has an important effect on processing time.

STRONG For resistant hair, a solution containing 10% of ammonium thioglycolate at pH 9.6 is advised. If solutions stronger than 10% are used, they may cause irritation to the scalp or a complete breakdown of the hair structure.

NORMAL For normal hair, a slightly weaker solution of "thio" is used, about 8% at pH 9.6.

WEAK For damaged or porous hair the weakest professional solution of "thio" must be used, 5% to 6% at pH 9.4.

There are still weaker solutions available, however, these take too long for professional use. (Even weaker solutions can cause considerable damage, if left to process in the hair for long periods of time.)

ADDITIVES

Besides the "thio" or other waving chemical, permanent wave solutions contain a number of other important substances.

WETTING AGENTS For the purpose of getting the solution quickly into the cortex, all permanent wave solutions must contain a good wetting agent, which is a non-foaming product, as well as a good cleansing agent.

ACTION OF WETTING AGENTS ON HAIR WAVING SOLUTIONS

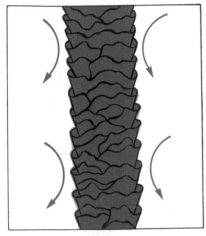

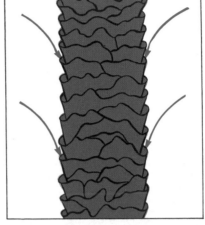

a. Solution without wetting agent.

b. Solution with wetting agent (note penetration).

ANTI "FLYAWAY" AGENT Waving solutions often contain special substances to reduce the electrostatic charges in the hair, which can be produced in excessive amounts during the final brushing out of the waves. These chemicals are absorbed into the cuticle and tend to give the hair a sheen in addition to a soft texture.

POROSITY CONTROLLERS Other chemicals in the solution help to control the porosity of the hair. Some newer plastics are put in the permanent wave solution to combine with the cuticle of the hair. This helps give the cortex a more controlled protection from the damage which may be caused by the solution.

Before applying the solution, the porous hair may also be given a re-conditioning treatment. Keratin type (protein) fillers or pastes are especially beneficial for this purpose.

HAIR CONDITIONERS The alkaline permanent waving solution has a tendency to remove natural oils from the hair, causing it to dry out rapidly through loss of its essential moisture. Mineral oils, lanolin, or lanolin esters are used in the solution, or in a separate application, to replace these natural oils. By remaining in the hair after the permanent wave solution has been rinsed out, the moisture content is protected.

Older solutions of this type were usually cloudy or turbid. New conditioners are available which remain clear in solution and this counteracts the tendency of some conditioners to settle out of the permanent waving solution on standing.

CLOUDING AGENTS   Some firms prefer to market a cloudy type permanent waving solution, because they believe it looks more attractive to the practitioner and to the patron. Chemicals known as clouding agents are added to the waving solutions. Pearly flakes can be included with certain conditioning agents as well.

THICKENING AGENTS   The permanent wave chemicals can be thickened into foaming "creams" by *special* substances. A thickened cream, however, may actually be weaker than a liquid type permanent waving solution. Nevertheless, it looks stronger to the inexperienced person and so can influence sales.

PERFUMES   Fragrance in all hair preparations is very important but, *in permanent wave solutions it is essential.* In permanent wave processing solutions there are strongly alkaline odors. It is very difficult to find a perfume that is not itself affected by the solutions and loses its effectiveness. Newer, more stable perfumes are becoming available to mask the characteristic "thio" odor.

PROCESSING

The period during which the permanent wave solution is left in contact with the hair is called the processing time. The actual processing of the hair proceeds in three separate ways:

SOFTENING   The main purpose of the solution is to soften the hair cortex. This softening is made possible by:

1. Breaking S-bonds and
2. Breaking H-bonds.

The softening action of permanent solutions can be very rapid. Porous hair can be completely softened in about 2 to 4 minutes, but more resistant hair may take as long as 30 to 45 minutes, or even longer.

Note:

There is evidence to suggest that some of the H-bonds in the cortex are protected by certain of the more stable S-bonds. After these S-bonds have been broken by the wave solution, the "thio," or even water, is then able to break the remaining H-bonds, producing a much greater softening effect upon the cortex. The broken S-bonds are also heavily dehydrated, thus softening the keratin even more.

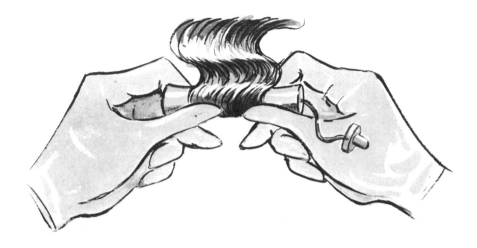

Method of taking a test curl to determine processing time.

REARRANGEMENT OF KERATIN CHAINS The resulting alterations or "slip" of the keratin chains is caused by the physical tension and pressures generated by winding the hair on the rods. The slip must be sufficient to get satisfactory permanent waves from the curl formation. However, the slip must not be excessive, as this will produce exaggerated curls which result in frizziness and overly tight waves.

ACTION OF REARRANGEMENT Proper rearrangement cannot take place unless:

1. *Processing time is sufficient.* When the S and H-bonds have been broken, rearrangement or slip of the keratin (polypeptide) chains takes place rapidly on the rods (within 5 to 10 minutes or less).
2. *The hair is correctly wound on the rods.* Pre-dampening with permanent wave solution softens the cortex but does not form any curl. Slipping of the chains MUST take place on the rods before any curl can form in the hair.

Hair which is not wound on rods but saturated with permanent wave solution will not form a curl. Despite this absence of a curl, end-bond damage and *loss of strength will take place whether the hair is wound or not.* Therefore, the rearrangement of the keratin chains in the cortex, which is only possible as a result of the breaking of the cross-bonds, takes place in the later stage of processing.

BREAKDOWN Depending on circumstances such as strength of solution, length of processing, porosity and textures of the hair, the wave will vary from a negligible one to a strong one within a given period of time.

But, proceeding somewhat behind this softening and rearrangement could be an undesirable breakdown of the end-bonds (peptide bonds) of the cortex. As a result, the hair left in longer contact with the permanent wave solution will slowly lose its strength. Hair damage, caused by the breakdown of the end-bonds, finally leads to complete loss of wave and elasticity.

CHANGES IN HAIR CORTEX
DURING PERMANENT WAVING

In naturally straight hair all cross-bonds—sulphur (S) and hydrogen (H) bonds—are in a straight position across every peptide chain. It is necessary to break both of these types of bonds to permanently wave the hair.

But it is equally essential that the same cross-bonds be reformed to hold the wave. It is also desirable that the scalp and hair not be damaged during these changes.

As these are two entirely opposite reactions, two different solutions must be used:

(a) one solution to break S and H bonds (waving lotion),
(b) another solution to reform these cross-bonds (neutralizer).

The penetration of solutions into the cortex must be fairly rapid and uniform. Therefore, removal of all foreign matter (including excess shampoo) is essential for success.

Preparation

Shampooing not only cleans hair but prepares it for processing as well. Excess rinsing water evens out the porous areas which are often present in the cortex.

Proper wetting of the hair, followed by towel drying, increases the rate of absorption of the permanent wave solution. (For example, it is far better to use a damp cloth, not a dry one, for soaking up spilt milk.)

Processing

Permanent wave processing solution may be applied before or after winding on the rods. This depends on the speed of the practitioner, the texture of the hair and the strength or type of permanent wave solution. The action of this solution breaks the H-bonds and the majority of S-bonds in the cortex. The hair is then in a very softened condition and must be handled carefully.

CHANGES IN HAIR CORTEX DURING PERMANENT WAVING

1. STRAIGHT HAIR
(Both H and S Bonds in Straight Positions.)

S-BOND
H-BOND

2. HAIR WOUND ON RODS AND SOFTENED BY SHAMPOOING AND COLD WAVE SOLUTIONS.
(H Bonds and Nearly all S Bonds Broken.)

3. HAIR AFTER NEUTRALIZING.
(Some H Bonds and many S Bonds Reformed.)

4. HAIR ON ROLLERS AFTER PROPER DRYING.
(Most H Bonds Reformed as well as S Bonds.)

5. HAIR AFTER UNWINDING.
(Original S Bonds Stretched into Waved Positions.)

The hair is allowed to process for varying periods. During processing, the broken S-bonds allow slipping of the keratin chains on the rods. The amount of slip is very small for each chain, but it is vital for the success of the wave.

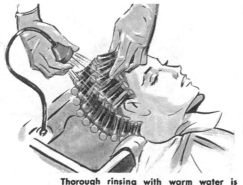

Thorough rinsing with warm water is essential to remove all traces of excess cold waving solution from the hair.

Rinsing or blotting

When processing has reached a satisfactory stage (as shown by test curls), the excess waving solution is quickly rinsed from the hair. (Some manufacturers delete the rinsing and rely on towel blotting to remove the excess lotion.)

Neutralizing (oxidizing)

When rinsing is completed, the neutralizer is carefully applied to the hair *on the rods*. There are many examples of neutralizers, but all have the same purpose.

The function of these solutions is to restore S-bonds between adjacent keratin or polypeptide chains in the cortex. But each individual S-bond must be altered to hold a waved position, giving the waves a permanent basis. However, the processing solution is unable to break all the straight S-bonds. Therefore, the neutralizer cannot convert all S-bonds into wave holding bonds. The reformed S-bonds are weaker than the original, unbroken cross-bonds. But, as wave holding bonds are very numerous, this has no immediate effect on the waves.

Some new H-bonds are formed by the neutralizer. The reason for this is that neutralizing solutions always contain mild acids. Some shrinking and hardening of the cortex take place as a result.

There are always small amounts of strongly alkaline permanent wave solution (pH 9.6) left in the cortex. The neutralizer can destroy these traces of alkali because it is an acid (pH 3.0 to 4.0). Neutralizing this alkali stops the action of the "thio," and thus prevents the slow weakening of the fiber by the continuing action of the permanent wave solution on the end-bonds of the hair.

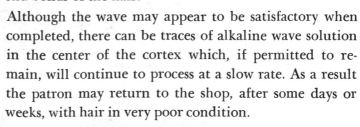

Plastic containers force neutralizers more efficiently into hair on rods.

Although the wave may appear to be satisfactory when completed, there can be traces of alkaline wave solution in the center of the cortex which, if permitted to remain, will continue to process at a slow rate. As a result the patron may return to the shop, after some days or weeks, with hair in very poor condition.

Drying

The hair is carefully unwound from the rods after proper rinsing. It is usually wound onto rollers for setting. Careful drying reforms the broken H-bonds into a shape built around the altered S-bonds.

Finally, the hair is removed from the rollers and brushed or combed out into a predetermined style.

Note that some S-bonds are not able to find suitable S-partners and so remain broken. In addition, a percentage of S-bonds keep their original straight form. But these S-bonds are stretched into the newer waved position of the hair.

In fact, research has shown that normal permanent waving alters only half the original S-bonds into a wave. For this reason even permanent waving methods do not result in a "permanent" wave but must be repeated at intervals.

CHEMISTRY OF PERMANENT WAVING

There are two main types of permanent waving solutions. These are identified by the difference in the chemicals employed and by the pH of their solutions.

FUNCTION OF ALKALINE PERMANENT WAVE SOLUTION

Alkaline waving solutions usually contain ammonium thioglycolate and excess ammonia. The typical pH range is 9.4 to 9.6.

In virgin, naturally straight hair, the cystine or S-bond (sulphur) forms across parallel strings of amino-acids in the polypeptide chains. The amino-acids themselves are held in position by end-bonds. "Thio" type waving solutions, unfortunately, attack these end-bonds as well as the S-bonds, thus weakening the hair structure and the waves.

Ammonium thioglycolate solutions are strong reducing agents in an alkaline condition. Thus ammonium thioglycolate (thio) is rich in hydrogen (H) atoms. In contact with S-S bonds, "thio" solutions can break these chemical bonds. It does this by substituting its excess H atoms, thus forming S.H.-H.S. bonds. In this way, S-S bonds are broken, allowing the keratin chains to slip into suitable waved positions on the rods.

FUNCTION OF THE NEUTRALIZER

Neutralizers are rich in oxygen. In fact, most of these neutralizers contain hydrogen peroxide—a strong oxidizer. Hydrogen peroxide breaks down to form water and releases an active oxygen atom.

$$H_2O_2 \rightarrow H_2O + O$$

hydrogen peroxide   water   oxygen

Active oxygen has a very strong attraction for hydrogen (H) atoms, especially when they are joined to sulphur (S) atoms.

Therefore, the oxygen (O) atom bridges the gap between the previously reduced sulphur atoms (S.H.).

HAIR — S.H. — O — H.S. — HAIR

(KERATIN)   (KERATIN)

CHEMISTRY OF COLD WAVING

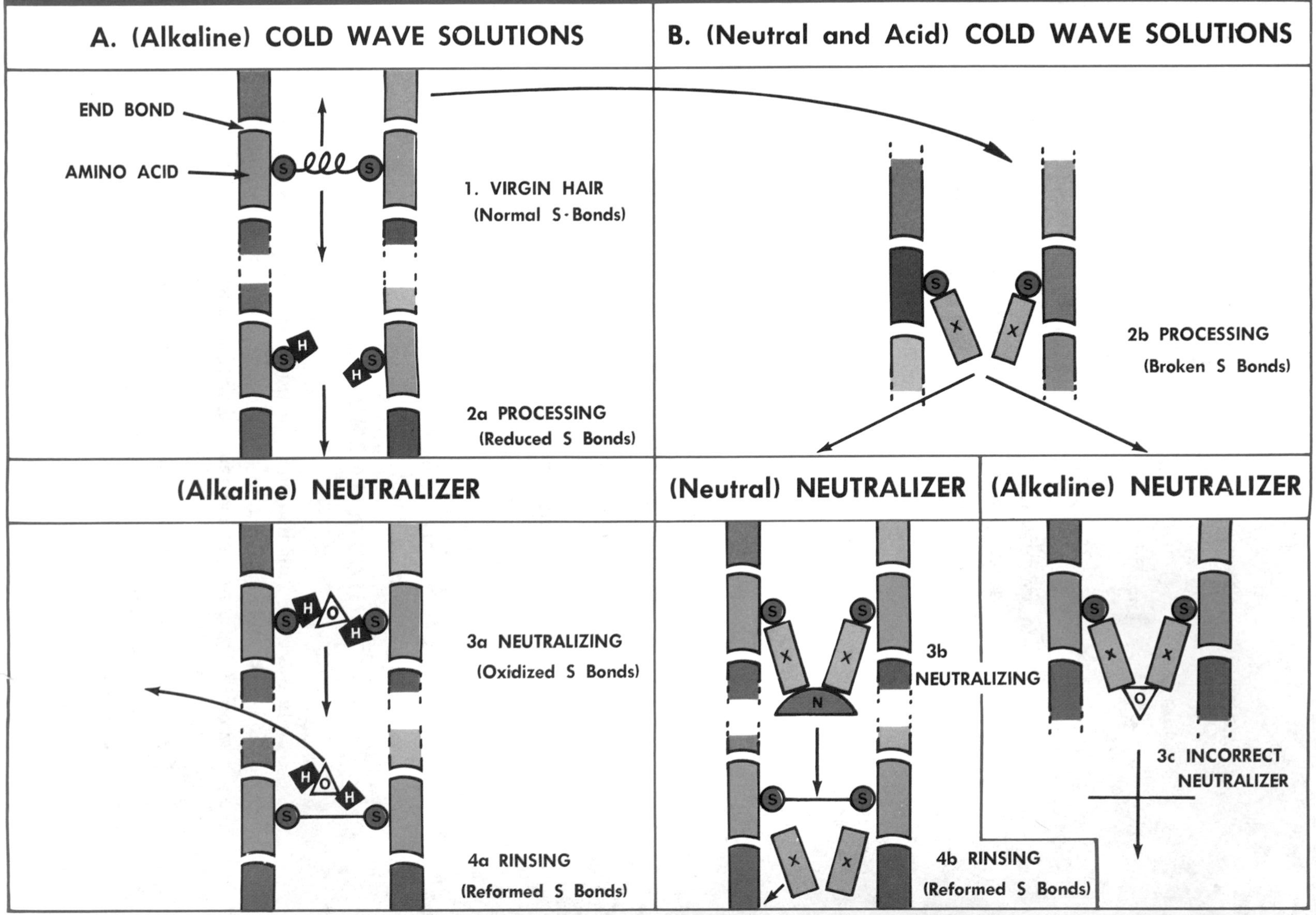

A. (Alkaline) COLD WAVE SOLUTIONS
END BOND
AMINO ACID
S
S
1. VIRGIN HAIR
(Normal S-Bonds)
S
H
H
S
2a PROCESSING
(Reduced S Bonds)
(Alkaline) NEUTRALIZER
S
H
O
H
S
3a NEUTRALIZING
(Oxidized S Bonds)
H
O
H
S
S
4a RINSING
(Reformed S Bonds)
B. (Neutral and Acid) COLD WAVE SOLUTIONS
S
X
X
S
2b PROCESSING
(Broken S Bonds)
(Neutral) NEUTRALIZER
S
X
X
S
N
3b
NEUTRALIZING
S
S
X
X
4b RINSING
(Reformed S Bonds)
(Alkaline) NEUTRALIZER
S
X
X
S
O
3c INCORRECT
NEUTRALIZER

This long bond is soon broken to form H-O-H or H_2O (water). This leaves behind the S. atoms, which are also active. They link up with other S. atoms, whenever possible, to again form S-bonds.

Therefore, the cystine or S-bonds are reformed. If the keratin chains have moved into new positions in the meantime, the new S-bonds will keep them there (waved). *Most "thio" type neutralizers are mild acid solutions* (pH 3.0–4.0), and thus shrink the keratin chains together, making the reforming of S-bonds between adjacent chains easier.

Furthermore, the acid present in the neutralizer causes the cuticle to press down tightly and the natural sheen and luster of the hair is then regained.

CHEMICALS IN THE NEUTRALIZER

In order to carry out its functions the neutralizer contains:

MILD ACIDS Many mild acids can be used to give the desirable pH range (3.0 to 4.0). These acids neutralize the alkali in the wave solution, especially the acetic, citric or tartaric acids.

OXIDIZERS The reforming of the S-bonds is caused by the oxidizing action of the neutralizer. There are a number of oxidizing agents that can be used.

Hydrogen peroxide neutralizers

Hydrogen peroxide (H_2O_2) is a convenient solution for oxidizing and thus reforming the S-bonds. It is used in the stabilized acid state and so has little lightening action on the hair.

About 2 to 5 volume peroxide is used as a "splash" neutralizer. Because of its weaker oxidizing action it takes about 10 minutes to reform all the S-bonds in all parts of the cortex. Several applications of "splash" neutralizers are advisable in order to assure thorough hardening of the hair.

Neutralizers termed "instant" are stronger peroxide (approximately 20 to 25 volume) and will act very quickly on the cross-bonds. The word "instant," however, is very misleading. Although it is certainly much faster than the splash types, the action of the stronger neutralizer is certainly *NOT* an instant one.

The neutralizing time is *reduced,* not entirely eliminated. The neutralizer must still penetrate through the wrapped hair to the rods.

The acid content of instant neutralizers also prevents the stronger hydrogen peroxide solutions from lightening the hair while it is in the process of neutralizing. However, if peroxide more powerful than 30 volume is used as a neutralizer, there is a serious danger of lightening and causing damage to the hair cuticle and cortex whether the hydrogen peroxide is acid or otherwise.

Powder neutralizers

Some neutralizers are supplied as a powder to be dissolved in warm water before use. These types are not very convenient for professional use and are often found in home kits.

Examples of powder neutralizers are: sodium perborate, sodium or potassium bromate, tartaric or citric acids.

Some of these powder compounds can be combined with hydrogen peroxide and used as a lotion or cream. Special purpose neutralizers usually have this type of formula.

Non-neutralizers (atmospheric oxidation)

A non-neutralizing wave is really a self-neutralizing wave. Because part of the job of neutralizing is an oxidation process, oxygen from the air will eventually harden the hair. The hot air from a dryer may help to produce the same effect in the ordinary permanent wave. This method of atmospheric oxidation is far too slow for professional use because it takes from 6 to 12 hours to form a "permanent" wave (with a sufficient number of S-bonds reformed).

Some permanent wave solutions used in home kits contain metallic salts in order to speed up the process. However, these salts can cause damage to the hair by prolonging the oxidation of the hair bonds. During this extended period a breakdown of end-bonds and loss of cortex strength and manageability may take place.

Another serious objection to this approach to neutralization lies in the failure to neutralize the alkaline condition of the hair. Simply relying on rinsing for removal of all permanent wave solution is not likely to bring the hair back to its normal condition (pH 6.5). Brittleness, excessive dryness, poor condition and poor texture are likely to follow. Many examples of such hair damage come to the attention of the practitioner as patrons expect a satisfactory wave, despite the fact that their hair is in a poor condition following the use of non-neutralizing home permanents.

WETTING AGENTS IN NEUTRALIZERS

PROFESSIONAL TYPE The problem of penetration of the neutralizer is critical and to assist entry into the cortex, it must contain a good wetting agent which, for professional use, is usually of a non-foaming type.

NON-PROFESSIONAL TYPES There are some wetting agents used which are high foamers. The foam is supposed to give greater control and permit easier application of the neutralizer. The wetting agent changes the normal liquid neutralizer into a non-running tight foam. But this foam may be difficult to rinse out and will penetrate the cortex much more slowly. For this reason, these neutralizers are not used professionally where time is important.

The presence of large amounts of foam will only hinder the job of the neutralizer, which should penetrate into the cortex quickly and evenly with sufficient strength to completely harden the hair. Besides, there is absolutely no need for a neutralizer to also have a cleansing function since the hair should already have been cleaned by the initial shampoo. They may simply be called "gimmick" type neutralizers which make a sales appeal to persons who do not properly understand their performance.

Whereas the hair cannot be over-neutralized, it can be under-neutralized with consequent ill-effects on the lasting qualities of the wave. Despite the importance of proper neutralizing there is no simple way of timing the neutralizer except by the practical experience of the practitioner. Many failures in permanent waving can be traced back to poor neutralizing and it is vital that this essential step should receive the maximum attention.

NEUTRAL PERMANENT WAVE SOLUTIONS

Neutral permanent wave solutions use different chemical compounds than "thio" type waving solutions. It is well known that alkalies have a harmful effect on lightened and damaged hair. Yet, "thio" solutions will not work efficiently unless they are strongly alkaline.

This problem has now been overcome by using permanent wave solutions having a pH of between 7.0 and 8.0 that tend to be "neutral" or very close to it. These are slow acting products; and in order to speed up the process, the hair is saturated before wrapping begins. This pre-saturation technique is performed on virgin hair only and is often undesirable in the case of damaged hair. Heat can also be applied to increase the speed of processing.

The wave formed by this type of product tends to be a soft wave. Many patrons on the other hand prefer a hard wave that is longer lasting and gives more value for their money.

In discussions based on alkaline type waving solutions and their associated neutralizers, it was a relatively simple matter for a person, without any formal training in chemistry, to understand the role of hydrogen and oxygen atoms in the softening (processing) and oxidation (neutralizing) processes. But, in the case of breaking and reforming sulphur bonds through the use of acid and neutral waving lotions, formulas become quite complex and should be explored as a special project if such information is required.

HAIRSTYLING AFTER PERMANENT WAVING

CORRECT WAVE SIZE The final stage in permanent waving is to set and dry the hair for a style. The wave that results is built around the permanent curl established on the rod, the curl itself being deliberately made tighter to allow for dressing or brushing out in the final wave.

The aim, in selecting the correct rod size, is to produce waves or curls which, when relaxed, are as compatible as possible with the finished hair-style, e.g., soft, loose waves, use large rods. For a tight set, narrow rods would be best.

DELIBERATE RELAXATION OF WAVE

COMBING OUT Natural relaxation of the curls commences as soon as the permanent waving rods are removed from the hair. Because the hair is still damp, not all of the H-bonds have yet been reformed. (The acid neutralizer only reforms a few of these in its action.) Therefore, further relaxation of the curl can be obtained by combing out before thoroughly drying the hair.

SPECIAL TECHNIQUES A thick, acid cream with a weakened neutralizing action is used to partially harden the cortex before drying. Some of the S-bonds in addition to the H-bonds are reformed by this "fixative" cream. Rearrangement of the hair into a wave form is possible because of the fixative nature of the semi-hardener, which allows the artisan to mold the partially hardened waves after unwinding from the rods. Further neutralizing and drying complete the formation of the permanent wave.

ACTION OF DRYING The total reformation of H-bonds in the cortex is not completed until ALL of the excess moisture is removed from the hair by the action of the dryer. The original shape of the permanent waves may only be seen when the hair is dampened. (Either by a water spray or moisture absorbed from high humidity in the atmosphere.)

CONCLUSIONS

Even after the procedure of permanent waving, we find that the resulting waves are really not "permanent" at all. Nevertheless, they are longer lasting, and so permanent waving has been a very important step towards perfect hair waving in the future.

NATURAL STRAIGHT HAIR Naturally straight hair cannot be successfully waved unless the straight position of both S- and H-bonds are altered. Previous information shows that special solutions are required which will penetrate into the cortex and break these bonds. With the cross-bonds broken, the keratin chains can be moved around by reason of physical forces generated by wrapping the hair on rods. Having first obtained this necessary rearrangement of the keratin structures, the "slip" is fixed by neutralizing the hair. The neutralizer is able to reintroduce sufficient S-bonds to hold the wave in approximately the curl diameter required.

HAIR SLIGHTLY OVERWAVED Smaller rods are used because slight relaxation of the waves always takes place when the hair is removed from the rods. One reason being that *it is simpler to comb out excessive wave than to put more wave in straight hair* after it has been neutralized. So the hair is slightly overwaved.

ARRANGEMENT OF KERATIN CHAINS IN WAVY AND STRAIGHT HAIR.

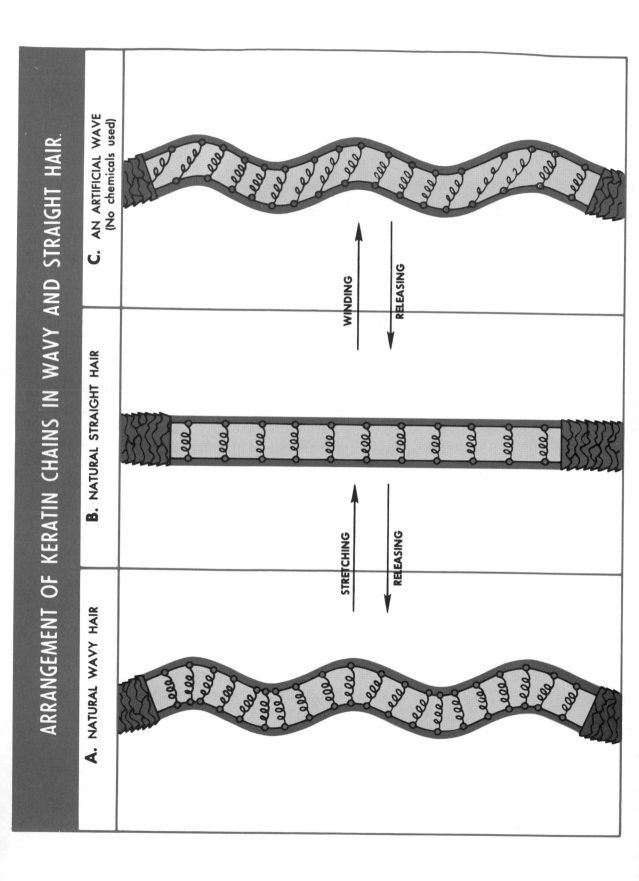

A. NATURAL WAVY HAIR

STRETCHING

RELEASING

B. NATURAL STRAIGHT HAIR

WINDING

RELEASING

C. AN ARTIFICIAL WAVE
(No chemicals used)

Alkaline permanent waving solutions are not overly efficient in breaking S-bonds. This means that some of the original S-bonds must be stretched in order to accommodate a change from straight to waved hair.

In fact, improvements in permanent waving formulations are mainly aimed at increasing the efficiency of breaking S-bonds without causing damage to the cortex or cuticle. Properly neutralized, the majority of S-bonds are providing strength to hold the waved position.

CORRECTLY WAVED AND SET Next the hair is carefully set on rollers. Drying the hair re-establishes the H-bonds into their newly waved form.

Therefore, following a recent permanent, we actually have two waves, one built around another. The task of the practitioner is to make the altered S-bonds (permanent wave) give the necessary foundation to the H-bond waves (produced by setting and drying, curling iron, blow waves, etc.) .

The H-bonds are dominant under normal circumstances (dry hair) and so will control the hair. Although the H-bonds are individually much weaker, they control the form of hair whenever their combined strength permits.

UNRULY STRAIGHT HAIR Hair is subject to many unruly or disturbing influences in the ordinary course of events. For example, strong winds, pressure from a hat or the pillow during sleep, moisture picked up in damp and humid conditions, strong rays of sunshine and outdoor activities. Then there is the daily attention of brushing and combing, not forgetting the frequent necessity for shampooing. Irregular rearrangement of the H-bonds follows such disarrangement and this untidiness in the hairstyle must be corrected by re-styling. The hair is shampooed and in the process the H-bonds are broken. Restyling techniques, followed by proper drying, reforms the H-bonds to hold the hair in a waved position, thus supporting the S-bonds once more.

EFFECT OF WAVE LOSS ON HAIR SETTING

Despite repeated attempts to reorganize the hairstyle by these physical changes, the method slowly brings less and and less success. This failure is brought about by relaxation of the altered S-bonds to a straighter form.

Thus it becomes increasingly difficult to establish a satisfactory curl depending on setting alone. The relaxation of permanent waves is the result of leaving a high proportion of the original S-bonds unchanged and in a stretched or stressed, straight form.

These S-bonds, which were reformed by the neutralizer, appear to have less strength on their own than the unreformed, natural S-bonds. Any factors causing S-bond breakage will first have their effect on these artificially waved or changed S-bonds. This will release the unaltered S-bonds to operate freely on the hair form (pull it straight) .

WAVE LOSS FROM SUNLIGHT

Sunlight is an important factor which can break the neutralized S-bonds. Sunlight contains 8% ultra-violet rays. These are high energy rays which can produce changes in the cortex. Here they break those S-bonds which were carefully altered during processing and neutralizing. Therefore, a permanent wave will have a shorter life in a harsh, dry climate than in cool, mild areas with average humidity.

As only the *altered* S-bonds are broken, this permits the stretched but straight original S-bonds to pull on the keratin chains, thus reducing their degree of "slip." This process does not take place steadily, but rather through a series of steps. Oxygen is able to rejoin S-bonds as a normal procedure. So the oxygen in the atmosphere quickly reforms the S-bonds which have been broken by sunlight.

But in the interval before this rebuilding takes place, the freed chains are pulled a little straighter by the stretched, unbroken S-bonds. These steps are repeated again and again and the waves are gradually weakened until they almost disappear.

OTHER CAUSES OF WAVE LOSS

Dandricides

Relaxation may also be caused by a patron using certain scalp dandricides. Many of these chemicals are based on sulphur or organic sulphur compounds. It is thought that the anti-dandruff properties of these treatments may be caused by the sulphur being changed to hydrogen sulfide gas. As this gas can also break S-bonds, it can be directly linked to wave relaxation.

Diet

The natural growth of the hair is under the influence of the diet, particularly with regard to sulphur-containing amino-acids. Some diets are low in these necessary A-grade proteins. If insufficient sulphur is available for proper growth, the hair may not be able to support the permanent as long as it would otherwise.

Medication

Sulphur is occasionally used in internal medicines and drugs. This sulphur in the blood circulation has long been known to affect the hair growth as well as cases of continued nervous tension and worry. These factors could easily disturb the normal S-bond characteristics of keratin.

Hormone Disturbances

In addition, there are unknown physiological conditions such as hormone disturbances, old age, expectant motherhood, long convalescence, etc., which produce unknown keratin differences in the cortex. Failure of permanent waves over a shorter period than usual may be caused by faults already present within the hair shafts of the patron.

Skin Secretions

There may be times when there seems to be nothing wrong with the hair, yet the permanent still does not hold. One suggested cause for this condition is that some individuals secrete hydrogen sulfide from their skin. While there is an insufficient amount of gas to smell, other evidence supports this claim. Some of these persons cannot wear silver ornaments as they turn black. Other metallic jewelry worn by them slowly becomes green, black or otherwise tarnishes. Some authorities believe that their permanent waves collapse from the same cause (hydrogen sulfide).

Poor Technique

On the other hand, it may be equally true that these waves quickly relax because they had not been properly formed from the beginning. These critics argue that even patients in hospitals can have good, lasting waves. They refuse to believe that drugs or anesthetics will cause artificial waves to relax any faster.

Whatever the reason, the truth is that permanent waving is not really "permanent." Depending on the texture of the hair, rate of growth and the needs of the patron, the practice must be repeated periodically (every 3–6 months). Then, once more, as many S-bonds as possible are rearranged into a waved position for the same cycle to be repeated.

CONCLUSION

Most of the strength of the permanent wave is due to the altered position of the S-bonds. Failure to slightly "overwave" the hair, by virtue of the position of the S-bonds, could result in a weak wave. In addition, failure to reform the H-bonds could also result in a poor appearance in the final style. Thus, there are actually two waves in their hair cortex, the permanent wave (S- and H-bonds) and the temporary wave (H-bonds).

H-BOND WAVE The form of this wave is only seen when the hair is dry, because the more numerous H-bonds overcome the form of the hair as introduced by the reforming of S-bonds on the rods during neutralizing.

S-BOND WAVE This wave form shows when the hair is wet, due to the reformed S-bonds which are free to cause the hair to take up the artificial waved position.

TIMING THE ALKALINE PERMANENT WAVE PROCESS

TEST CURLS

Alkaline permanent wave solutions penetrate through the cuticle and enter the cortex. These processing solutions break S-bonds allowing the keratin chains in the cortex to slip on the rods.

The amount of slip of these chains must be carefully monitored by test curls. Test curls are useful indicators of processing time, provided that the following points are kept in mind:

1. Allowance is made for the time taken to observe the test curl and then rinse and neutralize the remaining curls.
2. Consideration of the test curl when heavy and wet against curl formation when hair is normal.
3. Test curls are taken properly. The biggest error made when taking test curls occurs as the practitioner pushes a wave into the test curl rather than unwinding the curl a sufficient number of turns to show that an actual curl exists.
4. The test curl represents the overall picture of average curl formation on the head.

UNDERPROCESSED HAIR   Curl formation must wait for solution penetration into the cortex and the breaking of S-Bonds before any "slip" can take place. Thus rearrangement of keratin chains proceeds very slowly at first. *If the neutralizing process is begun at this point, the hair will be underprocessed.*

Gradually the degree of curl begins to increase as more S-bonds are broken. This rate depends, of course, on the porosity of the cuticle. Porous hair develops waves rapidly but resistant hair is much slower to process.

Just before the desired wave is reached the excess processing solution is rinsed or blotted away and the neutralizer applied. This period is to allow for rinsing away excess solution and the "working" time of the neutralizer.

OVERPROCESSED HAIR If processing is not stopped, the slip of the keratin chains on the rods becomes more exaggerated (leading to frizziness) and the solution begins to weaken the end-bonds.

Processing must not be allowed to reach this point. If hair has reached this stage already, it is essential to stop the processing immediately.

After neutralizing and unwinding from the rods, excess frizz can be removed by combing a little processing solution through the curls. Applying fresh neutralizer will harden the now looser waves into position.

DAMAGED HAIR Continued processing causes the excess curls to fall away rapidly. Although the curls may return to a desirable shape, the hair is irreversibly damaged.

Still further processing will lead to the hair becoming straighter. *Alkaline permanent waving solutions can break peptide or end-bonds if left too long on the hair and these are not repairable.*

Even though this necessary rearrangement or slip of the keratin chains has taken place, reforming of altered S-bonds cannot hold these chains in a waved position . . . the keratin chains move under the weight of the hair, for their peptide bonds (end-bonds) are broken at various points.

Most serious damage occurs within fifteen minutes or less, depending on the hair. Breaking more peptide bonds increases the weakness of the hair and leads to loss of elasticity and texture. Cuticle scales are shed and the hair breaks very easily when it is combed or pulled.

Many of these problems can be overcome by using neutral or acid permanent wave solution. The chemical action of these improved permanent waving solutions is more specific. Their action is more confined to breaking S-bonds. They do not cause excessive swelling or damage to the hair. For these reasons, acid or neutral permanent wave solutions are more suitable for lightened and damaged hair than alkaline processing solutions. But, as mentioned previously, these products work very slowly and have not gained popularity in this country. There are two positions on the processing graph (see illustration) which will give the required wave. The first position is recommended, as the desired wave develops without loss of texture or elasticity.

But, there is no way of predetermining the exact point on the processing curve which each winding has reached. Test curls are helpful, but must be unwrapped and checked at frequent intervals while the hair is still under-processed and *in the act of developing a curl.* It is important to recognize that this curl pattern may also be due to a previous permanent still in the hair.

TIMING THE ALKALINE COLD WAVE PROCESS

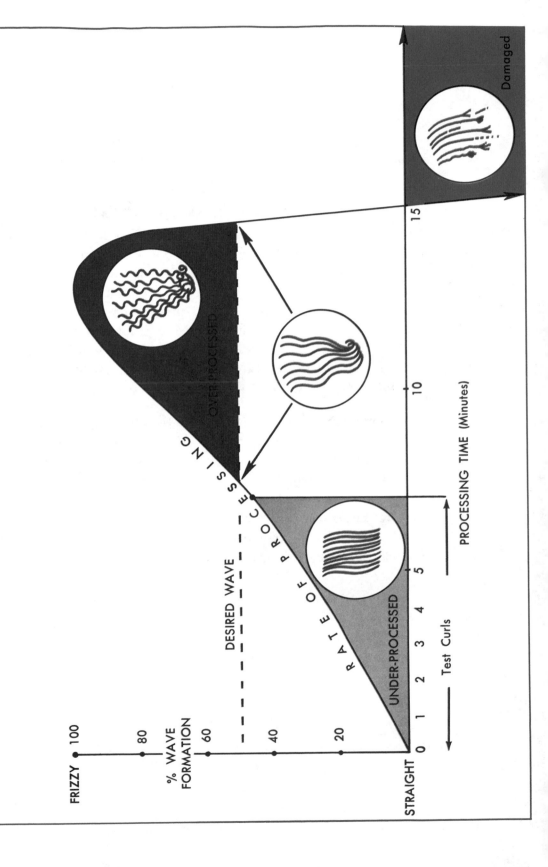

Note:

This chart represents a hypothetical situation and actual processing time will vary according to the texture and condition of the hair.

Failure of waves caused by a breakdown of the keratin chains may be due to the additive effect of this and other treatments, particularly towards the tip of the hair, which may already be damaged by chemicals.

These factors may cause too-rapid processing, which in turn, often leads to failure of the permanent wave process. Curls may be formed, but the practitioner has taken test curls too late to show them. For example, damaged hair, overporous hair, poorly lightened or badly tinted hair.

OTHER TIMING FACTORS

TEMPERATURE Chemical processes are speeded up by heat and slowed down by cold. If it is a winter's day and the salon is cold and drafty, the normal processing and neutralizing times may be inadequate. Failure of the hair to take a wave may be due to insufficient allowance for these climatic or weather factors. It may be better to process the hair under the steamer, processing machine or other heat source for a few minutes. This procedure would be very helpful in cases of resistant, wiry hair. A hairdryer, although creating a rise in temperature, will also rapidly evaporate the permanent wave solution and stop processing.

POOR PREPARATION The hair may be in a soiled condition or covered with hair lacquer or setting sprays. All of these can hinder normal processing. A soap shampoo may have coated the cuticle with soap scum which prevented easy entry of the waving solution into the cortex.

Metallic dyes and hair color restorers may have smothered the cuticle thus preventing easy penetration of solutions.

The qualified professional must take these factors into consideration if he/she hopes to perform permanent waving successfully.

CHAPTER 16

PROBLEMS IN PERMANENT WAVING

MISUSE OF TERMS

There are a number of problems associated with permanent waving. In order to discuss them without confusion the following terminology must be clarified.

"SOLUTION"—"LOTION" The solution or lotion should always be called the permanent wave solution or the permanent wave processing solution. (A solution is *ANY* substance which has been *dissolved* in a liquid.)

NEUTRALIZER The term, "neutralizer," is very bad, but since it is so popular, it is doubtful that it can be changed now. The most correct name would probably be "oxidizer."

The neutralizer does have some neutralizing action, but only on alkaline type permanent waves. The real function of the "neutralizer" is to oxidize the broken S-bonds and thus reform them.

HAIR PROBLEMS

CORTEX-CUTICLE RATIO The hair texture is an important factor in assessing the expected processing characteristics of certain types of hair.

Unfortunately, a casual examination does not always indicate the real texture or condition. One problem is that *only the cuticle is visible* on the outside of the hair shaft, while the waving action of permanent wave processing solution takes place entirely within the cortex. Therefore, the amount of cortex in relation to the cuticle will determine the holding power of the wave. In other words, the more the cortex predominates the better are the chances of a good wave.

This cortex/cuticle ratio is more important as the hair diameter becomes less. Fine hair is often hard-to-wave hair because it has a low cortex/cuticle ratio.

Such fine hair can be waved only with difficulty and will have a tendency to relax or straighten more rapidly after waving.

Note:

It is important to bear in mind that the thickness of the cuticle layer does not depend on the diameter of the hair. Thus, there might be much more cuticle in fine hair than in coarse hair.

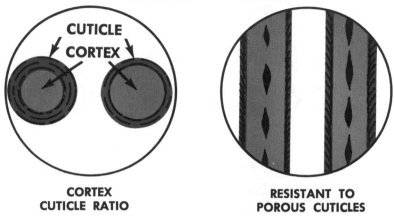

**CORTEX
CUTICLE RATIO**

**RESISTANT TO
POROUS CUTICLES**

POROSITY OF THE CUTICLE   The cuticle is on the outside of the hair shaft, so all solutions must first pass through this layer before they can work on the cortex.

If the imbrications are far apart the hair will have a porous condition. Hair may also have a high porosity if the cuticle has been damaged. The excessive porosity may be treated by applying fillers before waving.

However, the imbrications may be tightly closed around the hair shaft, or the hair may be coated with lacquers, sprays, grease or dyes.

In these cases, the solutions will penetrate slowly into the cortex, and the processing takes longer unless some steps are taken to reduce this resistant condition, such as, removing lacquer, shampooing excessively oily hair or pre-dampening with processing solution.

DIFFERENCE IN POROSITY OF HAIR CORTEX   The hair cortex may have areas of low and high porosity. In older hairs there may be air spaces present in the cortex.

If undiluted processing solution enters these spaces it will process too rapidly. Furthermore, it will cause a rapid breakdown of the keratin as there are fewer S-bonds where the spaces are located.

One method of evening out the porosity is to leave the hair towel-dry after rinsing with warm water. The porous part of the cortex holds more water and so dilutes the permanent wave solution where it is most desirable.

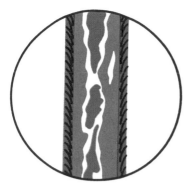

DIFFERENCES IN POROSITY OF HAIR CORTEX

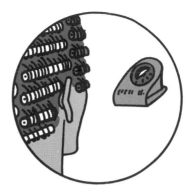

TIME OF PROCESSING

TIME OF PROCESSING One of the most important factors in permanent waving is the length of time the processing solution is left on the hair. This time must be sufficient for the cross-bonds to be broken and the keratin chains to be rearranged.

If the wave solution is rinsed and neutralized too soon, then the hair is underprocessed. On the other hand, leaving the processing solution on too long will cause overprocessing and hair breakage.

TEMPERATURE OF PROCESSING The permanent wave process is not carried out at cold temperatures. Rather, it is more effectively a "warm" process. Rising body heat from the scalp, captured by a processing cap, will increase the temperature.

The chemical action of the processing solution will itself cause a rise in temperature on the rods. Chemical changes take place quicker as the temperature goes up.

Consequently, resistant hair may be processed under a steamer, processing machine or other heating device to shorten processing time. On the other hand, if hair is processed in a cold draft or in an unheated or overly air conditioned salon or shop, the time for proper processing will be lengthened.

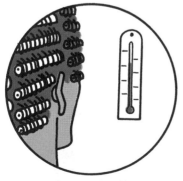

TEMPERATURE OF PROCESSING

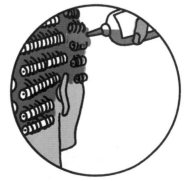

STRENGTH OF WAVING SOLUTIONS

Note:

The average rate of chemical change is altered by 10% for every degree (rise or fall) of temperature.

This works both ways, with cooler temperatures lengthening the processing time and warmer temperatures shortening the processing time. This means that if certain hair will achieve the desired wave in 10 minutes at 72°, at 73° the wave will be achieved in 9 minutes. On the other hand, if the temperature were 71°, the processing time would be 11 minutes. Thus you can see that the temperature factor can have an important bearing on effective waving.

STRENGTH OF WAVING SOLUTIONS   The strength or activity of permanent wave solutions also influences processing to a great extent. For resistant hair a 10% stronger solution of active waving agent is used to accelerate the rate of processing. Although normal solution strengths could be used, the resulting chemical action would be too slow for professional use.

But porous hair would be seriously damaged by these stronger solutions. Therefore, processing solutions for lightened and damaged hair only contain some 4% to 6% active waving agent. The slower chemical action of these weaker solutions allow normal test curls to be taken as with other types of hair.

WETABILITY OF SOLUTIONS   Hair is made of hard keratin covered with a thin layer of natural oils. Both of these substances are hydrophobic (water haters). So virgin hair is wet only with difficulty. Therefore, permanent wave solutions are slow to penetrate into the cortex.

For this reason, most processing and neutralizing solutions contain wetting agents. These agents allow faster and more efficient wetting of the hair with consequent easier entry into the cortex.

These improved solutions are more efficient because they have a reduced surface tension. Some neutralizers may also contain "foamers" to produce a rich foam. These additives are supposed to prevent runoff and dripping of solutions from the wrappings, but the claim that they improve neutralizing is debatable.

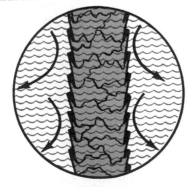

**WETTABILITY OF
SOLUTIONS**

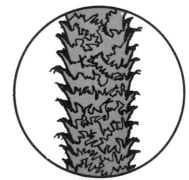

DAMAGED CUTICLE

DAMAGED CUTICLE The cuticle may be damaged by previous alkaline treatments, mainly over-lightening and tinting. Removal of or damage to this natural protective barrier (the cuticle) creates excessive porosity. The damage to the cuticle causes the permanent wave solution to be taken up too quickly, giving further reason for more damage.

A damaged cuticle can be treated by combing various fillers or conditioners through the hair strands before processing. These fillers may contain substances such as cholesterol, lecithin, polypeptides, etc., which cling to the damaged cuticle or exposed cortex and help protect the hair from more chemical attack.

Courtesy: Gillette Company Research Institute, Rockville, Maryland

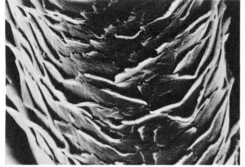 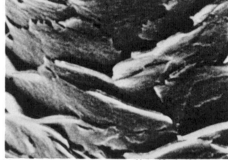

Magnified 2100 times   Damage to cuticle caused by permanent waving   Magnified 4200 times

NATURAL WEAKNESS IN HAIR SHAFT Despite proper wrapping and processing, the hair may break off. One of the causes could be a natural weakness of the hair itself.

Hair growth is governed by the many nutritional and health factors of its owner. During long periods of ill-health, there may be a serious interference with the natural formation of hair in the follicle. *Taking drugs or other medication and treatments can prevent normal hair growth.*

The hair shows this loss of activity by lack of a medulla and by growing finer in diameter. After a period of convalescence a return to the normal diameter of the hair may follow.

You must remember that a single hair can have a life of up to six years (well beyond the average). Few patrons realize this and will fail to connect an illness over twelve months ago with any subsequent hair breakage.

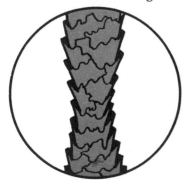 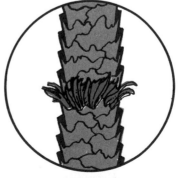

NATURAL WEAKNESS IN HAIR SHAFT   **EFFECT OF OVER-LAPPING OF CHEMICALS**

EFFECT OF OVERLAPPING OF CHEMICALS This is a result of poor technique. Most professional hair products can be safely used for at least one application. Trouble usually appears when several applications are required during the life of the hair strand.

This situation frequently is found in hair damaged by home perming, tinting or lightening. Furthermore, tests on this hair has shown that there is an additive effect. In other words, the damage caused to hair exposed to any two treatments is far in excess of damage to similar hair which has been treated only once. Hair breakage following a permanent wave will usually occur at the point where chemicals used in previous treatments were overlapped.

Many chemicals contain special thickeners or use plastic squeeze bottles to direct their contents just to the regrowth of untreated hair. A further difficulty is keeping these chemicals away from the soft keratin of the scalp (skin).

DIFFICULTIES IN RINSING EXCESS SOLUTIONS FROM THE HAIR Another problem is the removal of excess waving solutions from the hair wound on the rods. Most of this processing solution is found trapped within the wrappings. Thorough rinsing with warm water is mainly directed at removing this excess permanent wave solution but there is more solution present inside the cortex. In fact, without this processing solution entering the hair there would be no chemical change or permanent wave.

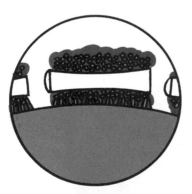

DIFFICULTIES IN RINSING EXCESS SOLUTIONS FROM HAIR

But it is almost impossible to remove the entire quantity of waving solution which is inside the cortex by rinsing with water. A very important task of the neutralizer is to "neutralize" or inactivate this internal waving solution.

If the external waving solution is not properly rinsed from around the hair strands, the activity of the neutralizer is seriously impaired.

Many examples of faulty permanent waves are due to this failure to rinse or blot away the excess waving solution, followed, in turn, by incomplete or under-neutralizing. Collapse of the wave is inevitable.

COARSE HAIR This is hair that has a larger diameter than average or normal hair. Penetration of the permanent wave solution is slower and so processing time is longer. Coarse hair can be three times as thick as fine hair. Therefore, there can be nine times as many bonds to alter and this explains why this hair is regarded as being "strong." *However, the porosity of the cuticle may drastically change this situation.*

THICK HAIR   This is hair that is thick or abundant on the scalp. The follicles are more numerous and closer together, so there is more hair to be waved. Because of this fact, it is necessary to take smaller and narrower blockings in order to get sufficient penetration of permanent wave solution into each curl. In addition, large, wide blockings would cause bulky wrapping that would result in excessively wide waves.

SULPHUR CONTENT   Some hard-to-wave hair has a higher sulphur content, which means that more S-bonds have to be broken and reformed in order to create the wave.

Some types of natural red hair shows this difficulty as the sulphur content is usually high. However, once having formed the wave, red hair has more lasting power and gives stronger waves.

FEWER S-BONDS   While many of the broken bonds can be reformed during neutralization, 100% success is never achieved. Only about 50% of the original S-bonds can be reformed in a changed position no matter how effectively neutralization is carried out.

Permanent waving solutions leave approximately 30% of the natural S-bonds unchanged during processing. More could be broken but the risk of hair damage due to end-bond breakage is the real reason for limiting processing time.

In natural waves it is believed that all of the S-bonds are linked together, thus providing great strength. In artificial waves only 50% of them are changed, but they provide sufficient strength to overcome the stretched, unchanged S-bonds (30%). This 30%, however, will eventually cause the chains to slip back into their former straight position.

MISCELLANEOUS PROBLEMS

H-BONDS   Not all the H-bonds are broken by ordinary alkaline "thio" solutions and these unbroken H-bonds also tend to weaken the wave.

For this purpose special H-bond breaking salts have been tested in some "thio" permanent wave solutions and have been found to give a more lasting wave than permanent wave solutions without this extra action on the H-bonds.

EVAPORATION OF PERMANENT WAVE SOLUTION   One cause of wave unevenness is the tendency of the "thio" to dry out and lose strength through evaporation.

Alkaline permanent waving solution always contains excess ammonia which is an easily vaporized gas dissolved in water. When this gas escapes from the waving solution, while on the hair, the pH will drop below 9.4 and the action of "thio" will be slowed.

Evaporation occurs mostly on the outside of the wrapped hair and so waving action slows down in this area. However, a processing cap or steamer will keep the solution moist and active as well as warmed by body heat.

SWELLING OF CORTEX If the winding on the rods is too tight the hair may be overstretched during processing. This can be exaggerated because of the excessive swelling of the hair that takes place when a strongly alkaline solution of "thio" is left in contact with the hair.

METHOD OF WINDING The partings and blockings must also be of the correct width and depth. Stretching of the hair to fit on the rods may create excessive tension and result in poor waves or hair breakage.

DIAMETER OF RODS As the curl will tend to follow the diameter of the rods, selection must be made carefully. If the rods are too slender in diameter or, contain only a small amount of wound hair, then the curl will be too tight, provided, of course, that the softening and rearrangement of the cortex is completed.

WINDING ON ROD The wave will gradually get larger as the previously wound hair increases the actual size of the winding until it reaches the last curl near the scalp. Spiral winding is the only way that the waves can be made uniform all along the hair shaft, but of course this is not as convenient as croquignole winding.

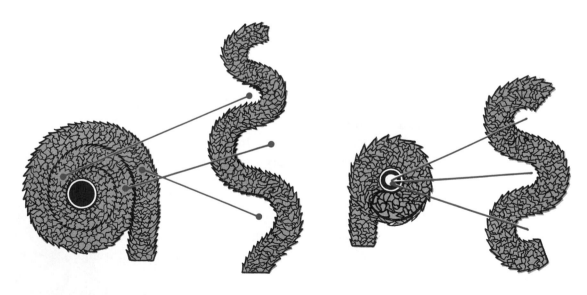

Hair croquignole wound on larger rod, giving larger, looser wave.

Hair spiral wound on small rod, giving tight, even wave.

"THIO" PROBLEMS

Permanent wave solutions based on ammonium thioglycolate have a number of disadvantages.

1. ALKALINITY

The solutions have to be highly alkaline in order to soften the hair but, alkalies may cause excessive swelling. Therefore, if the hair is not wound correctly on the rods, the swelling, caused by the strong alkali, will create excessive tension in the hair with risk of damage and breakage.

2. EFFECT ON END-BONDS

Ammonium thioglycolate solutions are not confined in their action to breaking S and H-bonds and no other bonds. In the excessive alkaline condition, the "thio" also breaks end-bonds or peptide bonds. This action leads to progressive weakening of the hair, especially in the outer part of the cortex, where the waving solution has a longer time to act on the end-bonds.

3. HAIR DISCOLORATION

REACTION WITH IRON The "thio" will also react to traces of iron in the hair, producing undesirable purple discolorations. The presence of this iron in the hair may be caused by:

1. Special types of hair with high iron content.
2. Rusty flakes of iron from metallic objects used in the hair.
3. Hard water (with iron contamination) used to rinse or shampoo the hair.
4. Metallic dyes (iron base) .

OTHER DISCOLORATIONS In addition to the reaction to traces of iron, "thio" cold waving solutions may cause other discolorations in hair treated with:

Various metallic based hair colorings.
Color rinses.
Medicated scalp ointments and lotions.
Left-over residues in the hair from swimming pool chemicals, etc.

EFFECTS Discolorations are more pronounced in lightened, grey or white hair than in hair of normal color.

4. HAIR DAMAGE

RESULTS Alkaline permanent waving solutions tend to damage the structure of the cuticle and also tend to remove the last traces of natural oils from within the imbrications. Both of these protective layers are necessary to maintain the condition of the hair and when damaged, the new, extra porous nature of the cuticle makes the hair more receptive to staining from perspiration, smoke or chemicals.

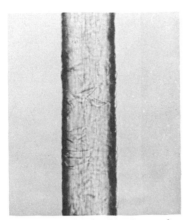

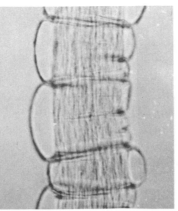

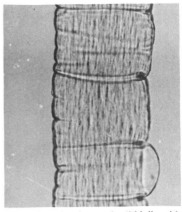

1. Lightened hair after shampooing and rinsing.

2. Same hair after 5 minutes in ammonium thioglycolate (pH 9.4). Gross swelling of cuticle has detached scales from hair shaft.

3. After 8 minutes in "thio" cold waving solution. Cortex has swelled excessively. Severe damage occurs when using alkaline waving solutions on lightened hair.

TREATMENT This problem may be met by reconditioning treatments or made less severe by "thio" solutions containing conditioners or modifiers which slow down their strong action.

COLOR FADING Certain natural pigments in the hair may become lighter after permanent waving and this color fading is most noticeable on the ends of the hair (although oily or wavy hair may look lighter than dry or straight hair due to light reflection). The fault may lie in using strong (highly alkaline) wave solutions, over-processing or the neutralizer assuming a high pH (the alkalies react with the hydrogen peroxide in the neutralizer to create bleaching conditions). Porous hair will show color fading more readily. Some stripping of color from tinted hair may also result from harsh permanent waving chemicals.

DANGERS IN USING "THIO" SOLUTIONS

DERMATITIS A serious problem with alkaline thioglycolate solutions is the effect they have on the skin, since the skin is made of soft keratin and is more readily broken down than the hard keratin of the hair. Furthermore, if there are abrasions on the scalp, the permanent wave solution may enter and cause severe dermatitis and scalp inflammation. Some countries will not permit thioglycolate to be used at all for permanent waving because of the possibility that it may cause injury to the scalp.

EYE INJURY "Thio" permanent waving solutions can also cause serious damage to the cornea if accidentally splashed into the eye.

ACTION ON HANDS The nails and skin of the fingers of the practitioner may soften and discolor due to the corrosive action of the "thio" solution. The wearing of gloves will provide protection, but because gloves cause sweating of the hands and seem to interfere with movements of the fingers, many professionals refuse to wear them.

PREVENTIONS Permanent wave solutions should be kept away from the skin. If spilt on the skin or in the eye, it should be washed away as quickly as possible. The use of creams, sponges, absorbent papers and gloves will help prevent many injuries, both to the patron and to the practitioner. Some practitioners are even allergic to the fumes of waving solutions and if possible, other work should be arranged for them.

NEWER WAVING SOLUTIONS

NEUTRAL AND ACID To overcome the disadvantages of alkaline ammonium thioglycolate solutions, both neutral and acid type permanent wave solutions have been developed.

ADVANTAGES

WILL NOT OVERPROCESS Acid type wave solutions are especially valuable in the case of damaged, lightened, over-porous, weakened hair. Newer type chemicals are used to break the S-bonds and it is believed that acid wave solutions will not overprocess any hair under any circumstances because of their milder action.

PLEASANT SMELL Another distinct advantage is in the range of fragrant perfumes that can be used with them. A common complaint with ordinary "thio" solutions is the smell but, because of their highly alkaline state, very few perfumes are stable in them. However, in acid and neutral solutions there is a wide range of usable, pleasant perfumes and very little risk of breakdown.

IMPROVED WAVE The wave also contracts or tightens on drying instead of loosening up as with alkaline solutions. The lower pH also means less swelling of the hair and it therefore leaves more lustre and body in the hair after waving.

HAIR STAYS STRONG There is no action on the end-bonds of the hair and therefore the hair is not weakened during the waving process and it maintains its quality and strength.

DISADVANTAGES

COST Acid and neutral solutions are relatively expensive to buy.

SLOW ACTING The processing time involved is extremely long and the busy modern patron seems unwilling to extend the time now spent for professional services. The processing time can be shortened somewhat through the application of heat.

NEUTRALIZER   They require a special neutralizer because if a neutralizer designed for the alkaline type wave is used, it will leave the hair in a rubbery, limp condition. The reason is that S-bonds are not reformed by hydrogen peroxide type neutralizers. If used, another type of cross-bond forms which is not very satisfactory.

CONCLUSION

THE FUTURE   It is quite likely that in the near future, there will be a decline in the use of ammonium thioglycolate in favor of the more advanced types of acid or neutral permanent waving solutions. Nevertheless, it will still be essential for practitioners to follow manufacturer's directions, especially in regard to the hardening of the waves by the neutralizer.

Whenever it becomes difficult to obtain a good permanent wave the blame is usually laid on the condition of the hair. Such an easy excuse is often used to cover up poor workmanship. Some professionals maintain that nothing can be done to improve results and in this way they hope to avoid their responsibilities to the patron.

The solution to the problem lies in a proper understanding of hair, its properties and deficiencies. A patron expects that professionals have this information and that a professional service will give beautiful, lasting, "natural" waves.

The beneficial knowledge of hair waving is now available to *ALL* practitioners. Application of this knowledge will maintain the high standards of professional services which play a major role in the proper grooming and well-being of the community.

PRACTICAL WORK

Tests for different types of waving solutions may be made in the following way:

1. pH TEST

Solution	Typical Reaction
Alkaline	Blue/purple
Neutral	Green
Acid	Pink/red

pH is readily determined by using chemically treated test paper as prepreviously described.

2. TEST FOR IRON

Add a few crystals of ferrous sulphate (or any solution of an iron salt) to the cold waving solution.

Solution	Indication
Ammonium thioglycolate	Stable, deep purple
Neutral	Fleeting reddish color
Acid	No reaction

CHEMICAL HAIR STRAIGHTENERS OR RELAXERS

Introduction

It is a recognized psychological theory that we often desire the opposite appearance from what we have. Individuals with naturally curly hair often go to great lengths to have it straightened, while those with straight hair spend hours with the professional artisans to have it waved or curled.

For many years, "permanent waves" have been given to patrons with naturally straight hair. Opposite to this is the desire of those with tight waves or over-curly hair to have it relaxed or straightened.

Now that more is known about the nature of chemical compounds and solutions that can soften or break the internal bonds of the hair and rearrange them into a new pattern, chemical hair straightening has become very popular. In order that the public be better protected and better served, it has become necessary that this knowledge be made available to the professional.

HOW HAIR TAKES ITS FORM

HEREDITY Whether our hair be straight, wavy, curly or tightly curled, the nature of the hair with which we are born depends, to a large degree, upon our ancestors. It has been said facetiously that if you desire straight hair you should have picked yourself parents with that kind of hair. Of course, children don't always follow the hair patterns of their parents. Sometimes it is the hair form of the grandparents or the great-grandparents that appears. But, taken overall, if you have a long line of Chinese ancestors, it's fairly predictable that your hair will be straight. This same statement can be made about almost every other type of hair texture and form.

The same heredity pattern is seen, but to a lesser degree, in hair coloring. We have come to expect people of Scandinavian descent to be mostly blond and blue-eyed. Many people of Celtic descent have very fair, sensitive skin and red hair. Among people of such genetic background it would be unusual to find a dark-skinned child with dark brown, tightly-curled hair.

Physiologists have put forward various theories to explain how the hair follicles that produce straight hair differ from those which give rise to tight, kinky curls.

CYCLICAL THEORY   Biochemists propose that the control of hair waves and curls can be found in the germinal matrix. It is thought by these scientists that the increased concentration of amino-acids (or uneven rate of cell division) first on one side of the germinal matrix and then on the other side, alternating with a decrease on the first side, is the most probable explanation.

It is an observed fact that over-curly hair has an unusually rapid growth. Perhaps this is caused by the rapid release of amino-acids first on one side of the growing hair, then on the other. Because the amino-acid supply is in excess of that found in straight hair, the curl is more tightly sprung.

If you were to undo a hand-knitted garment, you would find the yarn to be very crinkly. If you proceeded to cut the wool into tiny segments one-eighth inch in length, it would be impossible to detect a kink or curl in the wool. As only one-eighth inch of any hair follicle is embedded in the dermis, skin sections do not indicate curl within the skin. So it is practically impossible to determine, while in the follicle, the way over-curly hair grows. But we know by *external* observation that it grows in an incomplete circle, implying that the keratin chains receive uneven amounts of amino-acids on the longer, outside curve of the hair.

THE PRACTICE OF HAIR STRAIGHTENING

Manufacturers, practitioners and the general public are all very interested in the practice of hair straightening or chemical hair relaxing. The practitioner, especially, should understand not only why it is possible to change the form of curly hair, but how it is achieved. In this respect, the advantages, as well as the dangers of using strong chemicals on the keratin of the hair, must be understood.

DEFINITIONS

Chemicals used to permanently straighten over-curly hair have two functions:

1. *The relaxer* or straightener is used during the processing step, breaking both S- and H-bonds in the cortex which softens and changes the form of the hair.
2. *The neutralizer* (fixative) stops the action of the relaxer and, by oxidation, rehardens the hair and reforms the newly positioned and recently broken S-bonds.

Just as in the case of permanent waving, *hair straightening is a chemical change*. It must also be remembered that *most chemical changes that take place in the hair weakens the hair*. Therefore, a thorough understanding of the kind of hair to be straightened is necessary in order to minimize possible damage to the patron's hair or scalp. As professionals, we must be able to detect the differences between the following types of hair and the action to be expected of the chemical hair straightener:

FINE HAIR   The part of the hair that is to be straightened is the cortex. If the hair is fine and, therefore, has a smaller diameter than normal or average hair, the amount of cortex will be less. Therefore, if the cuticle of the hair is not overly resistant, penetration of the relaxer will be quicker and processing time shorter.

POROUS HAIR   This kind of hair, because of rather widely spaced cuticle scales, absorbs solutions more rapidly than normal hair and is naturally quicker to process. Less processing time should be allowed.

COARSE OR STRONG HAIR   This type of hair usually has a larger diameter than normal hair and this results in a greater area of cortex. Thus, there are many more sulphur bonds to be broken and processing will be slower. Furthermore, if the cuticle is of the resistant type, processing time will be lengthened still more.

ABUNDANT HAIR   This kind of hair thickly covers the scalp. As the follicles are numerous and closely clustered together, there are more hairs to be straightened. The practitioner must use great care in applying sufficient amounts of the chemical to insure that all hairs are exposed equally to the straightener.

RESISTANT HAIR   This type of hair is less likely to be damaged by over-processing with the straightening chemical because the cuticle scales, being closer together, slow the rate of its penetration.

SULPHUR CONTENT   Some hair, usually red and black, has a higher sulphur content. This means that there are more sulphur-bonds to be broken and reformed during the straightening process, thus lengthening the time required.

DEGREE OF PERMANENCE

Natural regrowth of adult hair takes place at about the rate of $\frac{1}{2}$ to $\frac{3}{4}$ inch per month. Therefore, the patron who wishes to keep her friends guessing as to whether her hair is naturally straight or chemically achieved will be required to have the regrowth straightened every six weeks to two months.

This technique is a vast improvement over the heat method (hot thermal iron or pressing comb) which was developed in the early 1900's. The heat method temporarily straightened over-curly hair. The heat, applied directly to the hair, softened the S-bonds and, at the same time, the physical (H) bonds were broken. This permitted the hair to be smoothed and straightened to some degree.

This change was primarily a physical change which was only of a temporary nature. In approximately two weeks the hair reverted to its original curly form. This process of reversion was further accelerated by exposure to humidity, rain or moisture in any form.

DISULFIDE OR S-BONDS

In hair straightening as in permanent waving, the most important factor involved is the breaking and reforming of the S-bonds of the cortex. To fully understand the importance of these bonds, it is necessary to briefly review their role in the hair.

Recall that the structure of the hair strand is similar to that of rope in which each main strand consists of many smaller strands, each of which is wound closely round other strands for tensile strength. We must have a picture in our mind's eye of all these long strands, or poly-peptide chains of amino-acids in the hair, not only twisted round each other but connected to each other horizontally as well. Between each *amino-acid unit* of the poly-peptide chain is an *end* bond. But, connecting the chains crosswise are *disulfide (sulphur)* bonds of great strength and *hydrogen* bonds of a weaker nature.

The role of the various softening creams used in hair straightening is to break the chemical S-bonds or to relax them, so that their position and that of the poly-peptide chains can be permanently shifted. This permits curly hair to be straightened and to assume a permanently straight position.

HAIR DAMAGE If the cream formula is too strong, too abundant, or left on too long, not only will the S-bonds be affected, but the END bonds may be weakened or dissolved. The outward visible sign of this chemical reaction is destruction or a breaking off of the hair. This also may result in:

1 Complete loss of elasticity.
2 Breakdown of hair strength.
3 Roughness and dryness of the hair.
4 A tendency of the hair to tangle or mat, resulting from the raising and/or removal of cuticle scales.
5 Complete loss of cuticle scales, if hair damage is severe. The hair would then be very dry, brittle and, without doubt, in a "fly away" condition.

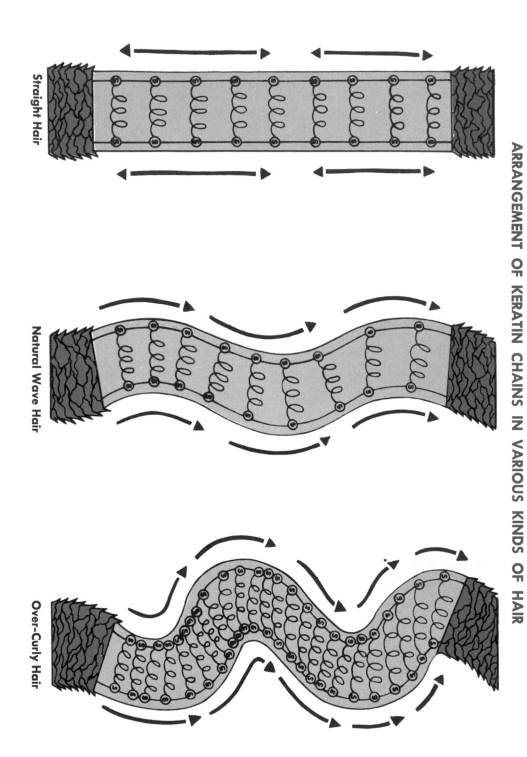

ARRANGEMENT OF KERATIN CHAINS IN VARIOUS KINDS OF HAIR

Straight Hair

Natural Wave Hair

Over-Curly Hair

THE STRAND TEST

A practitioner who has the interest of the patron at heart will give a strand test before proceeding with the straightening process.

A strand test presents the overall reaction of hair in its normal state. It may be made on the head 'or by taking samples from the head and treating them separately with straightener of different strengths and for different periods of time. A series of test tubes can be used for this purpose, with the tubes marked with the strength of straightener used and the time noted. Rinsing and neutralizing will follow treatment with the relaxer. This method avoids any chance of damage to the entire head and can be used to compare the dangers and efficiencies of various brand products.

When planning to provide services for patrons who have a hereditary pattern of over-curly hair, it is important to remember that all over the world people seek professional services to improve their appearance and, perhaps, get a boost in morale. Of course, the treatments that are used to improve a patron's appearance may differ, but the aim is the same. People know that attractive and fashionably styled hair is one of the most outstanding features of a well-groomed appearance. Therefore, strand tests are designed to help insure that the treatment produces the proper results.

MAIN TYPES OF CHEMICAL RELAXERS

It is no longer necessary to apply a heavy oil to the hair and then mechanically pull it straight in order to remove excess curl. Nor do people have to tolerate the unpleasant appearance of flattened, greasy hair. Today, there are three separate relaxing formulas available to those who wish to change the appearance of their hair from over-curly to straight. As practitioners, we can contribute to the happiness of many millions of people . . . providing we give service that recognizes the possible dangers to patrons' hair if the straightening procedure is not properly carried out.

While many different firms produce chemical straighteners, there are only three primary ingredients used in these hair straightening products. One of the most frequently used is the well known cold wave solution AMMONIUM THIOGLYCOLATE, a strong alkali in which the word "THIO" refers to the presence of SULPHUR. The two other preparations are SODIUM HYDROXIDE and AMMONIUM SULFITE.

AMMONIUM THIOGLYCOLATE

Before proceeding to the technique of hair straightening with a "thio" based chemical, it is best to first understand what happens internally when this relaxer, in either cream or liquid form, is applied to the hair. While the cream is in contact with the cortex, the strong alkali softens and swells the hair and causes the original S-bonds to be broken. This action permits the removal of excess curl from the hair by combing through the softened hair and manually straightening each strand.

However, only about fifty per cent of the broken S-bonds are reformed in the act of neutralization. This means that the reformed S-bonds that were previously holding the original curved position will now be holding the hair straight. If straightening is improperly carried out, there may be some relaxing of the newly positioned S-bonds and the hair could revert to the waved or curly position. It also must be remembered that there is a limit to the length of time the chemical can remain in contact with the hair; otherwise, permanent end bond breakage may result.

FORMULA   The Thioglycolate (Thio) straighteners are formulas of Thioglycolic Acid or Monoethanolamine Thioglycolate adjusted to the proper pH level (above 9.0) with Ammonium Monoethanolamine. The formula is contained in a heavy cream base which is required to hold the hair in a straight position while it is being processed.

There is a great similarity between the THIO action in permanent waving and in hair straightening. In both cases, the S-bonds of the keratin are broken down in the softening process. But in waving, the hair is wound on rods to induce the softened hair to take up a curled or waved position, while in straightening, the objective is directly opposite. The poly-peptide chains of the cortex are unlinked cross-wise by the bond breaking action of the Thio and are then rearranged into a straight position by the mechanical action of the comb and/or hands. The heavy cream aids the process by maintaining hair in a straight position.

There are available to the practitioner a number of Thio hair straighteners produced by different manufacturers. Since each producer has developed his own formula, we cannot present any single product table. However, set forth below is a list of the chemical components usually found in a Thio cream or liquid formula. The exact quantity of each ingredient employed is part of each manufacturer's guarded formula, and is slightly different for each product.

Thioglycolate Straightener—Ingredients

1 Thioglycolic acid
2 Sodium lauryl sulphate
3 Ceresin
4 Stearic acid
5 Ammonium hydroxide
6 Distilled water
7 Paraffin
8 Glycerol monostearate
9 Perfume

These formulas are designed with a pH of between 9.2 and 9.6.

CHEMICAL HAIR STRAIGHTENING - AMMONIUM THIOGLYCOLATE

1. VIRGIN CURLY HAIR
Virgin polypeptide chains show original position of cystine disulfide links between them.

2. PROCESSING
Reduced S-bonds (breaking of cystine disulfide links).

3. NEUTRALIZING
Prepared neutralizer poured through hair, after smoothing and straightening.

4. RINSING
Excess neutralizer and water removed leaving hair in a straightened position.

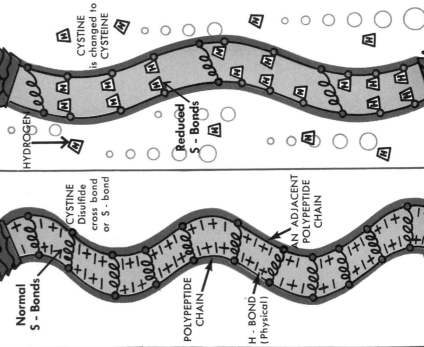

Normal S - Bonds

CYSTINE Disulfide cross bond or S - bond

AN ADJACENT POLYPEPTIDE CHAIN

POLYPEPTIDE CHAIN

H - BOND (Physical)

HYDROGEN

CYSTINE is changed to CYSTEINE

Reduced S - Bonds

Oxidized S - Bonds

OXYGEN

WATER MOLECULE

Reformed S - Bonds

DRYING REFORMS THE H - BONDS

NEUTRALIZATION After the Thio has remained in the hair a sufficient period of time to properly straighten the hair, the neutralizer (fixative) is applied. The fixative compound (an oxidizer) is thoroughly applied to completely penetrate into the cortex and stop the action of the Thio compound. It really has two major functions:

1. It prevents further bond breaking action of the Thio solution and neutralizes (to a degree) the alkalinity.
2. It reforms the broken S-bonds in their new position in order to hold the hair in its newly straightened position.

It is important for the practitioner to have a thorough understanding of the product being used and its method of application. The neutralizer (fixative) may be applied after the hair has received a water rinse intended to remove surplus softener, or when the surplus has been removed by blotting. The time required for complete neutralization may vary from 5 to 20 minutes. In every case, the manufacturer's instructions must be followed implicitly.

Most of the Thio type neutralizers (fixatives) are mild acid solutions with a pH from 3.0 to 4.0, and therefore, shrink the keratin chains together, making the reforming of the S-bonds between the polypeptide chains easier.

Furthermore, the acid present in the neutralizer causes the imbrications of the cuticle to press down tightly and helps restore the natural sheen and lustre to the hair.

THIO HAIR STRAIGHTENING PROCESS The Thio process of hair straightening is divided, for all practical purposes, into two chemical actions: (1) the processing or softening action, and (2) the neutralizing and hardening action.

Processing or Softening Action:

Hair-S-S-Hair → Add: Thio Hair → Result: Hair swells and
(Cystine links or   Straightener   softens
S-bonds intact)   (Cystine change
                                                     to cysteine—S-bonds
                                                     åre broken)

Neutralizing—Hardening Action:

Hair Soft and → Add: Neutralizer or → Result: Hair reduces in
Swollen   Fixative (an   diameter, hardens
(S-bonds are   oxidizer)   in new form
broken)   (Cystine links
                                                     or S-bonds
                                                     reformed)

Some of the most suitable chemicals used in neutralizers are Potassium Bromate, Sodium Perborate and Hydrogen Peroxide.

ADVANTAGES Thio hair straighteners are especially useful in reducing waves in hair which has been over-processed in permanent waving. They also have a basic advantage due to the fact that they exhibit a low level of skin irritation when properly used. They appear to have very little or no systemic effects upon most patrons.

While it may be affirmed that if Thio preparations are used properly they present little or no hazards to most patrons, there are some people whose eyes are sensitive to them. It is, therefore, wise to question patrons as to allergic reactions to cosmetic hair preparations or to take some sort of test to determine a patron's reactions. Patrons who at first show no sensitivity to a product may later become sensitive to it either on the skin or in the eyes.

DISADVANTAGES The most important disadvantage of this type of straightener, in addition to the fact that it is capable of breaking end bonds, is the pulling of the comb or the hands through the cream on the hair. Excessive pulling on the weakened end bonds of the cortex contributes to the likelihood of breakage.

PRE-ANALYSIS FOR ALL HAIR STRAIGHTENERS:
1. Examine scalp. If patron has scalp sores or abrasions, DO NOT APPLY CHEMICAL RELAXER.
2. Examine hair. If hair is dry, hard, brittle, over-porous or stretches too easily, a strand test should be given.

Note:

For dyed, tinted or lightened hair, most manufacturers have specific instructions for the use of their straightener. It is always advisable to perform a strand test.

PROCEDURE FOR THIO PREPARATIONS

PROCESSING Always follow manufacturer's specific instructions. However, the following is a generalized procedure for THIO type straighteners.

1. Thoroughly shampoo hair with a soapless shampoo (detergent type).
2. Refrain from rubbing or massaging scalp.
3. Rinse and towel dry (*Do not apply heat in the drying process.*)
4. Section hair.
5. Apply hair straightening cream $\frac{1}{4}$ to $\frac{3}{4}$ inch from the scalp of each section. Repeat performance over the whole head including the scalp area. Do not apply cream to ends at this time.
6. Work cream smoothly over and into the hair. Arrange hair in a straight position through manipulation by the hands. (The heavy cream will help keep it in place.)
7. Leave on for 5–10 minutes.

8 Comb through to the ends of each section of the hair once.

9 Allow to process for time recommended by manufacturer.

10 Smooth. For resistant hair, allow the process to continue for 5 additional minutes. Examine the hair at 2-minute intervals until it has reached the desired degree of straightness.

11 Do not process longer than 30 minutes after the straightening cream has been applied.

12 Rinse thoroughly, using warm water, until the cream has been completely removed from hair. Blot out excess water.

13 Neutralizing:

(a) Prepare neutralizer; pour into a plastic container, and set in the shampoo basin.

(b) Pour the prepared solution through the hair, collecting it in the bowl and reapplying 6 or 7 times. Smooth and straighten while rinsing to assure complete neutralizing of all strands.

(c) Rinse thoroughly to remove neutralizer.

14 Set hair in desired style.

SODIUM HYDROXIDE RELAXERS

The fastest and most effective chemical hair straightening products are the Sodium Hydroxide relaxers.

Sodium Hydroxide, in solution with Glycerine Monostearate or Stearic and Oleic Acids, plus a number of additives, makes a very effective hair straightener. These products are noted for their very high pH of from 10 to 14. They are compounds with varying percentages of Sodium Hydroxide, ranging from 5% to 10% in different formulas.

In general, it may be stated that the higher the percentage of Sodium Hydroxide, the faster the chemical reaction on the hair. However, it also is true that the higher the pH factor, the more danger of hair damage or breakage.

These products react on the hair by causing the fibers to swell and break the S-bonds which hold together the polypeptide chains. The entire softening process should be completed within a maximum time of 8 minutes. If it is not, the action should be stopped immediately by rinsing and neutralization.

CAUTION: Extreme care must be taken to KEEP THE CHEMICAL FROM CONTACTING THE EYES AND EARS. This is particularly important when the hair is being rinsed. Caustic Soda will burn the skin and scalp, and it should never be applied over cuts, burns or abrasions. Other possible side effects are:

a. If Sodium Hydroxide is left on too long, the hair may turn red.

b. Hair may become brittle and break off.

c. *If left on longer than 10 minutes, the hair may dissolve.*

1. CURLY HAIR

Both H and S bonds holding polypeptide chains in position.

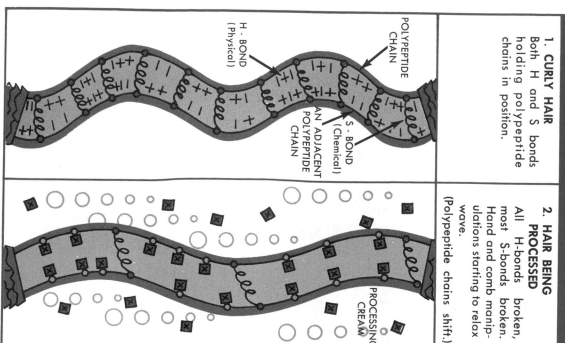

POLYPEPTIDE CHAIN

H - BOND (Physical)

S - BOND (Chemical)

AN ADJACENT POLYPEPTIDE CHAIN

2. HAIR BEING PROCESSED

All H-bonds broken, most S-bonds broken. Hand and comb manipulations starting to relax wave.

(Polypeptide chains shift.)

PROCESSING CREAM

3. HAIR BEING NEUTRALIZED

The neutralizer fixes polypeptide chains in a straight position after hair has been fully relaxed.

NEUTRALIZER

4. STRAIGHTENED HAIR . . .

after rinsing and proper drying. LANTHIONINE cross links now exist between polypeptide chains, keeping the hair in a permanently straight form. Drying reforms the physical bonds.

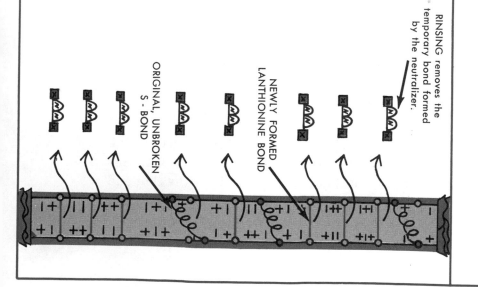

RINSING removes the temporary bond formed by the neutralizer.

NEWLY FORMED LANTHIONINE BOND

ORIGINAL, UNBROKEN S - BOND

FORMULA   As is true in the case of Thio products, Sodium Hydroxide straighteners are prepared by a number of manufacturers. While Sodium Hydroxide is the most important base ingredient for all these straighteners, the various formulas are closely guarded secrets. However most of these formulas contain the following ingredients in various percentages:

Sodium Hydroxide
Stearic Acid
Oleic Acid
Glycerine Monostearate
Glycerol
Water
Perfume

With the pH adjusted from 10 to 14.

STRAND TEST   Most manufacturers do not recommend the use of this product on previously processed hair. However, some manufacturers have lowered the hydroxide content and the pH value to permit their product to be used on tinted as well as lightened hair. In each case, a strand test is always advisable.

PROCESSING   Always follow the manufacturer's instructions in addition to the following:

PROCEDURE

1. Do not shampoo. Do not rub or otherwise irritate the scalp.
2. Do not use hot or warm combs or irons.
3. Apply protective cream evenly and completely in order to cover the scalp.
4. *Put on protective gloves.*
5. Apply the preparation at the nape of the neck first. Section the hair with the fingers and apply the product to hair close to the scalp.
6. With previously straightened hair, the product should only be applied to the curly regrowth. Begin to straighten hair at root area and hairline by smoothing action. *It is important that the hair should not be pulled or stretched during the application.*
7. The approximate time for straightening hair is as follows: For fine hair—two to three minutes; for medium hair—three to five minutes; for coarse hair—five to seven minutes. The maximum time for the most resistant hair should not exceed 8 minutes.
8. Rinse with a strong force of warm water. Start at hairline and hold hose 4 to 5 inches from head. Do not use hand to remove the cream from the hairline; let the force of water remove it.
9. Shampoo the hair with a non-alkaline shampoo (soapless or detergent type). The hair must be "squeaky" clean.
10. Towel blot hair. Do not comb.
11. Neutralize and style.

AMMONIUM SULFITE AS A HAIR STRAIGHTENER

The third type of product used for chemical hair straightening employs an Ammonium Sulfite base. Although this product is not new and has been tried by manufacturers, there still does not seem to be any demand for it by professionals. The long period of time required to obtain any degree of hair relaxation has discouraged its use.

The Ammonium Sulfite method requires a long waiting period, with the patron sitting under a plastic turban cap designed to trap heat needed to assist the process. This use of excessive time, in order to be effective, has made "Ammonium Sulfites" economically unsound for professional services.

The same principle of softening the keratin chains takes place with the use of this chemical as with the THIO preparations.

The ammonium sulfite functions at a nearly neutral pH in the range of 7 to 7.5 in a moderately viscous base. Rinsing, and the use of a neutralizer after the softening step, permit the disulfide cross-bond or S-bonds to reform. Thus, the hair has been substantially rebuilt to its original chemical state but in a straightened form.

PROCEDURE

DYED, TINTED OR LIGHTENED HAIR Do not use this product immediately after giving a hair tint or lightener. For hair that has been treated in any of these ways, there is a special formulation. In addition, it is important to perform a strand test.

PROCESSING Follow manufacturer's instructions, which should be similar to the following:

1. Prepare mixture. Mix lotion and allow to stand 10 to 15 minutes.
2. Shampoo hair thoroughly with a soapless shampoo (detergent type).
3. Rinse and towel dry.
4. Apply relaxer. Begin at the neckline area. Then apply throughout the rest of hair, working towards the front of the hair until all the hair is covered. Use ¾ of the bottle, saving the remainder for step 6.
5. Pile hair on top of head and tie plastic cover around head. It is important that cover is tied on the forehead and not on the hairline. For virgin hair, the cover is left on for a maximum of 20 minutes; for lightened or tinted hair, only 10 minutes. Timing will vary somewhat according to the texture and condition of hair.
6. Remove covering and apply remainder of lotion. Section hair into 4 quarters with a *large comb*. Smaller sections are then made within each quarter and the hair is continuously hand straightened all around the head.

    Do not use excessive pressure. Your strand test will help you to judge how much guiding is necessary. Do not process virgin hair for more than 20 minutes; tinted or lightened hair for more than 15 minutes.

7 Rinsing. Thoroughly rinse hair with lukewarm water. To assure complete lotion removal, one light washing with a mild shampoo is recommended. Keep hair straight while shampooing. Rinse out shampoo.

8 Mix and apply neutralizer.

9 Set and style in normal way.

CONCLUSION This particular service, "hair straightening," plays an important role in society. The psychological reasons for changing one's appearance are to progress with fashion and thus maintain social acceptance.

HEREDITY

The patron will benefit from an understanding that heredity establishes limits as to what can be done to change the appearance of the hair. Another point is that although hair can be straightened, we cannot defeat nature and new growth will be curly. We can however, with the help of science, run parallel with nature and make temporary adjustments.

GROWTH OF CURLY HAIR The theories associated with the growth of tightly curled hair are a prerequisite for any attempts to change the hair from the natural growth pattern. If the practitioner understands the CYCLICAL THEORY of natural wave formation thoroughly, the role which he/she can play becomes more important.

THE NATURE OF HAIR ITSELF Before the practitioner can proceed to the art of hair straightening, it is essential that he (she) can recognize different hair types. Timing is one of the fundamental principles of satisfactory processing and it is closely tied to the nature of the hair. The professional must be able to recognize instantly:

1 Fine hair
2 Sparse hair
3 Porous hair
4 Coarse or thick hair
5 Abundant hair
6 Resistant hair

INTERNAL CONTROLS The student must also understand the internal chemistry of the hair in order to know what controls the changing of the hair from the curly to the straight form.

UNDERSTANDING THE PROCESS

DISULFIDE OR S-BONDS Hair straightening pre-supposes an understanding of the process of permanent waving. This procedure depends upon knowing the basic internal structure of hair, the positioning of the amino-acid, polypeptide chains, the role of the S-bonds, and the importance of the peptide or end bonds. Every professional, while understanding the external and internal structure of hair, must be continuously aware of the dangers of overprocessing in relation to hair straightening. This is important not only because of the danger to the patron's hair but also because the artisan who wishes to continue in business must preserve his (her) good reputation. The patron may bring a lawsuit in case of injury or, if no such drastic action is taken, may look elsewhere for professional services.

STRAND TEST: A wise artisan who wishes to protect himself or herself as well as the patron should always give a strand test before attempting to chemically straighten hair.

SALESMANSHIP

This area is very important. Patrons like to feel that special attention is paid to them by businessmen, promoters and practitioners. Any person who wishes to increase sales and clientele should always keep this in mind.

HISTORICAL BACKGROUND An understanding of the hair straightening methods of the past is basic in order to inform the patron of the great advances made in the process. There is universal interest in the "Facts of Science," even among those with little scientific backgrounds.

THE FUNDAMENTAL REASON FOR HAIR STRAIGHTENING The artisan also must be a psychologist, always remembering that the real reason the patron came to have the form of his/her hair changed has to do with HOPE. The artisan has the ability to make a person not only LOOK BETTER but FEEL BETTER.

HAIR COLORING —THE NATURE OF COLOR AND LIGHT

Introduction

The last decade has produced many new hair care techniques, the most numerous of which are in the field of hair coloring. Each year the demand for hair coloring services has grown 10% to 15%.

Most of the early objections to hair coloring came from reasons such as:

1. Lack of professional skill in giving hair coloring services.
2. Unsuitable products.
3. Fear of family disapproval.
4. Expense (including retouching).
5. Doubts about reaction of friends.

The popularity of hair coloring has swept aside most of these fears. Development of newer, improved products, scientific investigation into color problems and proper training of coloring experts are some reasons for the wide acceptance of hair coloring by the public today.

Once patrons have been pleased with a professional hair coloring treatment they are more loyal to the shop or salon. There evolves a greater dependence upon the professional and this assured "repeat business" makes hair coloring an extremely profitable service.

COMPONENTS OF NATURAL HAIR COLOR

Before examining the technique and processes used in hair coloring, a brief look into the mysteries of color itself, will be helpful.

The colors actually seen in the hair are due to:

1. Nature of light
2. Source of light
3. Reflection of light
4. Absorption of light
5. Function of the eye.

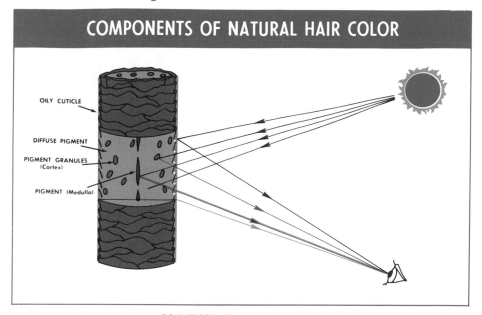

COMPONENTS OF NATURAL HAIR COLOR

OILY CUTICLE

DIFFUSE PIGMENT

PIGMENT GRANULES
(Cortex)

PIGMENT (Medulla)

NATURE OF LIGHT

LIGHT WAVES   Light travels in the form of waves at the tremendous speed of 186,000 miles per second.

COMPOSITION OF LIGHT   White light (sunshine or artificial light) is made up of a mixture of colors.

Under certain conditions (e.g., rainbow or prism) these colors are separated. When the colors from light are separated in this manner they form the colors of the visible spectrum.

COLOR EFFECTS OF NATURAL LIGHT   A person with normal vision can see many more colors in the spectrum than the official list of colors. This is because each of the six spectrum colors blends gradually with its neighbors to form intermediate hues of great beauty, e.g., tomato, tangerine, lemon, etc.

The red glow of the rising or setting sun shows the colored nature of white light. When the sun is high in the sky, the same light is a dazzling whiteness, although we can see only 12% of its rays.

A further example of the nature of sunlight is the lovely and delicate colors found in a soap bubble. Oil floating on the surface of water reveals yet another example of this separation of sunlight into its various colors.

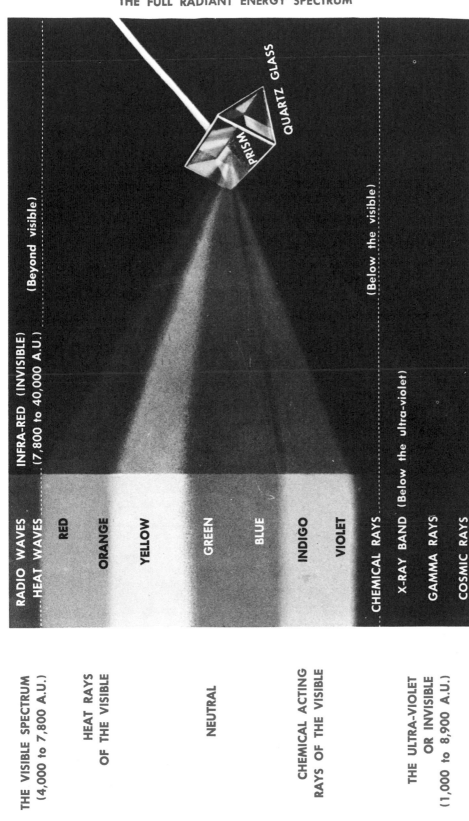

THE VISIBLE SPECTRUM
(4,000 to 7,800 A.U.)

HEAT RAYS
OF THE VISIBLE

NEUTRAL

CHEMICAL ACTING
RAYS OF THE VISIBLE

THE ULTRA-VIOLET
OR INVISIBLE
(1,000 to 8,900 A.U.)

PRIMARY COLORS

The primary colors of the spectrum are red, yellow and blue. By mixing these three colors together we can obtain all the other colors.

$$\left.\begin{array}{l} \text{Red} + \text{yellow} \\ \text{Yellow} + \text{blue} \\ \text{Blue} + \text{red} \end{array}\right. \left[\begin{array}{l} \rightarrow \text{orange} \\ \rightarrow \text{green} \\ \rightarrow \text{violet} \end{array}\right] \text{Secondary Colors}$$

Different mixtures of these pairs can give all other shades required.

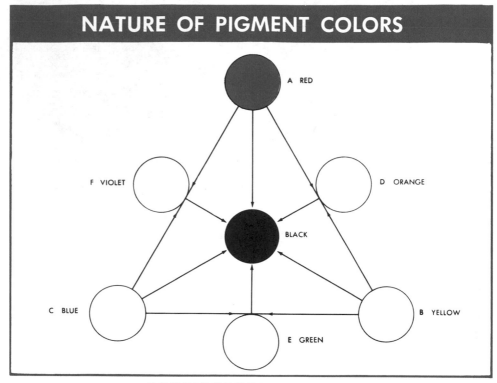

NATURE OF PIGMENT COLORS

A RED

F VIOLET

D ORANGE

BLACK

C BLUE

B YELLOW

E GREEN

COMPLEMENTARY COLORS

These are colors which are contrasting or directly opposite to each other.

red — green
orange — blue
yellow — violet

When blending lights rather than pigments, mixtures of each pair of colors form another color which appears to be white. Although, in the case of complementary pairs, this color would not be exactly white but tends toward grey.

PRACTICAL EXPERIMENT

Effects of colors may be studied by using colored chalk board chalks. Grind the chalk into small pieces and sprinkle them into shallow glass dishes (such as used for mixing a bleach) and place them on white paper. Various effects can be achieved by mixing different colored chalks into the dishes.

USE OF COMPLEMENTARY COLORS

Complementary pairs of colors are very important in hair coloring, e.g., to mask the yellow appearance of lightened hair, a purple or violet rinse can be used. However, if there is an excessive amount of yellow in the hair, *a blue rinse can produce a greenish cast.* This is caused by the primary color effect of the blue and excess yellow turning green.

TO OVERCOME A GREEN CAST, a red toner is used. The red in the toner and the green in the hair are also complementary colors and together they reflect a whitish light to the eye.

The best way to handle the problem of excess yellow in the hair is to use a mauve or violet rinse. This forms a direct complementary pair of colors with the background straw-yellow of lightened hair. A violet rinse gives a silvery white cast which is very attractive in the hair.

IF THE HAIR THROWS UP PURPLE when using a red tint (all tint colors are mixtures) then a gold or yellow toner will overcome it, as these are also complementary colors.

OTHER COLOR FACTS

Black is *NOT* a color but is a total absence of color.

White is a full mixture of all the spectrum colors.

Hues are full strength spectrum colors.

Tints are hues lightened by adding white.

Shades are hues darkened by adding black.

Pastels are hues mixed with black and white.

Tone refers to depth of each color ranging from light to full strength.

Warm colors are orange, red and yellow.

Cool colors are blue, green and violet.

SOURCE OF LIGHT

SUNSHINE OR DAYLIGHT The most natural light is daylight, which of course, comes from the sun about 93,000,000 miles away. It takes each ray of light approximately eight minutes to make this journey travelling at 186,000 miles per second.

The temperature of the sun is over 1,000,000°F. and from this fantastic amount of energy the following rays reach the earth:

    A. Ultra-violet rays
       (very short waves)   = 8%
    B. Infra-red rays
       (very long heat waves) = 80%
    C. Visible light rays   = 12%

The colors of the spectrum are found within the range of visible light received from the sun.

THE NATURE OF LIGHT

NATURAL LIGHT

WHITE
(From Sun)

GLASS PRISM

SPECTRUM COLORS

INFRA-RED

RED
ORANGE
YELLOW
GREEN
BLUE
VIOLET

V S
I P
S E
I C
B T
L R
E U
  M

ULTRA VIOLET

LONG
WAVES

SHORT
WAVES

ARTIFICIAL LIGHT

INCANDESCENT
LIGHTING

FLUORESCENT
LIGHTING

ARTIFICIAL LIGHT

NEED Natural light is available only during the daytime (apart from a small amount of light reflected by the moon and from the stars). So, in most parts of the world there are long periods when there is not enough natural light.

METHOD OF MAKING ARTIFICIAL LIGHT If metal is heated, the temperature gradually increases. As the metal gets hotter it begins to glow or to give off visible rays of light. At first the light is dull red (warm) —then red—yellow —blue white—white (very hot). If a toaster or electric radiator is switched on, this change can be clearly seen. But of course the toaster and radiator do not get very hot for if they did they would burn out. Therefore, they only give off a dull red form of light.

Early man discovered that burning oils or candles made a light but these materials do not burn very well and the light they gave was yellow and smokey.

INCANDESCENT LIGHT

A much higher temperature can be obtained by passing an electric current through a delicate filament inside a vacuumed light bulb. Despite the apparent efficiency, the light from an electric light bulb appears to be white but this light is actually yellow-white.

This can be proved by switching on an outside light during the daytime. The contrast of sunlight and artificial light shows the light to be weakly yellow.

In order to produce blue rays in artificial light, in an effort to overcome the yellowness, the filament must be made much hotter. However, it is not possible to make the electric light operate efficiently at very high temperatures, since less than 10% of the power used by an electric bulb is converted into visible light. The cost of creating and maintaining the great temperature required would be excessive and the life of the bulb would be greatly shortened.

Besides, it would be impossible to get bulbs to work at the temperature of the sun (1 million degrees). Thus, the incandescent light cannot be made to imitate natural daylight and these bulbs give off mainly a red and yellow form of white light.

FLUORESCENT LIGHT

Instead of heating a filament inside a bulb, an electric current can be passed through a tube coated with special powders. The electricity causes these powders to vibrate rapidly making them "fluoresce" or give off light.

By using different powders and colored glass in the tube, the modern fluorescent tube is able to supply light in a wide range. Still, not all fluorescent tubes give the same type of light (whereas incandescent lamps all produce light of the same quality and only vary in amount of light produced).

CONCLUSION

In selecting artificial light, the practitioner must take into account the following:

1. Cost of operation.
2. Intensity of light output.
3. Purpose of the light required.

Fluorescent tubes are cheaper to run continuously than ordinary lighting and therefore shops have installed them. However, not all of these tubes produce the same light output or the same type of light. Artificial lighting can vary from warm colors (containing more yellow) to cool colors (containing more blue) .

REFLECTION OF LIGHT

SCATTER OF NATURAL LIGHT Light tends to travel in straight lines, but everyone knows that we cannot look at the direct light from the sun because it is much too strong for our eyes. Consequently, most of the natural light we see arrives by reflection. (Some of the sun's rays are reflected by dust particles in the atmosphere producing the blue of the sky.) On account of this scatter, natural light gives a more even background of light, especially in a room well equipped with windows.

DIRECT REFLECTION Another part of the light that reaches our eyes is reflected directly from other objects. A mirror will reflect the rays of the sun and this will dazzle you the same as direct sunlight, because none of the rays are changed by the mirror.

Light is also reflected from a very flat or smooth surface in the same way, e.g., by calm water, polished metal or gloss paint. However, a person cannot see the object or surface itself if all the light falling on it is directly reflected back to the eyes.

LIGHT REFLECTION FROM HAIR In the case of hair it is known that the cuticle has a rough, scaly surface. Now rough surfaces tend to absorb rather than reflect light and so the cuticle of the hair could be expected to appear dull and drab. However, normal cuticle is also covered with a layer of natural oils, which smooths out some of the roughened scales and adds to its ability to reflect light. This added reflection produces the natural lustre or sheen of the hair.

DIFFERENCES IN CUTICLE If the hair is dry or dirty it will look dull, due to lack of reflection of light and when the hair is too oily or sprayed with lacquers, it will reflect too much light. Any hair coloring or cosmetic used on the hair should attempt to maintain the light reflection properties of the cuticle surface.

A curved surface will reflect more light to the eye than the same surface which is straight. So wavy hair will look lighter and shinier and this is another reason why wavy hair is preferred to straight hair.

ABSORPTION OF LIGHT

EFFECTS OF COLORED SURFACES   In normal circumstances some of the light falling on an object will be absorbed. In fact, we cannot see the object at all unless it does absorb some of the light. A white substance absorbs very little light and seems cool; a colored surface absorbs a great deal of light and seems warmer. The actual temperature will be higher as well.

TINTS AND PIGMENTS   Certain chemicals (tints and pigments) have exceptional ability to extract certain colors from light (the color of the tint or pigment being that of the *unabsorbed* part of white light) .

Thus, a pigment which absorbs violet, blue, blue-green, green and yellow rays will reflect orange and red rays. Accordingly, the pigment will be orange-red in color.

PIGMENTS IN HAIR   The natural pigments in hair are colored:

> black—absorbs all light
> brown—absorbs almost all light
> yellow—absorbs all except yellow
> red—absorbs all except red

Note:
Some light will be reflected directly by the cuticle as sheen, lustre or highlights and will not be absorbed in the hair.

NATURE OF TINTS AND PIGMENTS

Science does not know how tints and pigments are able to absorb one part and yet not another part of the spectrum.

COLORED MOLECULES

It is known that colored molecules in the tints or pigments are very special molecules which have the following features:

1. THEY ARE LARGE   All tints and pigments are made of very large molecules. However, not all large molecules are necessarily colored.

2. THEY HAVE A SPECIAL STRUCTURE   Colored molecules are also very active and so they are able to absorb or alter some of the light that falls on them because of their special structure.

FUNCTION OF THE EYE

STRUCTURE OF THE EYE The human eye is a wonderful organ of sight and converts light falling on the retina (at the back of each eye) into nervous sensations. These sensations pass to the brain and are recorded as vision or sight by a special area in the brain.

COLOR VISION

SPECIAL NERVE ENDINGS The retina can detect white light and absence of light (black). In addition, it has special nerve cells that can receive colored light. These cells pick up sensations from all colors of the spectrum. Combinations of these colors produce the never ending range of colors that it is possible to see.

COLOR-BLINDNESS However, in some individuals there may be a lack of certain cells for seeing specific colors. Because of this lack, *about one person in every twelve is partially color-blind.*

Other persons, though not color-blind in a strict sense, find it difficult to distinguish slight differences in colors in the yellow-red range. *In hair coloring this could be a serious handicap.*

EFFECT OF LIGHT SOURCE

COLORS SEEN IN NATURAL LIGHT The human eye can only see what it considers as ordinary colors in natural sunlight. Because of the absorption of different lights by colored objects the use of artificial lights may change the apparent color of the objects.

COLOR MATCHING PROBLEMS Lighting the shop by artificial lights should receive a great deal of attention from the practitioner because of the problematic changes in hair color that can take place. The source of light is *critical* especially for tinting and color matching. *A perfect match of colors under artificial light may appear quite different in daylight.*

INTENSITY OF LIGHT

EFFECT ON EYE The amount of light that falls on the eye has another effect on color vision. Color vision is best in sunlight and full daylight, but the intensity of daylight varies greatly. It is subjected to changes because of time of day (morning, mid-day, afternoon) weather (clear, cloudy) and the season (summer, winter).

In the dim light of dusk color vision is nearly gone and in the light of the half-moon, color vision is completely gone.

EFFECT ON PATRON Direct, clear sunlight is at least a hundred times brighter than artificial lighting at night, therefore, it is the best for viewing colors, although a bit unkind to persons with greying hairs. Many patrons take care not to look at their hair in strong light as they may not want to admit to themselves that their hair is losing its natural pigmentation.

SPECIAL INSENSITY EFFECTS For color matching of dark colors (e.g., dark browns) the intensity of illumination should be more than twice the intensity used for light colors (e.g., blondes).

PROFESSIONAL COLOR WORK

DISTRACTIONS Distraction of a competing color in the shop can upset your judgment about hair color.

AFTER-IMAGES Competing colors often cause after-images in the eyes. Therefore, *the walls in the working area, where tinting is done, should be in a neutral or pastel color with a mat or semi-gloss finish.* The haircolorist should wear a light colored or neutral grey uniform.

The color looked at last also influences color vision and staring at two colors, which are very close shades, will tend to blend them as one. *To contrast close colors the first reaction to their differences should be recorded.*

THE LIGHTING IN THE SHOP is a most important factor. Some hair coloring experts prefer to exclude daylight as its ever changing qualities make color work very difficult. Furthermore, they claim that the patron sees his or her own hair color only under indoor lighting. Therefore, the desired *color is judged in these conditions and should show up best under artificial lights rather than under natural lighting.* In the office or the main part of the shop, the lighting should be strong, without shadows. In the area set aside for hair coloring and tinting, the color composition of the lighting is most important.

COMPLEMENTARY COLOR EFFECTS ON SKIN The most popular fluorescent tubes produce an excess of blue light and this gives a ghastly appearance to the face and skin because there is a complementary color effect. The normal warm tones (pink to red) of the face and skin are drowned by the cold blue light and as a result are turned to a pale whitish, grey, unhealthy color.

Naturally, this has a very bad effect on patrons seeing themselves in the mirror. As a general rule, lighting in the shop should improve and emphasize the natural appearance of patrons and make them feel that they look their best. Therefore a warm light is most desirable.

RANGE OF TUBE LIGHTING

To overcome the cold blue effect of the normal tube, newer tubes are now available. These tubes have a yellow-pink or red component and will produce a warmer more flattering light.

Type of fluorescent tube	Light produced
Daylight (stamped on outside of tube)	*Cold light*—commonly used Suitable for reception areas only *NOT* suitable for hair coloring work
Warm White or warm white deluxe (stamped on outside of tube)	Restful, warm light Most suitable for color work Can be used with ordinary lighting to give harmonized color rendering

PROPER CHOICE OF LIGHTING

In order to select the correct lighting, the colorist should not rely solely on the advice of an electrician. The artisan should contact an illuminating engineer for consultation and up-to-date information on all aspects of lighting. The correct lighting costs no more to install or operate than inefficient lighting, but it will more than pay for itself in increased satisfaction to the patron.

COLOR MATCHING

A most important aspect of lighting in hair color work is the task of matching previously tinted hair with new growth (retouching). *As the older tint itself has changed color in the meantime, the exact same tint cannot always be used on the new growth in order to match.*

Matching of the older tint may be perfect under artificial light, yet show up in sharp contrast under another type of lighting or under natural conditions. So the lighting must be selected for proper color matching conditions with the correct balance of all the different wave lengths in the right proportions.

A balanced mixture of incandescent with color-corrected fluorescent lighting plus a natural sky illumination is probably the best compromise.

METHODS OF
LIGHTENING (BLEACHING)

Introduction

"Lightening" or "Bleaching" is the process by which the natural color in the hair is decreased. These terms will be used interchangeably throughout this chapter.

Lightening of the hair occurs under:

1. Natural conditions.
2. Artificial conditions.

NATURAL LIGHTENING

SUNLIGHT contains 8% of ultra-violet rays, which are intense, penetrating rays that affect the skin and hair. These rays falling on the skin and hair may have the following effects:

1. Production of the protective pigment, melanin, in the skin.
2. Relaxation of permanent waves.
3. Lightening of natural pigment in the hair.

In hotter climates, the intensity of ultra-violet radiation is quite high. In the summer, especially, the hair may be lightened and severely dried by sun and wind, particularly on the beach.

OTHER CAUSES Limited lightening may occur in the hair from the effects of water in swimming pools. Most pools are chlorinated in order to kill bacteria and this chlorine can cause lightening and other color effects (green discoloration) on the hair as well.

ARTIFICIAL LIGHTENING (BLEACHING)

The most general and convenient way of lightening the hair is through the action of special chemical lighteners. There are two main methods by which lightening of the hair is achieved:

1. ETCHING AWAY OF PIGMENT GRANULES Chemical lightening causes severe chemical changes in the hair. One technique of lightening the hair uses special products which slowly *etch* away the pigment granules in the cortex and the dissolved pigment spreads throughout the cortex. There is less light absorbed by the smaller areas of color and so the hair appears lighter. Although, of course, it is possible to lighten the hair color only slightly by this process.

2. CHEMICAL CHANGES OF HAIR PIGMENT A more drastic effect is caused by the action of chemical lighteners on the pigment granules, changing melanin to oxymelanin and in some cases breaking it down completely. Some of the chemicals used on the hair cortex for lightening are the following:

Hydrogen peroxide
Ammonia
Ammonium hydroxide
Ammonium persulfate
Percarbonate
Sodium peroxide

HYDROGEN PEROXIDE

NATURE Hydrogen peroxide (H_2O_2) is a light-blue liquid with unpredictable, explosive properties and in the pure form is a most dangerous material.

SOLUTIONS For professional use, hydrogen peroxide is broken down with pure water, after which it becomes most useful in the salon.

PROFESSIONAL USES

Hydrogen peroxide can be used for a number of purposes:

1. NEUTRALIZING (reforming) the S-bonds of the hair cortex during permanent waving.

2. LIGHTENING the natural pigment of the hair. (Either to lighten dark hair or to even out grey hair.)

3. MORDANT EFFECT (improved color fastness) Reacting on the resistant cuticle to increase its porosity for tinting.

4. DEVELOPING THE COLOR of the oxidation hair tints in permanent hair coloring.

5. STRIPPING excess tint from the hair under strong alkaline conditions.

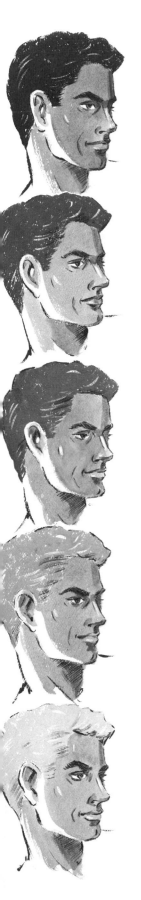
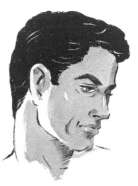
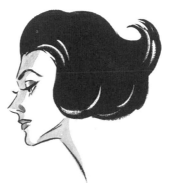
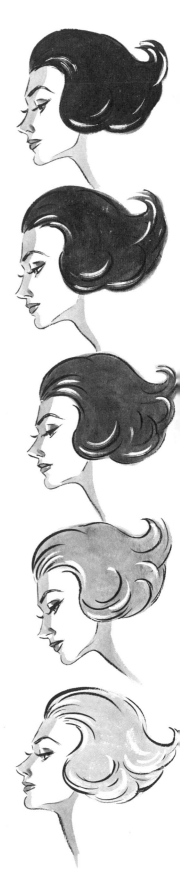

SEVEN STAGES IN LIGHTENING FROM DARK HAIR TO ALMOST WHITE
(Pale Yellow)

A virgin head of dark hair passes through seven stages before it arrives at the almost white stage.

The change in the color depends upon the type of lightener chosen and the length of time that it remains on the hair.

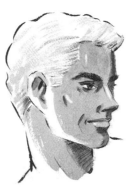
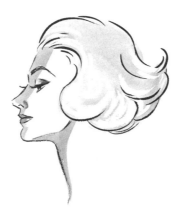

STRENGTH OF HYDROGEN PEROXIDE SOLUTIONS

The strength of hydrogen peroxide solutions is usually given in volumes or percentages.

EXAMPLE: 5   10   20   30   50   100 Vol.

              1.5%   3%   6%   9%   15%   30%

This means for every volume of hydrogen peroxide solution, there can be set free

5,   10,   20,   30,   50,   100 Vols. of oxygen gas.

This also means that hydrogen peroxide will further break down to leave only water on the hair. Thus it has the distinct advantage that no dangerous product is formed and left behind in the hair.

$$H_2O_2 \rightarrow H_2O + O$$

hydrogen   water   oxygen gas
peroxide

STABILIZED HYDROGEN PEROXIDE

Unfortunately, hydrogen peroxide breaks down very readily and it's possible to lose its strength long before reaching the shop. Therefore, the hydrogen peroxide solution must be stabilized. Certain protective chemicals (phosphates), may be added, together with diluted acid in order to accomplish the objective of stabilization.

Stabilized hydrogen peroxide is able to maintain its strength over longer periods but there is still no guarantee that it will keep fresh.

For example, the bottle must always be kept cool and in a dark place. If it "pops" when the stopper is removed, this indicates it is getting weaker (not that it is extra strong), because oxygen gas is being set free prematurely.

PRECAUTIONS Once opened, the bottle of hydrogen peroxide should be used within two days and the remainder thrown away. Do *NOT* pour the small, left-over amounts into stock bottles as this is false economy. One reason being that dust in the air will fall into the hydrogen peroxide which has been left in an open dish. If this is poured back into the bulk container this dust will cause it to break down more rapidly.

Hydrogen peroxide solutions are packed into brown bottles as light and heat will also cause it to break down more rapidly.

PREPARING HYDROGEN PEROXIDE LIGHTENERS

To activate the hydrogen peroxide for lightening, the practitioner can use two methods:

1. Add activators or boosters.
2. Increase strength.

ACTIVATORS

AMMONIA The addition of 5 to 10 drops of ammonia to each fluid ounce of hydrogen peroxide solution will increase the pH to 10.0 (approx.). Hydrogen peroxide is more unstable in alkaline conditions and it will then lighten the pigments in the hair cortex more rapidly.

This method of adding ammonia to hydrogen peroxide solutions was the basis of the old, clear liquid lighteners. But, since watery liquids run easily they are difficult to apply to the hair. This is especially true when retouching or lightening the new growth at the roots.

Furthermore, bleaching action ceases when bleach dries out and watery solutions are inclined to dry out before lightening is complete. Since lightening takes from 1/2 to 2 hours for each stage, this drying action produces unevenness of lightening along the hair shaft.

Liquid hydrogen peroxide and ammonia is useful as a "mordant" since the time of contact with the hair is shorter and a mordant effect can be achieved. This usage usually precedes coloring hair with temporary colors in an effort to make them longer lasting.

PREPARED ACTIVATORS Because of the problems associated with liquid lighteners, it is now common practice to use powder or emulsion cream activators. These mixtures, together with the hydrogen peroxide solution, form a paste for lightening the hair. The powders or creams contain the following:

1. *A measured amount of alkali* to neutralize the acid in hydrogen peroxide (the consistency of the mixture, serving as a guide to strength, ensures that excess alkalies cannot be added).
2. *Boosters* to de-stabilize or activate the hydrogen peroxide so as to get the maximum lightening action. Boosters give the effect of doubling the strength of the hydrogen peroxide solution (20 vol. becomes equivalent to 40 vol.).
3. *Colored toners* to overcome undesirable color casts (e.g., blue or red toners) formed by hydrogen peroxide.
4. *A thickening agent* to form a paste or cream. A cream lightener is easier to apply and also slows down the loss by evaporation. The action of the lightener continues for a longer period as a result.
5. *Conditioning and filling agents* to reduce risk of hair damage.
6. *Modifiers* to slow up the breakdown of the hydrogen peroxide. (Ammonia activates the hydrogen peroxide too quickly and its lightening action ceases in 20 minutes.) But actually, depending on the type of hair being lightened, 1/2 to 2 hours is required for each application of a lightener. The emulsion formed by the prepared activator and hydrogen peroxide will last nearly 2 hours, in most cases.

BIOLOGICAL ACTIVATOR Another method uses an enzyme for activating hydrogen peroxide solutions. It is claimed to be successful without making the hair cortex alkaline or causing damage in the hair.

INCREASING THE STRENGTH OF HYDROGEN PEROXIDE

The effectiveness of the hydrogen peroxide depends on its strength, so solutions of 20 vol. and under require an activator to speed their action. Although hydrogen peroxide solutions stronger than 30 vol. may be applied directly to the hair, the utmost care is required when lightening with such strong solutions. Their action is so fast that over-decolorization and hair damage is invariably the result. Only the best and fastest technicians can use these strengths.

DISADVANTAGES OF HYDROGEN PEROXIDE

STABILITY Hydrogen peroxide must be stabilized for storage in order to insure its strength because it can break down prematurely, releasing the oxygen that it contains. However, no guarantee can be given that even stabilized hydrogen peroxide will keep its strength over a long period. Moreover, there is no satisfactory way for the practitioner to test the hydrogen peroxide solution for stability.

Therefore, supplies should be purchased fresh, properly stored (in the refrigerator during hot weather) and bottles of hydrogen peroxide should not be kept if there are any doubts about their potency.

EFFECT OF METALS Hydrogen peroxide solutions react vigorously in the presence of metals. Therefore, metal bowls or implements should be kept away from the solutions. It is preferable to use wood, glass or plastic containers or bowls.

Hydrogen peroxide will react with metal salts which may have been used to tint the hair. For example, hair colored with "hair restorers" will cause a violent chemical change if lightened with hydrogen peroxide. The hair can be seriously damaged in the lightening process, therefore, a strand test must be made if metallic dyes are suspected.

INACCURATE FORMULA When activating a liquid bleach, the practitioner has a tendency to add excessive amounts of ammonia to hydrogen peroxide solutions, since consistency does not serve as a guide to strength as in the case of the cream type lighteners.

EFFECT ON CUTICLE The ammonia used in the hydrogen peroxide mixture will strip the natural oils from the cuticle because it has a chemical effect on the oils, turning them into a form of soap. Hence, the oils are easily washed out of the hair during the rinsing of the lightener. Hydrogen peroxide itself will react on these natural oils, with the result that lightened hair becomes dry and brittle (especially when atmospheric humidity is low).

Damage to hair cuticle caused by hair lightening
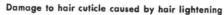

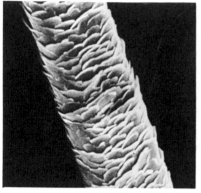
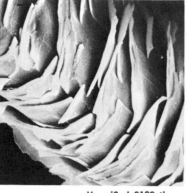
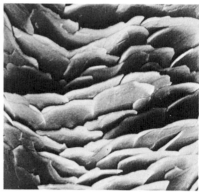

Magnified 1080 times   Magnified 2100 times   Magnified 2100 times

Courtesy: Gillette Company Research Institute, Rockville, Maryland

CONTROL OF ACTION Conditioners are often used in the cream or emulsion type lighteners which include hydrogen peroxide, but their effect is very poor. The strongly alkaline oxidizers required for lightening, practically defeat any attempt to modify its severity. *Hair conditioners are best applied after the lightening process is completed.*

ALKALIES IN LIGHTENERS Excess alkali causes too much swelling of the hair shaft and can leave it in a weakened, alkaline state even after thorough rinsing.

Traces of alkaline lightener, left in the cortex, results in "creeping oxidation." This means that the action of the lightener continues long after the client has left the salon (3 to 4 months).

Although, at the time of the lightening service, the patron's hair is left in a fairly good condition, afterwards, there is a steady weakening and breakdown of the hair. Large amounts of hair may come away in the brush or comb even weeks later.

Modern research has shown that all lighteners suffer this disadvantage.

PREVENTION OF CREEPING OXIDATION

To overcome this continued oxidation of the lightener, and at the same time restore "body" to the hair, apply a mild acid rinse. Special acids, in powder form, are sold for this purpose and are dissolved in water, then rinsed through the hair. Commercial preparations such as an acid cream rinse are satisfactory for both conditioning and neutralizing the traces of alkali.

These cream or acid rinses are applied through the hair after excess lightening solution is thoroughly removed by warm water. Hence, the normal acid condition of the hair is restored. Furthermore, a better hairstyle can be achieved when the lightened hair is finally styled.

INCREASING BLEACHING SPEED

Lightening of the hair is inclined to be a slow process. To lighten a virgin head of dark hair to pale yellow could take 10 to 12 hours. This is not only too long, but the hair may be severely damaged at the same time.

Most decoloring is thus properly confined to lightening the hair a few shades at a time. The total number of visits required depends on the original color of the hair and the degree of lightening desired by the patron. Practitioners can speed up the time considerably by using heating devices such as processing machines and steamers.

Steaming of the lightener will assist it to work faster, as heat and moisture are two requirements for effective lightening action.

THE DANGERS OF APPLYING HEAT However, care should be taken to be certain that there is enough lightening strength left while the hair is being heated. Heating the lightener shortens the active period of decolorization. The possibility of damage to the hair and scalp may also be aggravated by heating.

DANGER OF HYDROGEN PEROXIDE SOLUTIONS

EFFECT ON BODY Strong hydrogen peroxide solutions are very dangerous to handle. Hydrogen peroxide can be increased to 100 vol. for special purposes but, even at 20 vol. the solutions are still not safe. Hydrogen peroxide solutions react instantly when splashed on the skin or in the eye and they should be washed off immediately with plenty of water.

SPECIAL HANDLING Because of the unstable nature of these strong solutions they require special handling. For example, they should be only lightly capped, to save explosive breakage of the container, and on hot days it is good practice to store them in the refrigerator.

When pouring 100 vol. solutions practitioners are advised to wear protective gloves and a face mask of clear plastic. *NEVER* mix strong hydrogen peroxide solutions with strong ammonia solutions.

OFF SHADES

Hydrogen peroxide with ammonia as a lightening mixture is inclined to produce stubborn red to yellow shades in the hair. The reddish casts are very persistent and very difficult to remove.

CAUSE BY AMMONIA Some authorities claim that excess ammonia (sometimes added by practitioners) causes the red to appear in the hair. If the amount of ammonia is reduced, it is believed that the development of the red is not as intense during decolorizing. In any case, excess ammonia causes highly alkaline lightening conditions, which may result in damage to the hair.

CAUSE BY IRON Other experts say that some types of hair contains small amounts of iron (up to 0.1%). The iron is supposed to throw up the red shade during lightening, or the water used to shampoo the hair may gradually build up deposits of iron in the hair. Therefore, these experts claim that ammonia has nothing to do with the throwing up of red during lightening.

REMOVAL OF OFF SHADES The red color can be removed by prolonged lightening, reducing the quantity of ammonia, or increasing the strength of hydrogen peroxide without the use of ammonia.

The strawlike color can be neutralized by using its complementary color, violet. If the violet contains too much blue and the hair is still strongly yellow, then the result will be a fatal green discoloration.

However, as previously indicated, a red toner can solve the problem of removing a tell-tale green cast. Of course, the actual colors are not removed by this procedure, but the eye is deceived into thinking that they are, and that the color of the hair is now really silvery-white.

OTHER TYPES OF LIGHTENERS

Because of the problems associated with hydrogen peroxide solutions, newer, powder lighteners have been developed. These are oxidizing agents which lighten the hair pigments in exactly the same way as hydrogen peroxide. Their advantage is that they are more stable and will keep their strength much longer, thus, costly bottles and risk of hydrogen peroxide explosions are avoided. For convenience this type of lightener comes as powders, tablets or creams.

EXAMPLES Urea peroxide is a very popular oxidizing agent for the powder type of lightener. Its action is very similar to hydrogen peroxide and is closely related to it, chemically. Urea peroxide picks up moisture from the air very quickly and therefore is often sealed in tubes. In appearance it looks very much like damp sugar crystals (if not already ground into a powder). It is often labelled as the "activator."

FORMULA Many blonding or highlighting creams use powder lighteners (urea peroxide) together with various conditioners, toners, or modifiers, in emulsion form, in order to produce special effects.

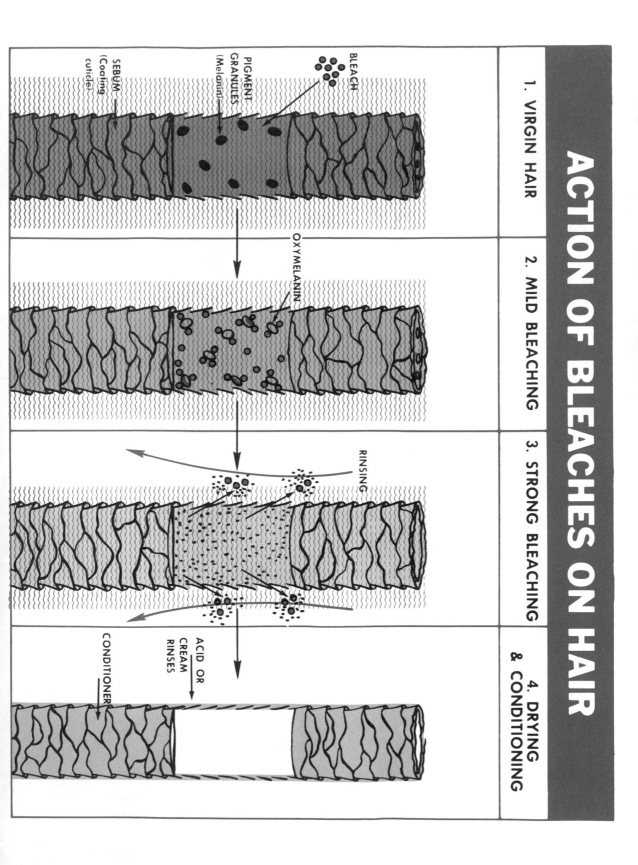

ACTION OF BLEACHES ON HAIR

1. VIRGIN HAIR

BLEACH
PIGMENT GRANULES (Melanin)
SEBUM (Coating cuticle)

2. MILD BLEACHING

OXYMELANIN

3. STRONG BLEACHING

RINSING

4. DRYING & CONDITIONING

ACID OR CREAM RINSES
CONDITIONER

DISADVANTAGES However, many of these products are not suitable for professional hair lightening as they are very slow. Despite its many disadvantages, hydrogen peroxide still remains as the primary lightening agent used by professionals. Nevertheless, it is likely that new and improved formulas will eventually replace hydrogen peroxide as the professional lightening agent.

CHEMISTRY OF HAIR LIGHTENING

Whereas many bleaches are now well-known, scientists are not able to give much information as to the exact manner in which these materials decolorize the natural hair pigments. Much more information must be gathered before the picture is complete.

NATURAL PIGMENTS

There are two main groups of hair pigments:

Melanin —gives black to brown shades.
Oxymelanin —gives red to yellow shades.

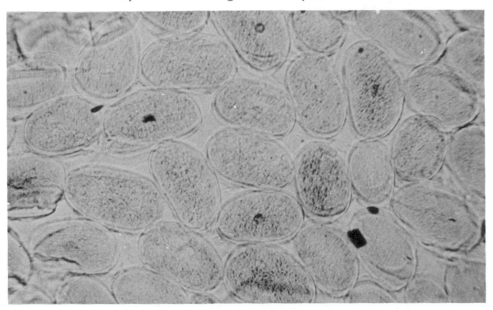

Cross-section of hairs showing natural pigments in auburn hair. (Note absence of color in cuticle)—
Courtesy: C. V. Stead, I.C.I. and American Perfumer

ACTION OF BLEACH ON NATURAL PIGMENTS

The action of hair lightening is believed to take place in two stages. The melanin molecules are first oxidized into the oxymelanin form.

$$\textit{Melanin} \;\rightarrow\; \textit{Mild} \;=\; \textit{Oxymelanin}$$
$$\text{(Black or Brown)} \quad \text{Oxidation} \quad \text{(Red or Yellow)}$$

This oxidation is very easy, causes little damage and usually proceeds smoothly because the mild agent applied to the hair will only oxidize the dark melanin into the lighter shades of oxymelanin.

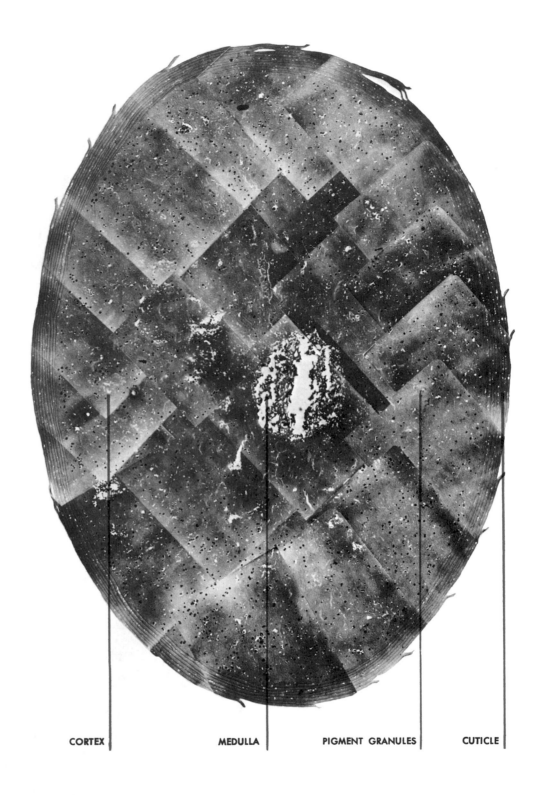

CORTEX | MEDULLA | PIGMENT GRANULES | CUTICLE

A cross section of an entire hair fiber; formed by taking a series of photos which were assembled to create a composite picture, magnified 1400 times. Note especially the layers of the cuticle, the cortex and the medulla, all clearly defined. Of special interest are the thousands of pigment (color) granules which are so important in hair lightening. *Courtesy: Gillette Company Research Institute, Rockville, Maryland*

ACTION ON OXYMELANIN The large oxymelanin molecule (red or yellow pigment) cannot be easily oxidized any further. Total destruction of the large molecules are required for any more decolorization to take place in the hair. This total destruction of the large molecules requires a much stronger treatment. It can readily be seen that it is fairly easy to lighten the black or brown shades, however, it must be noted that the mildly oxidized pigment throws up red or yellow shades, red in particular, when liquid ammonia-peroxide lighteners are used.

TOTAL LIGHTENING Stronger hydrogen peroxide (above 20 vol. and without added ammonia) will cause destructive oxidation of the oxymelanin. The large oxymelanin molecule is split into smaller fragments. These small pieces of the molecules are not colored and so the cortex is whitened to give perfectly lightened hair.

As the colorless fragments of the pigment are extremely small, they are relatively easy to rinse out of the cortex through the cuticle scales. Rinsing off the excess lightener also removes some of these particles from the hair.

KERATIN DAMAGE Hair melanin reacts much more rapidly with peroxide than does hair keratin. This is quite fortunate, otherwise an extensive amount of damage would be done to the hair keratin itself during the bleaching process. However, the melanin pigment represents only a very small fraction of the hair (usually about 2%) and thus it is only reasonable to expect that in the process of bleaching this 2% of the fiber, some chemical attack (hair damage) will also occur on the remainder of the hair. Hair keratin contains many different chemical bonds that can theoretically be broken by peroxide.

THE NATURE OF BLEACHING DAMAGE

Chemical analysis shows that the main point of attack of strong peroxide on hair keratin is the disulfide crosslinks (S-Bonds) :

Disulfide Crosslink + Hydrogen Peroxide → Oxidized disulfide
(Cystine)   (Cysteic acid)

Analysis of the building block amino acids making up hair keratin reveals that the change produced is a decrease in the disulfide crosslinks (cystine) and a corresponding increase in cysteic acid, the oxidized form of this amino acid.

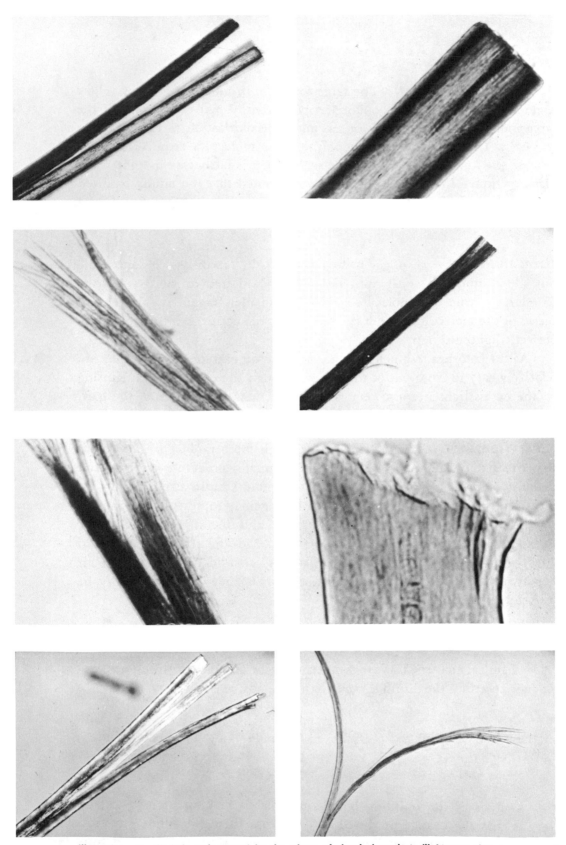

Illustrations of split hair ends caused by the misuse of chemical products (lighteners, tints or permanent wave solutions) in the performance of hair services.

PEROXIDE SHAMPOO Lightening has been considered by professionals as a separate service. But sometimes there is just a need for lightening or lifting the hair color a few shades. Peroxide shampoos are often used for this purpose. Because of their low hydrogen peroxide content, they only lighten the hair a little.

PRE-LIGHTENING Formerly, the hair was pre-lightened before it was tinted to a lighter color than the natural shade. A more common practice is to use stronger hydrogen peroxide as the tint developer. This stronger oxidizing solution can lighten the natural pigments and develop the required shade of tint at the same time.

Needless to say, there is little tint shade developed in the hair; otherwise it would produce a darker shade than the natural pigment in the hair. As a result, *these tint shades must be in the warm (red or blonde) color range.*

PRACTICAL WORK

pH OF LIGHTENERS

1. Take a few ounces of hydrogen peroxide and some drops of Universal Indicator solution. Then add, drop wise, 880 ammonia water.
   A. Note the rapid pH change.
   B. Record the number of drops of 880 ammonia required for a safe lightening solution (deep blue).
   C. Add more drops and see how quickly unsafe lightening conditions may develop (purple).
2. Take a prepared lightening powder and add required amounts of hydrogen peroxide. Then test pH of the resulting lightening emulsion. Note that conditions are safe for lightening (blue-deep blue) when the emulsion has the correct consistency.

REACTIONS OF LIGHTENERS

1. Add a few crystals of a metal salt (e.g., ferrous sulfate) to a hydrogen peroxide solution. Note vigorous reaction, heat and gas evolved in the process.

   (*Stand clear during this test for safety reasons.*) *This shows how hydrogen peroxide is affected by metals.*
2. To a diluted solution of potassium permanganate add:
   a) Hydrogen peroxide solution
   b) Urea peroxide (or "activator")

Note lightening of purple color and the faster action of the hydrogen peroxide.

IRON TEST

1. Take a small quantity of hair and dissolve in boiling potassium hydroxide. Cool and acidify with acetic acid. Then add a few crystals of potassium or ammonium thiocyanate.

   A pink to red coloration indicates iron. (This test may also be conducted on tap water after acid has been added to show presence of iron.)

MICROSCOPIC EXAMINATION Examine hair under a low powered microscope (40x to 100x) or a hand lens. Mount the hair strands on a glass slide with one drop of water/glycerine or tap water.

Tints, color rinses, pigments, cortex, medulla (if present) and hair damage, are easily seen. (Note that hair lacquers and sprays may be clearly visible but broken fragments are often confused with the cuticle scales. However, more specialized techniques are necessary to observe fine details of hair structure.)

CHAPTER 20

METHODS OF
HAIR COLORING

Introduction

Hair coloring has proven to be one of the most dramatic and profitable advancements in hair care, in recent times.

Since the dawn of history various materials have been employed to change the color of hair. However, only recently have advances been made in the science of hair coloring which now offer a vast range of superior colors and shades to the artisan. These materials and their methods of application compose the subject of professional hair coloring.

DESIRED PROPERTIES OF A HAIR COLORING PRODUCT

1. It should not injure the hair or scalp.
2. The color should be natural looking and attractive to the eye.
3. The hair should not lose its ability to be set and waved and the texture and sheen must be retained after coloring.
4. The color should not fade when the hair is exposed to long periods of sunlight, wind, salt water or heat.
5. The color must not strip out when using hairdressings, conditioners, setting lotions, hair sprays and shampoos.
6. There should be no discoloration when the hair is treated with alkalies, acids, cold waving solutions, etc.
7. It should not cause an allergic reaction.
8. The color must be developed safely, yet rapidly, so that only one application is required.
9. Dermatitis or dandruff should not appear after the coloring treatment.

10 The range and depth of color must cover all possible wishes of the patron.

11 When required, the color should be capable of being easily stripped or removed from the hair.

12 The hair coloring should be cheap and simple to apply.

Needless to say, the foregoing requirements for hair coloring products are very strict. There are *NO* coloring agents, at present, which meet all of these requirements and few which meet most of them.

CLASSIFICATION OF COLORING PRODUCTS

There are three general classifications for hair coloring products:

1 Temporary colors.
2 Semi-permanent colors.
3 Permanent colors.

1. TEMPORARY HAIR COLORINGS

COLOR RINSES OR WATER RINSES Some temporary hair colorings are also known as color rinses or azo-dyes. And, since they are acid, they leave the hair in fairly good condition. But, unfortunately, since color rinses are acid and harden the cuticle, they fail to penetrate the cuticle and only a very small amount of color is adsorbed on the surface.

Moreover, because they are quite soluble in water, the color which is left on the cuticle is easily rinsed out afterwards. In addition, since they do not pass into the cortex there is very little color and the natural pigments (if present) are still visible through the slightly colored cuticle. On the positive side, they have a very wide range of colors.

USEFUL FEATURES Water rinses are available in a wide range of colors and despite their handicaps, are very popular. Most of the color is removed with the next shampoo and therefore this may appear to give poor value for the money. However, many patrons prefer variety. The color rinses give them an opportunity to try out a new color before making it a permanent feature. They may also like the opportunity to wear a flamboyant, extravagant color on special occasions without being stuck with it for months afterwards.

Water rinses are also useful as complementary colors for removing off-shades in the hair.

DISADVANTAGES Some rinses are affected by the physical condition of the cuticle and as a result this may cause unevenness of coloring along the hair shaft. Bleached hair tends to take up more color than virgin hair; and, therefore, bleach may be used as a mordant on virgin hair.

COLORING SHAMPOOS Color rinses are also used in shampoos or wetting agents. However, the color intensity is very slight with this type of coloring material. Tints are very expensive substances, hence it would be much too costly to manufacture a shampoo with enough soluble tint in it to give good coverage.

PROBLEMS OF TEMPORARILY COLORING THE HAIR

In order to appear natural looking the hair coloring must pass through the cuticle and enter into the cortex. This is necessary to avoid the heavy "painted" look that a coated cuticle gives.

However, hair coloring molecules found in non-permanent products are very large, and large colored molecules are notoriously:

     1 unstable — *liable to fade*
     2 insoluble — *require special solvents*
     3 slow acting — *penetrate into hair with difficulty*

For coloring to be effected, water soluble molecules are required which can quickly enter the hair cortex. Yet the same molecules must be colored, non-fading (fast) and resist being washed out by shampoos, rinses or cold waving solutions.

OTHER DIFFICULTIES

1. The cuticle is a restricting barrier to the passage of large molecules. The size capable of entry into the cortex is therefore very limited.
2. The cortex itself is made of hard keratin. Keratin is an unreactive substance and there are few places available for fixing (attaching) the colored molecule. But, color must be fixed in the hair by some means if the colored molecules are not to be removed by the next shampoo.
3. The hair must be colored only under cold to lukewarm conditions. Many colors will be fast to hair when boiled together. But, of course, this technique cannot be used on the scalp.
4. The skin and hair are, chemically, very closely related since they are but different forms of keratin. Colored molecules, which will join with the hard keratin of the hair, will also attach to the soft keratin of the skin which is more reactive than the hard keratin. Therefore, the scalp will stain more quickly than the hair will pick up color.

OTHER TYPES OF TEMPORARY HAIR COLORINGS

We can conveniently divide the usual temporary hair colorings into:

COLORING SPRAYS Temporary colorings are also used in hair sprays. They are applied directly from a pressure-pack can, giving a more even coating to the cuticle.

Some coloring sprays contain aluminum powders to give the hair a shimmering, exciting look. Unfortunately, they are inclined to flake off when in contact with pillows, hats, combs, etc.

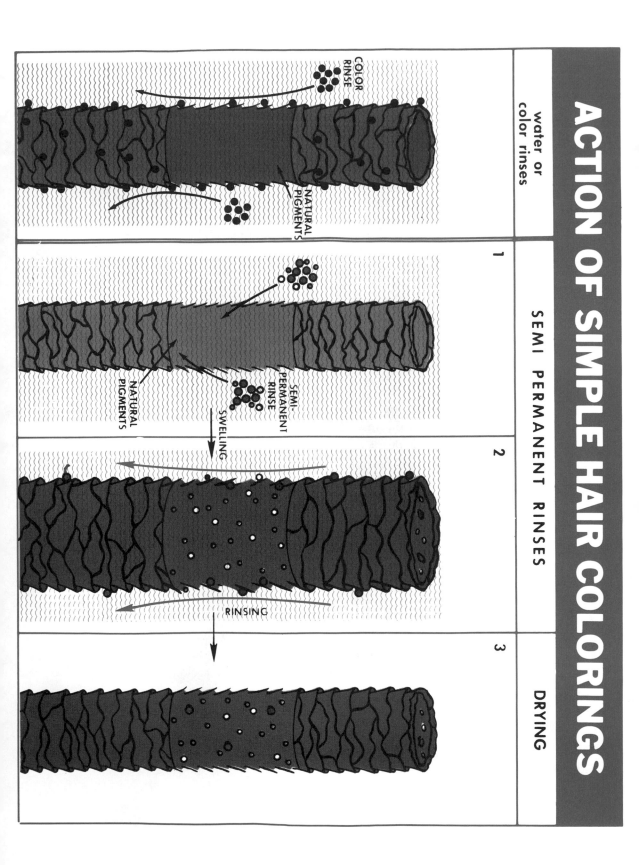

ACTION OF SIMPLE HAIR COLORINGS

water or color rinses

1

COLOR RINSE

NATURAL PIGMENTS

SEMI PERMANENT RINSES

SEMI-PERMANENT RINSE

NATURAL PIGMENTS

SWELLING

2

RINSING

3

DRYING

CRAYONS Another form of temporary hair coloring is colored crayons. These colors are massaged or brushed on with a special applicator. They are very useful for retouching new growth of hair to match previous treatments.

2. SEMI-PERMANENT HAIR COLORINGS

These are colors that persist a little longer on the hair. There are claims that they last up to 8 shampoos in the case of porous hair, but it is rare that they remain on normal hair for more than 3 or 4 shampoos. Semi-permanent rinses contain small colored molecules, although larger than those used for color rinses.

USE OF ALKALIES Many are mildly alkaline with a pH range around 8.0 to 9.0, and many also contain foaming, wetting agents. The alkali swells the imbrications of the cuticle and allows a limited number of the larger molecules of the semi-permanent rinse to pass into the cortex.

However, there is a limit to the swelling of the hard keratin caused by the mild alkaline shampoo. Stronger alkalies, furthermore, will excessively weaken the hair, so there is a limit to the size of the colored molecules that can safely penetrate into the cortex.

Recent developments in this field include products that use salt bonds to improve fastness to the hair. Thus the pH can be lowered to pH 7.0 to 8.0 and leave porous hair in a better condition.

USE OF "THIO" Some types of semi-permanent rinses use weakened ammonium thioglycolate together with the color. The "thio" allows the keratin chains to separate even further and by this means more color can pass into the cortex within the time permitted.

The "thio," of course, causes the breaking of S-bonds and the subsequent weakening of the hair. The colorist would have to carefully set and dry (for the purpose of atmospheric oxidation) the hair afterwards or the hair will tend to lose its wave. A mild acid rinse would be needed to neutralize the alkali.

COLOR FASTNESS is achieved because the colored molecules of tint, once having passed into the cortex by the swelling process, are trapped. This is done by rinsing away the alkali and drying the hair. *Furthermore, the molecules combine with the salt bonds in the cortex to give added fastness.* Nevertheless, mild swelling of the hair takes place during every shampoo and the color tends to wash out of the cortex a little each time.

PROBLEMS ASSOCIATED WITH
SEMI-PERMANENT COLORINGS

BROWNS The color range is good, especially in the red and blonde shades. However, brown shades present problems. The browns are usually made of mixtures of red, yellow and blue colored molecules. The only *good* blue molecules are larger than the reds or yellows and this causes various color problems, depending on the porosity of the imbrications of the hair.

In addition, the formula usually has a large excess of the blue molecules in order to get enough of them into the cortex of normal or resistant hair. On the other hand porous hair might absorb too many blue molecules. This excess of blue tint could react with the residual yellow in lightened hair to give a disastrous green cast.

REDS The red molecules in the brown and auburn colored products tend to outlast the blue and grey colors. As a result, an uneven reddish discoloration can develop in the hair because of shampooing. The shampoo selectively washes out some molecules and not others.

ACTION ON GREY HAIR Semi-permanent rinses do not cover more than 10% of the grey hair. However, they are quite good on almost white hair for evening out the shade. With nearly white hair, it is necessary to use a bluish-violet toner to produce a silvery cast. If neutral grey or blue rinses are applied on the yellowish white hair, it could result in a pale green cast.

The white hair is often discolored from natural oils, scalp tonics, perspiration, hair dressings, smoke, etc., and therefore is often slightly yellowish. The action of sunlight seems to increase this yellowish tinge, particularly on the ends. The water used for rinsing off the shampoo may itself contain dissolved substances which leave a dingy yellow residue on white or grey hair.

3. PERMANENT HAIR COLORINGS

In general, most patrons prefer their hair coloring to last much longer than a few shampoos. Originally, hair tints were intended solely to hide greying hair. Today patrons of all ages choose to color their hair simply to enhance their appearance. Permanent hair tints may be found in a number of different types.

VEGETABLE DYES

HENNA Many of the older hair dyes took this form. Only henna remains as a hair coloring, but its usefulness is very limited. Henna powder is mixed with water and mild acid to form a paste. The method is messy and the range of colors is very small.

INTERFERENCE WITH PERMANENT WAVING Henna penetrates into the cortex and produces a lasting color effect. But it does this by combining with S-bonds. As a result these S-bonds are no longer available for permanent waving and this creates a serious disadvantage. In addition, excess henna slowly builds up on the cuticle to give a flat, hard, auburn color.

METALLIC DYES

These hair dyes also have little purpose today. The metallic film on the hair cuticle, which gives the color, creates serious limitations. Some of the metal salts enter the cortex and combine with the S-bonds. Again, as with henna, this interferes with permanent waving.

The metal salts (lead, silver, copper) are very poisonous. They also cause a violent reaction with hydrogen peroxide lighteners on the hair. (A strand test will show the presence of metals in the hair.) These metallic dyes are used as so-called "hair restorers." By slowly building up a color deposit on the hair they were believed to "restore" the natural color.

Claims are made that they can be stripped by special treatments, but in effect, these are unreliable. The only way to properly and completely remove metallic dyes is to cut off that part of the hair.

OXIDATION DYES OR TINTS

Because the word "dye" is associated with the former, unsatisfactory vegetable and metallic hair colorings, oxidation dyes are commonly known as hair tints.

Hair tints have been known since 1883, and originally were employed for coloring animal furs (itself a form of hard keratin).

Hair tints are called various names, but actually they all describe the same chemical product. Here are some of the terms used:

1. Synthetic or organic tints.
2. Para dyes or tints.
3. Aniline derivative tints.
4. Oxidation tints.
5. Color shampoos (certain types only).

Note:

If a hair coloring comes in two bottles which have to be mixed together or the hair coloring has to have hydrogen peroxide added to it, then it is really a hair tint or oxidation dye, regardless of what it is called.

ACTION OF HAIR TINTS

TINT BASE Hair tints act in a different way than color rinses. The molecules of the colored rinses are the largest size that can pass through the cuticle. Hair tints, on the other hand are applied in the form of small, colorless molecules. As tint bases or intermediates, these molecules pass easily into the cortex.

ACTION OF HAIR TINTS

TINT BASE PLUS DEVELOPER ON HAIR

1. TINT MIXTURE ENTERS INTO CORTEX.

2. TINT PIGMENTS FORMED.

3. SHRINKING OF CUTICLE SCALES TO TRAP PIGMENT.

DRYING AND CONDITIONING

CONDITIONER

DEVELOPER   Inside the cortex the action of the developer, usually hydrogen peroxide (20 to 30 vol.), *combines the colorless molecules of the tint base into giant colored molecules*. These large molecules are stable and being insoluble, give a permanent color to the hair.

ADVANTAGES OF HAIR TINTS   Hair tints cannot be shampooed out of the hair because their molecules are too big to pass through the cuticle. Furthermore, there is evidence that they form bonds with the keratin chains in the cortex and thus become firmly affixed. Unlike the older dyes, this bond is an acid bond, and so leaves the H-bonds and S-bonds free for various hair treatments. Thus tinted hair can be permanently waved and styled with a minimum of trouble to the practitioner.

OLDER FORMS OF HAIR TINTS

LIQUID HAIR TINTS   The chemical compounds which form the tint bases are not very soluble in water. Older liquid tints overcame this problem of insolubility by using alcohol and water mixtures as solvents. They were primarily used in the darker shades for covering grey hair. They were quite concentrated (3 to 6% of tint) and resulted in heavy, deep applications of color to the hair.

Modern liquid tints are water emulsions of tint bases, containing the same amounts as the cream tints.

DARK SHADES   Liquid tints used for bases are chemicals known as "para" tints. The term "para" is short for para-phenylene-diamine. This dyestuff gives deep black shades when it is fully developed into giant molecules by the mild oxidation of the developer.

LIGHTER SHADES   To lighten the tint shade, other oxidation tints are used as mixtures with phenylene-diamine. As the required shades become lighter, this dark form of "para" tint is reduced in the formula. In the blonde or light ash stage "para" tints are entirely left out of the tint base.

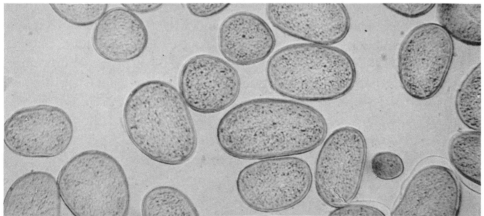

Auburn hair tinted by a mixture of phenylene and toluene diamines. (Note that color also occurs in cuticle)—*Courtesy: C. V. Stead, I.C.I. and American Perfumer*

NEWER OXIDATION TINTS

Most of the "para" tints are now replaced by newer types (which are not "para"). "Oxidation tints" is now a better term than the older one, "para" tints.

In any case, the "para" tints are not the compounds which form the color pigments inside the cortex because they are only the bases or intermediate substances.

CHEMICAL SHORTHAND FOR TINTS

The name of this substance, "para-phenylene-diamine," is really an example of chemical shorthand. Each term describes the exact nature of each molecule of the tint base or "parent" substance. For example—

"para" = prefix meaning "opposite" (as in *para*dox, *para*chute, *para*-llel, etc.)

"di" = prefix meaning "twice" or "double" (as in *di*vide, *di*lemma, *di*oxide, etc.)

This means that the tint base molecule (phenylene) has two (di) free arms (amine) which are opposite one another. This complete molecule is usually made from aniline which is a synthetic organic compound. The aniline molecule provides a ready source of the six-sided "ring" structure shown in the diagram (see illustration ⟶). This explains the reason for calling these hair tints aniline derivative dyes. The aniline molecule also has a six-sided ring, but it has only one amine group. But when another amine group is attached, the parent "ring" is called phenylene.

But even this substance (the para-phenylene-diamine molecule) is completely colorless and would be useless for a hair coloring. However, it can slip through the cuticle and enter the cortex. This action is aided by the swelling of the hair due to the excess alkali in the tint base formula.

THE DEVELOPER CHEMICALLY JOINS TOGETHER AMINE GROUPS or free arms from adjacent molecules. The developer will only work in alkaline conditions in the presence of excess ammonia and a pH 9.0–10.0. The coupling together of hundreds of the smaller colorless tint base molecules changes them into "giant" chains of colored pigment. As these pigments are much too large to pass out through the cuticle scales, they are trapped within the cortex making the tinting process a "permanent" chemical change. In addition, the tint pigments are joined to the keratin by salt bonds instead of cystine bonds as was the case in the metallic dyes.

CHEMISTRY OF HAIR TINTS

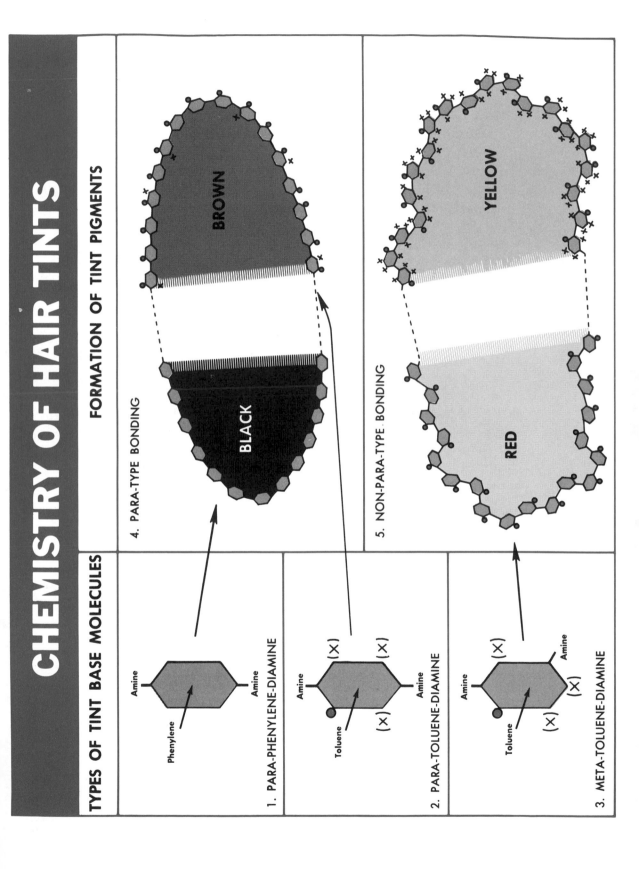

FORMATION OF TINT PIGMENTS

TYPES OF TINT BASE MOLECULES

4. PARA-TYPE BONDING

BROWN

BLACK

5. NON-PARA-TYPE. BONDING

YELLOW

RED

Amine

Phenylene

Amine

1. PARA-PHENYLENE-DIAMINE

Amine

Toluene

(X)

(X)

Amine

2. PARA-TOLUENE-DIAMINE

Amine

Toluene

(X)

(X)

Amine

(X)

3. META-TOLUENE-DIAMINE

FORMULA FOR LIQUID TINTS

Most of the liquid tints are formulas of alcohol and water (95%). This mixture has a tendency to run very easily, so it is not easy to apply to the hair without it running on to the scalp. Likewise retouching of new growth is particularly difficult. The use of the plastic squeeze bottle somewhat relieves the problem.

Furthermore, the alcohol makes the liquid tint dry out quickly and once dry, the action of developing and penetrating ceases. Because of this tendency to dry out in certain areas, the hair tint could end up with a moth-eaten or patchy look. Besides, the dried out tint is very difficult to shampoo from the hair and may create additional problems later on.

SOLUTION A—THE BASE You can identify this solution since it has to be kept in dark brown bottles in order to exclude light. In addition, the bottles have to be completely filled to keep out air. So small dark bottles packed in cardboard cartons is the container generally used.

FORMULA

Tint Bases

Para Tint 1	— black shade
Para Tint 2	— red shade
Non-Para Tint 3	— blonde shade

AMMONIA Since the tint base will only develop color in strongly alkaline conditions (pH 9 to 10) ammonia is required as an activator. The alkali also causes swelling of the hair and permits faster penetration of tinting chemicals into the cortex. Furthermore, it activates the hydrogen peroxide in the developer.

SOLUTION B—THE OXIDIZER This is mainly a stabilized (acid), 20 vol. (or 30 vol.) hydrogen peroxide solution.

NEWER CREAM AND LIQUID HAIR TINTS

Chemically, cream tints are identical to modern liquid tints but because of the difficulties with the liquid tints, these cream tints in collapsible tubes have grown to be quite popular.

FORMULA Because of the skin irritation caused by the para-phenylene-diamine (also known as phenylene diamine) there has been an attempt made to replace this tint with its nearest relative, para-toluene diamine (also known as toluene diamine or toluylene diamine).

PARA-TOLUENE-DIAMINE

First, by adding a special group to the "ring" structure (shown in red on the illustration) it is changed from a phenylene to a toluene base. This reduces the danger of dermatitis (although a patch test is still required by law).

The problem of having hair tints in a lighter color range is overcome to some degree by adding certain other groups at various places on the ring (shown in the diagram by X positions). This gives shades in a brown range without preventing the free arms joining to form an insoluble tint pigment in the cortex.

The practitioner can always check this information by looking at the label on the tint tube. Suppliers are required by law to indicate the para-dye used and the total concentration in each tube.

The toluene diamine tints do not color the hair as deeply as the phenylene diamines. Because of the harsh conditions of strong sunlight, drying winds, etc., it has been found necessary in some areas to use a stronger cream tint base than required in order to achieve the corresponding shade elsewhere. In general the para-phenylene series is less than 1.2% in concentration in the modern tint. (The old liquid tints were as high as 6% in strength of "Para" tint.)

CONCENTRATION OF SHADES . The "para" toluene series is more concentrated than the para-phenylene creams (but still less than liquid tints used to be).

EXAMPLE:

	Concentration
Dark Shades	Approximately
Black	1.7%
Brown	
Light Shades	Approximately
Blonde	0.4% to 0.1%
Red	

The net result is that the darker shades contain more tint bases. Therefore, they tend to be more sensitive to the skin than the lighter shades.

COLOR RANGE The new tints provide a wide variety of warm natural shades and are usually numbered for ease of identification. Mixtures of the tint bases by the colorist can meet almost any color requirement of the patron.

SALES APPEAL The older liquid tints were developed to hide greying hair by forming dark shades and were mostly intended for older patrons. But modern tints are used for changing hair color and therefore, they appeal to patrons of all ages.

EFFECT OF REDUCED CONCENTRATION The reduced concentration of the modern tint creates a problem in itself. The old "para" dyes could penetrate rapidly into the hair and then develop quickly. Nowadays, tint base molecules are bigger and so are slower moving (which has the effect of minimizing skin sensitivity).

SPEED OF APPLICATION

The development of color begins as soon as the liquid or cream tint base and the hydrogen peroxide are mixed together. This means that after mixing, the prepared tint must be applied to the hair as soon as possible because, once the giant colored molecules form, they are not able to penetrate the cuticle.

Also, particularly in the case of a light shade, there is much less tint base to develop into color pigment. Therefore, the colorist must not waste a moment of time during the tinting process, otherwise, the desired shade may not develop in the hair cortex.

META-TOLUENE-DIAMINE

For still lighter shades in the red to blond tints it is necessary to change the nature of one of the free arms (amine) to the "meta" site on the toluene ring.

"Meta" = prefix meaning "higher" or "change" (as in *meta*physical, *meta*center, *meta*morphose, etc.)

This means that we have to change the name of the compound in the chemical shorthand to meta-toluene-diamine. (This information is often carried on the label or pack of the product.)

The concentration of tint bases is also lowered in these lighter shades from 2.0% to less than 0.1% in some cases.

Nevertheless, even if the free arms have been changed from "para" to "meta" the developer or oxidizer can still link these molecules together to form giant tint pigments as before.

This is yet another reason for changing the name from "para tints" to "synthetic or oxidation dyes." This gives a more precise chemical meaning to the tint bases used today. Once again, there may be certain other groups substituted in the "X" position to give an almost endless range of permanent colors.

ADDITIVES

EMULSIFIER New emulsifiers have overcome the problem of getting the slightly soluble tint bases into solution. By using water as a carrier, the emulsion will not dry out as rapidly as when alcohol is used for dissolving the tint bases.

THICKENERS Other materials are added to thicken the cream in the case of tube packaging. As the emulsion creams contain about 90% water, the emulsion must be thickened. If the emulsion breaks down in storage to form a thin watery fluid, that tube or tint is useless and should not be used. This separation shows that the product was unstable and should be discarded.

WETTING AGENTS Wetting agents are required to remove excess sebum from the cuticle. Oils and greases can slow down the entry of the tint base molecules into the cortex. Consideration must be given to the fact that if the hair is excessively dirty or greasy, it requires a preliminary shampoo.

MODIFIERS Modifiers are often used to give special color effects to the hair. For example, the popular ash shades in tinting are created by special modifiers. This also overcomes the tendency of the tints to form brassy, unnatural colors in the hair.

CONDITIONERS Conditioners are also included in the cream to overcome any tendency of the strongly alkaline tints to damage the cuticle. Conditioners help prevent the drying effect of tints, which, before the addition of lanolin and other conditioners, was a common feature of tinting. But they still do not restore the normal condition of the hair, so reconditioning of the hair following a tint is still necessary.

LOSS OF TINT STRENGTH The tint base will slowly develop a color by picking up oxygen from the air. This can be seen around the screw cap on the opened tube or bottle. Sunlight itself will cause color to appear. For this reason creams are packed into tubes and liquid tints into brown bottles since once the tint pigment is formed it will not be able to enter the cortex.

DEVELOPER

HYDROGEN PEROXIDE The function of the tint developer is to join up the small, colorless tint base molecules into giant colored tint pigments. The most common developer is hydrogen peroxide solution. The excess alkali in the tint base supplies the activator for the normally acid solution of stabilized hydrogen peroxide. The color development begins immediately upon adding the hydrogen peroxide. The mild oxidizing conditions combine the small uncolored or weakly colored molecules together to form giant molecules within the cortex.

TIME OF DEVELOPMENT After 15 to 45 minutes all the tint bases are converted into insoluble tint pigment. Some products claim to stop at the desired shade, but careful monitoring of color development is still the best approach. Reducing the concentration of tint base however, will prevent darker shades from developing in the hair. The elimination of para-phenylene will prevent black shades from developing when only the lighter shades are required.

FORMING LIGHTER SHADES IN THE HAIR If stronger than normal hydrogen peroxide is used as the developer, there is a lightening action on the natural pigments at the same time. This saves the step of pre-lightening if a tint shade lighter than the original hair color is desired.

CREAM DEVELOPERS

Cream developers can be used instead of liquid hydrogen peroxide, because they contain other peroxides (e.g., urea peroxide) and tend to keep more stable than hydrogen peroxide does over a long period of time.

Use of a cream developer overcomes any possibility of the colorist using stale, ineffective hydrogen peroxide as a developer or oxidizing agent.

SPECIAL DEVELOPERS AND TECHNIQUES

TINTING TABLETS   The developer may also be put into the tint base itself. As the tinting process cannot proceed without the addition of water, this method uses hair tinting tablets. The action of dissolving the tablets in warm water begins the color development. Thereafter, the colorist makes up a paste and when ready, puts this on the hair in the usual way.

Firms which supply the tablets claim that this method gives a greater range of colors than the cream or liquid tints. By breaking up portions of different tablets and mixing them together, the normal range of colors can be extended to suit any requirement.

TINTING STICKS   Another variation is to make the tint bases in stick form coated with paraffin wax (similar to lip sticks in appearance). Warm water starts the tint color forming when the colorist is ready to apply it.

DEVELOPMENT ON HAIR   Another method is to moisten the hair with ammonia and hydrogen peroxide solutions. Then by rubbing a paste containing tint bases into the hair the permanent color develops in the usual way. With this method, the use of the steamer is advisable to speed up the process.

COMBINING TINTING AND WAVING

SEQUENCE   The tint should be applied to the hair before starting the permanent wave. After proper color development (allowing for color changes of wet hair and the stripping effect of permanent wave solutions) the hair is rinsed with warm water.

Rinsing removes the excess tint and the wetting agent in the tint supplies enough cleaning action to prepare the hair for the permanent wave. However, a shampoo should be given before normal permanent wave begins.

TINTING DURING NEUTRALIZING   Another method of combining tinting and waving is the following:

After the hair is softened with permanent wave solution, rinsed and made ready for neutralizing, a special neutralizer containing tint base together with hydrogen peroxide is used. Both neutralizing and tinting proceeds simultaneously.

COLOR STRIPPING

For the removal of previous tint or for lightening over-dark shades it is common practice to use a tint stripper. A tint stripper is a very strong oxidizing agent that acts on the giant colored molecules to reduce them in size. When the parts of the molecules are small enough to pass through the cuticle, these colorless fragments may be rinsed from the hair.

Sometimes the color does not strip out evenly because most tints are really mixtures of red, yellow and black molecules. The red molecules may be left behind to give red discolorations which persist for longer periods. The other colored molecules (yellow and black), are more easily removed from the hair.

EXAMPLES OF STRIPPING AGENTS

Hair strippers are chemical agents which are intended to strip out color with the least risk of damage to the hair. The chemicals used may be inorganic sulfites or organic reducing agents with moderating agents.

Hair tints can also be stripped using a liquid bleach (30 vol. hydrogen peroxide with excess ammonia to pH 10.0–12.0). The hydrogen peroxide solution may be boosted by sodium peroxide in tablet or powder form.

However, the action of stripping must be carried out under conditions which can only lead to hair damage, no matter what chemicals are used. Furthermore, the stripping rarely proceeds evenly, and resistant red pigments may be left behind to give unsightly streaks in the hair.

MILD STRIPPING

The action of the stripper is to break up the tint pigments into smaller colorless particles. These fragments can then be easily rinsed out through the cuticle imbrications. The excess alkali swells the imbrications even more than when that hair was being tinted. The alkali opens the keratin chains and weakens the salt bonds holding the tint pigment to the hair protein.

RINSING, DRYING AND CONDITIONING

Because the hair has been excessively softened during this process, it is essential that thorough rinsing be carried out to remove the excess stripper. After rinsing it is vital that the hair be reconditioned before styling. The acid in the reconditioning cream will restore some of the body and manageability to the hair and give the style more holding power.

Alkali strippers leave the hair cuticle in a very dry state. Although creams are included in the stripper itself, they will only help prevent excess hair damage, not really condition the hair. Mere rinsing of the excess stripper will not bring the hair back to its normal acid pH or reform all those S and H-bonds in the cortex broken by the alkali.

ACTION OF STRIPPERS ON HAIR TINTS

1. TINTED HAIR

2. MILD STRIPPING

3. RINSING

4. DRYING, SETTING AND CONDITIONING

STRIPPING METALLIC DYES

Certain "metal" strippers containing sodium sulfites are sold for reducing hair dyed with metallic dyes. As these dyes will react violently with tint strippers containing hydrogen peroxide; *the subsequent chemical reaction may cause so much heat that the hair is dissolved.*

Therefore, grey hair treated with so-called "hair restorers" (used by some older patrons) will contain metal salts (often lead sulfide, which darkens the hair). With this dyed hair the metallic or metal strippers are still not very effective. In fact the only real way to remove metallic dyes is to cut off that portion of the hair strands just as soon as sufficient growth has taken place.

DERMATITIS

No treatment of the oxidation hair tints would be complete without reference to the problem of dermatitis or sensitivity.

SYMPTOMS Dermatitis is caused by an allergy to the "para" tint, in certain individuals. It shows itself by the reddening of the skin, swelling of the face and fingers, sensations of burning and intense itching of the skin and scalp.

SENSITIVITY People in general, vary greatly in their reactions to the newer tints. For example, in an average 1,000 persons:

> 960 — are relatively safe.
> 25 — are mildly sensitive.
> 15 — are very sensitive.

OTHER CAUSES Dermatitis may be caused by a number of things other than "para" tints.

EXAMPLE:

Sunlight, X-rays, insect stings, detergents, cold waving solutions, poison ivy, certain gums (used in setting lotions and cheap hair sprays) .

PATCH TEST

In order to discover whether or not there is such a personal allergy to the "para" tints, it is important to give a patch test each time a hair tint is going to be used. In addition, the scalp should be thoroughly checked to see if it is free from scratches and inflammation.

The tint used for the patch test should be a portion of the tube or bottle (or the same number), as the one intended to be used on the hair. *Because "para" tints are really mixtures of different chemicals, proper patch testing with the preparation to be used is important.* A lighter shade may have little or no "para" tint present at all and if used for a patch test when a darker shade will actually be applied, results will not be valid.

In the latter case, the darker shade would contain a higher amount of the "para-phenylene-diamine" tint. This chemical appears to be the real cause of the danger and sensitivity in the oxidation tints.

To overcome the problem of sensitivity, some firms have changed to the less sensitive para-toluene-diamines. Furthermore, as lighter shades are now more popular with the public, the number of positive skin reactions are lower than when heavy dark shades were the fashion.

However, it is wise to continue patch testing, if only to protect the professional from dishonest individuals. Besides, the sensitivity of a person to the tint can suddenly develop even after many successful tintings.

CONCLUSION

Naturally colored hair has many advantages over artificially colored hair. Unfortunately, even with naturally colored hair, in the normal course of events the hair slowly loses its natural pigments. This greying process is a matter of much esthetic discomfort to many people.

Modern hair coloring provides everyone with an opportunity to emphasize or select their hair color, introduce warm shades into drab hair, brighten the hair with sparkling highlights, or remove brassy tones.

Finally, providing the colorist uses intelligence and suitable precautions, professional hair coloring services can produce a major portion of professional hair care income.

GLOSSARY ——————— Key to pronunciation is as follows: fāte, senate, câre, ăm, finâl, ärm, ȧsk, sofă, ēve, event, ĕnd, recent, evẽr, īce, ĭll; ōld, obey, ôrb, ŏdd, cônnect, sŏft, food, foot; ūse, unite, ûrn, ŭp, circus; those

GLOSSARY

---- A ----

absorption (ăb-sôrp′shŭn): assimilation of one body by another; act of absorbing.

acetic (ă-sĕt′ĭk): pertaining to vinegar; sour.

acetone (ăs′ĕ-tōn): a colorless, inflammable liquid, miscible with water, alcohol, and ether, and having a sweetish, ethereal odor and a burning taste.

acid (ăs′ĭd): 1) a substance having a sour taste; 2) a substance containing hydrogen replaceable by metals to form salts, and capable of dissociating in aqueous solution to form hydrogen ions.

acidic (ă-sĭd′ĭk): containing a high percentage of acid.

acne (ăk′nē): inflammation of the sebaceous glands from retained secretion.

activate (ăk′tĭ-vāt): to make active; to start the action of hair coloring products.

activator (ăk′tĭ-vā-tẽr): a substance employed to start the action of hair coloring products.

additive (ăd′ĭ-tĭv): a substance which is to be added to another product.

adsorb: to hold various substances on the surface of a solid.

adsorption: the taking up of a gas, vapor or dissolved material on the surface of a solid.

aerosol (â′rō-sōl): colloidal suspension of liquid or solid particles in a gas; aerosol container filled with liquified gas and dissolved or suspended ingredients which can be dispersed as a spray or aerosol.

affinity (ă-fĭn′ĭ-tē): 1) inherent likeness or relationship; 2) chemical attraction; the force that unites atoms into molecules.

after-image (ăf′tẽr-ĭm′âj): an image or sensation that stays or comes back after the external stimulus has been withdrawn.

albino (ăl-bī′nō): a subject of albinism; a person with very little or no pigment in the skin, hair or iris.

albumin (ăl-bū′mĭn): a simple, naturally-occurring protein soluble in water, coagulated by heat; found, in egg white (ovalbumin), in blood (serum albumin), in milk (lactalbumin).

alkali (ăl′kâ-lī): a class of compounds which react with acid to form salts, turn red litmus blue, saponify fats and form soluble carbonates.

alkaline (ăl′kâ-lĭn): having the qualities of, or pertaining to, an alkali.

alkalinity (ăl-kâ-lĭn′ĭ-tē): the quality or state of being alkaline.

allergy (ăl′ẽr-jē): a disorder due to extreme sensitivity to certain foods or chemicals.

amino-acid (ăm′ĭ-nō ăs′ĭd): 1) any one of a large group of organic compounds; 2) the end product of protein hydrolysis.

ammonia (ă-mō′nē-ă): a colorless gas with a pungent odor; very soluble in water.

ammonium monoethanolamine (ă-mō′nē-ŭm mō-nō-ĕth′ăn-ō-lă-mĭn): a combination of ammonia and ethanolamine (colorless, moderately viscous liquid), (ethylene oxide and ammonia).

ammonium sulfite (ă-mō′nē-ŭm sŭl′fĭt): a combination of ammonia and salt of sulfurous acid.

ammonium sulphide (ă-mō′nē-ŭm sŭl′fĭd): combination of ammonia and sulphur.

ammonium thiocylanate (ă-mō′nē-ŭm thī-ō-sīl′ă-nāt): a combination of ammonia and thiocyanic acid.

ammonium thioglycolate (thio) (ă-mō′nē-ŭm thī-ō-glī′kô-lāt): a combination of ammonia and thioglycolic acid to form the chemical; reducing agent used primarily in permanent waving and hair relaxing solutions and creams.

aniline (ăn′ĭ-lĭn, -lēn): a colorless liquid with a faint characteristic odor, obtained from coal tar and other nitrogenous substances; combined with other substances, it forms the aniline colors or dyes that are derived from coal tar.

anti-perspirant (ăn-tĭ-pẽr-spī′rănt): a strong astringent liquid or cream used to stop the flow of perspiration in the region of the armpits, hands or feet.

antiseptic (ăn-tĭ-sĕp′tĭk): a chemical agent that prevents the growth of bacteria.

antitoxin (ăn-tĭ-tŏk′sĭn): a substance in serum which binds and neutralizes toxin (poison).

aorta (ā-ôr′tă): the main arterial trunk leaving the heart, and carrying blood to the various arteries throughout the body.

aqueous (ā′kwē-ŭs): watery; pertaining to water.

arrector pili (â-rĕk′tôr pī′lī): plural of arrectores pilorum.

arrectores pilorum (â-rĕk-tō′rēz pĭ-lôr′ŭm): the minute involuntary muscle fibres in the skin inserted into the bases of the hair follicles.

atom (ăt′ŭm): the smallest quantity of an element that can exist and still retain the chemical properties of the element.

azo-dye (ā′zō-dī): a group of synthetic dyes derivable from azobenzene.

---- B ----

bacillus (bă-sĭl′ŭs): pl., **bacilli** (-ī); rod-like shaped bacterium.

bacteria (băk-tē′rē-ă): microbes, or germs.

bed hair (bĕd hâr): hair which has separated from the papilla and lies loosely in the follicle.

benzene ring: a ring of six carbon atoms joined to six (6) hydrogen atoms.

bleach (blēch): see: hair lightening.

bleaching (blēch′ĭng): see: hair lightening.

blocking (blŏk′ĭng): the act of dividing the hair into practical working parts.

bond (bŏnd): 1) the linkage between different atoms or radicals of a chemical compound, usually effected by the transfer of one or more electrons from one atom to another; 2) it can be found represented by a dot or a line between atoms shown in various formulas.

booster (bōōs′tẽr): oxidizer added to hydrogen peroxide to increase its chemical action; such chemicals as ammonium persulfate or percarbonate are used.

borax (bō′răks): sodium tetraborate; a white powder used as an antiseptic and cleansing agent.

bristle (brĭs′'l): the short, stiff hair of a brush; short, stiff hairs of an animal, used in brushes.

brittle (brĭt′'l): easily broken or shattered.

——————— C ———————

calcium (kăl′sē-ŭm): a brilliant silvery-white metal; enters into the composition of bone.

capillary (kăp′ĭ-là-rē): any one of the minute blood vessels which connect the arteries and veins; hair-like.

carbohydrate (kär-bō-hī′drāt): a substance containing carbon, hydrogen, and oxygen, the two latter in the proportion to form water; sugars, starches and cellulose belong to the class of carbohydrates.

carbolic acid (kär-bŏl′ĭk ăs′ĭd): phenol made from coal tar; a caustic and corrosive poison; used in dilute solution as an antiseptic.

carbon (kär′bŏn): a non metallic element widely distributed in nature; typical forms are: diamonds, graphite and charcoal.

carbon dioxide (dī-ŏk′sīd): carbonic acid gas; product of the combustion of carbon with a free supply of air.

carbonic acid (kär-bŏn′ĭk ăs′ĭd): a weak, colorless acid, formed by the solution of carbon dioxide in water and existing only in solution.

carbuncle (kär′bŭn-k'l): a large circumscribed inflammation of the subcutaneous tissue, similar to a furuncle, but much more extensive.

catalysis (kă-tăl′ĭ-sĭs): the process of change in the velocity of a chemical reaction through the presence of a substance which apparently remains chemically unaltered throughout the reaction.

catalyst (kăt′â-lĭst): a substance having the power to increase the velocity of a chemical reaction.

cation (kăt′ĭ-ŏn): an ion carrying a charge of positive electricity; the element which, during electrolysis of a chemical compound, appears at the negative pole or cathode.

caustic (kôs′tĭk): an agent that burns and chars tissue.

caustic potash (kôs′tĭk pŏt′âsh): potassium hydroxide.

caustic soda (kôs′tĭk sō′dă): sodium hydroxide.

cell (sĕl): a minute mass of protoplasm forming the structural unit of every organized body.

cell division (sĕl dĭ-vĭzh′ŏn): the reproduction of cells by the process of each cell dividing in half and forming two cells.

ceresin (kĕr′ē-sĭn): a white or yellow waxy cake, soluble in alcohol, benzene, chloroform, naptha; insoluble in water; used in cosmetics.

certified color (sûr′tĭ-fīd): a guaranteed safe commercial coloring product often used for temporarily coloring hair.

chemical change (kĕm′ĭ-kăl chānj): alteration in the chemical composition of a substance.

chemical symbol: a sign or emblem which identifies a particular chemical or combination of chemicals.

chlorinate (klôr′ĭ-nāt): to treat or combine with chlorine.

chlorine (klō′rĭn, -rēn): greenish yellow gas, with a disagreeable suffocating odor; used in combined form as a disinfectant and a bleaching agent.

cholesterol (kō-lĕs′tẽr-ōl): a waxy alcohol found in animal tissues and their secretions; it is present in lanolin, and used as an emulsifier.

citric acid (sĭt′rĭk ăs′ĭd): acid found in the lemon, orange, grapefruit; used for making a lemon rinse.

coiffure (kwä-fūr′): an arrangement or dressing of the hair.

colloid (kŏl′oid): particles having a certain degree of fineness and possessing a sticky consistency.

color filler (kŭl′ẽr fĭl′ẽr): a preparation used to recondition lightened, tinted or damaged hair.

complementary colors (kŏm′plê-mĕn′tẽr-ē kŭl′-ẽrs): any two colors of the spectrum which combine to form white or whitish light.

component (kŏm-pō′nênt): one of the parts of a whole (element).

compounds (kŏm′poundz): 1) made of two or more parts or ingredients; 2) in chemistry, a substance which consists of two or more chemical elements in union.

conditioner (kŏn-dĭ′shûn-ẽr): a sepcial chemical agent applied to the hair to help restore its strength and give it body in order to protect it against possible breakage.

configuration (kŏn-fĭg′û-rā′shûn): the arrangement and spacing of the atoms of a molecule.

corrode (kô-rōd′): to eat into or wear away gradually.

corrosive (kô-rō′sĭv): something causing corrosion.

cortex (kôr′tĕks): the second layer of the hair.

"cradle cap" (krā′d'l kăp): oily type of dandruff.

crayon (krā′ŏn): a temporary hair coloring, massaged or brushed on with a lipstick-like applicator.

cross bonds (krôs-bŏndz): the bonds holding together the long chains of amino-acids, which compose hair; the bonds holding together the parallel chains of amino-acids to form hair.

cuticle (kū′tĭ-k'l): the very thin outer layer of the skin or hair.

cycle (sī′k'l): circle; a complete wave of an alternating current.

cyclical (sī′klĭ-k'l): pertaining to or moving in a circle; having parts arranged in a ring or closed chain structure.

cysteine (sĭs′tĭ-ēn): an amino acid produced by digestion; it is easily **oxidized** to cystine; obtained by reduction of cystine.

cystine (sĭs′tēn): an amino acid component of many proteins, especially keratin; it may be **reduced** to cysteine.

cytoplasm (sī′tô-plăz′m): the protoplasm of the cell body, exclusive of the nucleus.

——————— D ———————

dandricide (dăn′drĭ-sīd): a chemical substance; counteracts the effects of dandruff.

dandruff (dăn′drŭf): pityriasis; scurf or scales formed in excess upon the scalp.

decolorize (dē-kŭl′ẽr-īz): see hair lightening.

degrease (dē-grēs′): to remove grease from.

density (dĕn′sĭ-tē): the quality or condition of being close, thick, compact or crowded.

deodorant (dē-ō′dẽr-ânt): a substance that removes or conceals offensive odors.

depilatory (dē-pĭl′â-tô-rē): a substance, usually a caustic alkali, used to destroy the hair; having the power to remove hair.

dermatitis (dûr-mă-tī′tĭs): an irritation of the skin; dermatitis resulting either from the primary irritant effect of the substance or more frequently from the sensitization to a substance coming in contact with the skin.

dermis, derma (dûr′mĭs, dûr′mă): the layer below the epidermis; the corium or true skin.

detergent (dē-tûr′jĕnt): a compound or solution used for cleansing.

developer (dē-vĕl′ŏp-ēr): an oxidizing agent such as 20-volume hydrogen peroxide solution; when mixed with an oxidation dye it supplies the necessary oxygen gas.

diameter (dī-ăm′ĕ-tēr): width or thickness of a thing; measurement across,

diffuse (dĭ-fūs′): scattered; not limited to one spot.

dilute (dĭ-lūt′; dī-): to make thinner by mixing, especially with water.

dispersion (dĭs-pûr′shŏn): 1) the act of scattering or separating; 2) the incorporation of the particles of one substance into the body of another, comprising solutions, suspensions and colloid solutions.

disulfide (dī-sŭl′fīd) (sulphur): a chemical compound in which two sulphur atoms are united with a single atom of an element, i.e., carbon.

——————— E ———————

elasticity (ē-lăs′tĭs′ĭ-tē): the property that allows a thing to be stretched and return to its former shape.

electro-static (ē-lĕk′trō-stăt′ĭk): pertaining to static electricity.

element (ĕl′ĕ-mĕnt): 1) a simple substance which cannot be decomposed by chemical means and which is made up of atoms which are alike in their peripheral electronic configurations and in their chemical properties; 2) any one of the 100 ultimate chemical entities of which matter is believed to be composed.

emulsifier (ĕ-mŭl′sĭ-fī-ēr): a substance, as gelatin, gum, etc., for emulsifying a fixed oil.

emulsion (ĕ-mŭl′shŭn): a product consisting of minute globules of one liquid dispersed through-out the body of a second liquid.

end bonds (peptide bonds) (pĕp′tĭd): the chemical bonds which join together the amino-acids to form the long chains which are characteristic of all proteins.

enzyme (ĕn′zīm): an organic compound, frequently a protein, capable of accelerating or producing high catalytic action that will promote a chemical change.

epidermis (ĕp-ĭ-dûr′mĭs): the outer epithelial portion of the skin.

epithelial (ĕp-ĭ-thē′lē-ăl): having the nature of epithelium.

epithelium (ĕp-ĭ-thē′lē-ûm): a cellular tissue or membrane, with little intercellular substance, covering a free surface or lining a cavity.

ester (ĕs′tēr): an organic compound formed by the reaction of an acid and an alcohol.

esthetic (ĕs-thĕt′ĭk): sensitive to art and beauty; showing good taste; artistic.

evaporation (ĕ-văp-ō-rā′shûn): conversion of a liquid or solid to vapor.

excrete (ĕks-krēt′): to separate (waste matter) from the blood or tissue and eliminate from the body as through the kidneys or sweat glands.

excretion (ĕks-krē′shûn): a substance that is produced by some cells, but in itself is of no further use to the body.

eye-shadow (ī′shăd′ō): a cosmetic applied on the eyelids to accentuate their brilliance.

——————— F ———————

fatty acid (făt′ē ăs′ĭd): an acid derived from the saturated series of open chain hydro carbons.

ferrous sulfate (fĕr′ûs sŭl′fāt): a salt of sulfuric acid derived from iron.

fiber (fī′bēr): a slender, threadlike structure that combines with others to form animal or vegetable tissue.

filler (fĭl′ēr): a commercial product used to provide fill for porous spots in the hair during tinting, lightening and permanent waving.

fission (fĭsh′ûn): any splitting or cleaving, **atomic f.**: the splitting of the neutrons of an atom in two main fragments.

fixative (fĭk′sà-tĭv): a hair dressing used to keep hair in place; in cold waving, it stops the chemical action of the cold waving solution and sets or hardens the hair; a chemical agent capable of stopping the processing of the chemical hair relaxer and hardening the hair in its new form; neutralizer, stabilizer.

fluorescent (flōō′ôr-ĕs′n′t): an ability to emit light after exposure to light, the wave length of the emitted light being longer than that of the light absorbed.

"fly away" (flī′à-wā): an excessive electro-static condition of hair which causes individual hair strands to repel one another and stand away from the head.

foamer (fō′mēr): a substance which creates an excessive amount of foam.

follicle (fŏl′ĭ-k′l): a small secretory cavity or sac; the depression in the skin containing the hair root.

fungus (fŭn′gûs): a vegetable parasite; a spongy growth of diseased tissue on the body.

furuncle (fū-rŭn′k′l): a small skin abscess (boil).

fusion (fū′zhûn): the act of uniting or cohering.

——————— G ———————

gel (jĕl): comprised of a solid and a liquid which exists as a solid or semi-solid mass.

gelatine (jĕl′â-tĭn): the tasteless, odorless, brittle substance extracted by boiling bones, hoofs and animal tissues, used in various foods, medicines, etc.

gene (jēn): the ultimate unit in the transmission of heredity characteristics.

genetic (jĕ-nĕt′ĭk): the genesis or origin of something.

germicide (jûr′mĭ-sīd): any chemical, especially a solution that will destroy germs.

germinal matrix (jûr-mĭn-âl mā-trĭks): an area of reproducing cells situated around the papilla at the base of the hair bulb.

germinative layer (jûr-mĭ-nā'tĭv lā-ēr): stratum germinativum; the deepest layer of the epidermis resting on the corium.

germ layer (jûrm lā'ēr): any of the three primary layers of cells from which the various organs and parts of the organisms develop by further differentiation.

gland (glănd): a secretory organ of the body.

globule (glŏb'ūl): a small, spherical droplet of fluid or semi-fluid material.

glycerin; glycerine (glĭs'ēr-ĭn): sweet oily fluid, used as an application for roughened and chapped skin; also used as a solvent.

glycerol (glĭs'ēr-ōl): see: glycerin.

glycerol monostearate (glĭs'ēr-ōl mŏn-ō-stē'rāt): pure white or cream colored, wax-like solid with faint odor; used as an emulsifying agent for oils, waxes and solvents; acts as a protective coating for various cosmetics.

glycine (glī'sēn): amino-acetic acid.

granules (grăn'ūlz): small grains; small pills.

gravity (grâv'ĭ-tē): the effect of the attraction of the earth upon matter.

H

---

hair bulb (hâr bŭlb): the lower extremity of the hair.

hair lightening (hâr lī'tĕn-ĭng): a chemical process involving the removal of the natural color pigment or artificial color from the hair.

hair stream (hâr strēm): the natural direction in which the hair grows after leaving the follicle.

H-bond: see: hydrogen bond.

henna (hĕn'ă): the leaves of an Asiatic thorny tree or shrub used as a dye, imparting a reddish tint; it is also used as a cosmetic.

heredity (hĕ-rĕd'ĭ-tē): the inborn capacity of the organism to develop ancestral characteristics.

hexachlorophenol (hĕks-ă-klō-rō-fē'nōl): white, free flowing, powder essentially odorless; used as a bactericidal agent in antiseptic soaps, deodorant products including soaps and various cosmetics.

homogeneous (hō-mŏj'ê-nûs): having the same nature or quality; a uniform character in all parts.

homogenizer (hō-môj'ĕ-nīz-ēr): serving to produce a uniform suspension of emulsions from two or more normally immiscible substances.

hormone (hôr'mōn): a chemical substance formed in one organ or part of the body and carried in the blood to another organ or part which it stimulates to functional activity or secretion.

humidity (hū-mĭd'ĭ-tē): moisture; dampness.

hydrolyze (hī'drō-līz): to decompose as a result of the incorporation and splitting of water; the two resulting products divide the water, the hydroxyl group being attached to one and the hydrogen atom to the other.

hydro carbon (hī'drō-kär'bŏn): any compound composed only of hydrogen and carbon.

hydrogen (hī'drō-jên): the lightest element; it is an odorless, tasteless, colorless gas found in water and all organic compounds. **h. acceptor:** a substance which, on reduction, accepts hydrogen atoms from another substance called a hydrogen donor.

hydrogen bond (physical bond) (hī'drō-jên bŏnd): that bond formed between two molecules when the electron of a hydrogen atom, originally attached to a fluorine, nitrogen or oxygen atom of a molecule, is attracted to the nucleus of fluorine, nitrogen or oxygen atom of a second molecule of the same or different substance.

hydrogen peroxide (hī'drō-jên pĕr-ŏk'sīd): a powerful oxidizing agent; in liquid form is used as an antiseptic and for the activation of lighteners and hair tints.

hydrophilic (hī-drō-fĭl'ĭk): capable of combining with or attracting water.

I

---

imbrications (ĭm-brĭ-kā'shŭnz): cells arranged in layers overlapping one another; found in cuticle layer of hair.

immerse (ĭ-mûrs'): to plunge into; dip; submerge in a liquid.

immersion (ĭ-mûr'shŭn): plunging or dipping into a liquid, especially so as to cover completely.

infra-red (ĭn'fră rĕd): pertaining to that part of the spectrum lying outside of the visible spectrum and below the red rays.

ingredient (ĭn-grē'dĭ-ĕnt): any of the things that a mixture is made up of.

insoluble (ĭn-sŏl'ū-b'l): incapable of dissolving in a liquid.

intensity (ĭn-tĕn'sĭ-tē): the amount of force or energy of heat, light, sound, electric current, etc., per unit area; the quality of being intense.

iodine (ī'ô-dīn dīn): a non-metallic element used as an antiseptic for cuts, bruises, etc.

ion (ī'ŏn): an atom or group of atoms carrying an electric charge.

irreversible (ĭr-ê-vĕr'sĭ-b'l): not capable of being reversed.

K

---

keratin (kĕr'ă-tĭn): a fiber protein characteristic of horny tissues: hair, nails, feathers, etc; it is insoluble in protein solvents and has a high sulfur content.

keratinization (kĕr'ă-tĭn-ĭ-zā'shŭn): the process of being keratinized.

L

---

lacquer (lăk'ēr): a thick liquid which forms a glossy film on the nail.

lanolin (lăn'ō-lĭn): purified wool fat.

lanthionine (lăn-thē'ô-nīn): a non-essential form of amino-acid.

lecithin (lĕs'ĭ-thĭn): a colorless crystalline compound, soluble in alcohol; it is found in animal tissues, especially nerve tissue, and the yolk of egg.

lever (lĕ'vĕr): a mechanical arrangement whereby a bar, acting over a fulcrum or pivot point, is capable of exerting a greater force.

lightener (līt"n-ēr) (bleach): the chemical employed to remove color from hair.

lightening (bleaching): see: hair lightening.

lipophilic (lĭp-ō-fĭl'ĭk): having an affinity or attraction to fat and oil.

lotion (lō'shŭn): a liquid solution used for bathing the skin.

lymph (lĭmf): a clear yellowish or light straw colored fluid, which circulates in the lymph spaces, or lymphatics of the body.

———————————— M ————————————

magnetism (măg'nĕ-tĭz'm): the power possessed by a magnet to attract or repel other masses.

manganese (măn'gă-nēs): a grayish-white, metallic chemical element which rusts like iron but is not magnetic.

marcel (măr-sĕl'): a series of even waves or tiers put in the hair with the aid of a heated iron.

matting (măt'ĭng): tangling together into a thick mass.

medulla (mĕ-dŭl'ă): the marrow in the various bone cavities; the pith of the hair.

melanin (mĕl'ă-nĭn): the dark or black pigment in the epidermis and hair, and in the choroid or coat of the eye.

melanocyte (mĕl-ân'ō-sīte): a pigment cell producing melanin.

metallic salts (mĕ-tăl'ĭk sôlts): a compound of a base and an acid.

meta-toluene-diamine (mĕt'ă-tŏl'ū-ēn-dī-ăm'ĭn): the name given to an oxidation dye used to provide lighter shades of red and blonde; it is an aniline derivative type.

micro-organism (mī'krŏ-ôr'gân-ĭz'm): microscopic plant or animal cell; a bacterium.

mixture (mĭks'tūre): a preparation made by incorporating an insoluble ingredient in a liquid vehicle; sometimes used to identify an aqueous solution containing two or more solutes.

modifier (mŏd'ĭ-fī-ēr): anything that will change the form or characteristics of an object or substance.

molecule (mŏl'ĕ-kūl): the smallest possible unit of existence of any compound; (consists of two or more atoms chemically combined).

mordant (môr'dânt): a substance such as alum, phenol, aniline oil that fixes the dye used in coloring.

mould (mōld): to form or to shape into a definite pattern.

———————————— N ————————————

nape (nāp): the back of the neck.

neutral (nū'trâl): exhibiting no positive properties; indifferent; in chemistry, neither acid nor alkaline.

neutralization (nū-trâl-ĭ-zā'shŭn): that process or operation that counter-balances or cancels the action of an agent; in chemistry, a change of reaction to that which is neither alkaline nor acid.

neutralize (nū'trâl-īz): render neutral; counterbalance of action or influence.

neutralizer (nū'trâl-īz-ēr): an agent capable of neutralizing another substance; (see fixative).

nitrogen (nī'trŏ-jĕn): a colorless gaseous element, tasteless and odorless, found in air and living tissue.

nucleus (nū'klē-ûs); pl., **nuclei** (-ī): the active center of cells.

———————————— O ————————————

oleic acid (ō-lē'ĭk ăs'ĭd): an oily acid used in making soap and ointments.

opaque (ō-pāk'): impervious to light rays; neither transparent nor translucent.

organic (ôr-găn'ĭk): relating to an organ; pertaining to substances derived from living organisms.

oxidation (ŏk-sĭ-dā'shŭn): the act of combining oxygen with another substance.

oxygen (ŏk'sĭ-jĕn): a gaseous element, essential to animal and plant life.

oxymelanin (ŏk'sĭ-mĕl'ă-nĭn): a compound formed by a combination of an oxidizing agent with the dark melanin (color) pigments in the hair; (generally found in the red to usually yellow shades).

———————————— P ————————————

papilla, hair (pă-pĭl'ă, hâr): a small cone-shaped elevation at the bottom of the hair follicle in the dermis.

para (păr'ă): see para-phenylene-diamine.

paraffin (păr'ă-fĭn): a white mineral wax.

para-phenylene-diamine (păr'ă fēn'ĭ-lēn dī-ăm'ĭn): a name given to the organic compound used as the basis for the older aniline derivative dyes.

para tint (păr'ă tĭnt): a tint made from an aniline derivative.

para toluene diamine (păr'ă tŏl'ū-ēn dī-ăm'ĭn): a variety of aniline derivative dyes commonly used in preparations compounded to provide red and blonde tones. (meta: prefix meaning higher, or change relating to the position of the amine free arm on the toluene ring.)

patch test (păch tĕst): see predisposition test.

penetration (pĕn-ĕ-trā'shŭn): act or power of penetrating.

pepsin (pĕp'sĭn): an enzyme which digests protein.

peptide (pĕp'tīd): a compound of two or more amino acids containing one or more peptide groups; continuous filaments in the case of fiber protein or keratin.

peptones (pĕp'tōnz): any of a class of diffusible and soluble substances into which proteins are changed by pepsin or trypsin.

peroxide of hydrogen (pĕr-ŏk'sīd of hī'drô-jên): a powerful oxidizing agent; in liquid solution is used as an antiseptic; used in tinting and lightening treatments.

perspiration (pûr'spĭ-rā'shŭn): sweat; the fluid excreted from the sweat glands of the skin.

percarbonate (pĕr-kär'bô-nāt): quantity of salts or esters of carbonic acid.

persulfate (pĕr-sŭl'fāt): a sulfate which contains more sulfuric acid than the ordinary sulphate.

pH: symbol used in expressing hydrogen-ion concentration; it signifies the logarithm, on the base of 10, of the reciprocal of the hydrogen-ion concentration.

pH number: a measure of the degree of acidity or alkalinity of a solution.

phenacetin (fĕ-nǎs'ĕ-tĭn): a compound in the form of white glistening crystals or fine white crystalline powder; without odor, it has a slightly bitter taste.

phosphorous (fŏs'fôr-ŭs): an element found in the bones, muscles and the nerves.

pigment (pĭg'mĕnt): any organic coloring matter of the body.

pliability (plī-ă-bĭl'ĭ-tē): flexibility.

polypeptide (pŏl-ē-pĕp'tīd): strings of amino acids joined together by peptide bonds, the prefix "poly" meaning many.

pore (pôr): a small opening of the sweat glands of the skin.

porosity (pô-rŏs'ĭ-tē): ability of the hair to absorb moisture.

porous (pō'rŭs): full of pores.

potassium bromate (pô-tăs'ĭ-ŭm brō'māt): a metallic element of the alkali group, used in medicines as a sedative.

potassium permanganate (pô-tăs'ĭ-ûm pĕr-măn'gâ-nāt): a salt of permanganate acid; used as an antiseptic and deodorant.

precipitate (prē-sĭp'ĭ-tāt): to cause a substance in solution to settle down in solid particles; to decrease solubility.

predisposition test (prē-dĭs-pō-zĭsh'ûn tĕst): a skin test designed to determine an individual's over-sensitivity to certain chemicals (patch test, allergy test, skin test).

primary colors (prī'mă-rē kŭl'ẽrz): pigments or colors that are, or thought to be, fundamental; red, yellow and blue are the primary colors in pigments.

primary hair (prī'mă-rē hâr): the baby fine hair that is present over almost the entire smooth skin of the body.

prism (prĭz'm): a transparent solid with triangular ends and two converging sides; it breaks up white light into its component colors.

processing (prŏs'ĕs-ĭng): the action of the chemical relaxer in softening the hair and relaxing the curl.

properties (prŏp'ẽr-tēz): the identifying characteristics of a substance which are observable; a peculiar quality of anything; i.e.: color, taste, smell, etc.

protein (prō'tĕ-ĭn): one of a group of complex nitrogenous substances of high molecular weight found in various forms in animals and plants; they are characteristic of living matter.

puberty (pū'bĕr-tē): the period of life in which the organs of reproduction are developed.

Q

---

quality (kwäl'ĭ-tē): the something special about an object that makes it what it is.

radiation (rā-dĭ-ā'shŭn): the process of giving off light or heat rays.

R

---

reducing agent (rê-dūs'ĭng ā'jênt): a substance capable of adding hydrogen; in cosmetology, a cold wave solution would be a reducing agent.

resilient (rê-zĭl'ĭ-ênt): elastic.

resistance (rē-zĭst'âns): the difficulty of moisture or chemical solutions to penetrate the hair shaft.

retina (rĕt'ĭ-nă): the sensitive membrane of the eye which receives the image formed by the lens.

reversible (rê-vẽrs'ĭ-b'l): capable of going through a series of changes in either direction, forward or backward, as a reversible chemical reaction.

S

---

sachet (sà-shā'): a perfumed bag or pad.

S-bonds: see: sulphur bonds.

scarf skin (skärf skĭn): epidermis.

science (sī'êns): knowledge duly arranged and systematized.

sebaceous glands (sê-bā'shûs glăndz): oil glands of the skin.

sebum (sē'bŭm): the fatty or oily secretions of the sebaceous glands.

secondary hair (sĕk'ûn-dâ-rē hâr): the stiff, short, coarse hair found on the eyelashes, eyebrows and within the openings or passages of the nose and ears.

secretion (sê-krē'shûn): a product manufactured by a gland for a special purpose.

selenium sulphide (sê-lē'nĭ-ûm sŭl'fīd): a non-metallic element resembling sulphur in its chemical properties.

shampoo (shăm-pōō'): to subject the scalp and hair to washing and rubbing with some cleansing agent such as soap and water.

shed hair (shĕd hâr): dead, detached hair which has been removed from the head.

singeing (sĭnj'ĭng): process of lightly burning hair ends with a lighted wax taper.

slippage (slĭp'âj): the shifting and changing of position of the sulphur bonds.

sodium (sō'dē-ŭm): a metallic element of the alkaline group.

sodium carbonate (sō'dē-ŭm kär'bŏn-åt): washing soda; used to prevent corrosion of metallic instruments when added to boiling water.

sodium hydroxide (sō′dē-ŭm hī-drŏk′sīd): a powerful alkaline product used in some chemical hair relaxers; caustic soda.

sodium lauryl sulphate (sō′dē-ŭm lô′rêl sŭl′fāt): a metallic element of the alkaline group, in white or light yellow crystals; used in detergents.

sodium perborate (sō′dē-ŭm pêr′bô-rāt): a compound, formed by treating sodium peroxide with boric acid; on dissolving the substance in water peroxide of hydrogen is generated; used as an antiseptic.

sodium sulphite (sō′dē-ŭm sŭl′fīt): a soft, white metallic salt of sulphurous acid.

solubility (sŏl-û-bĭl′ĭ-tē): the extent to which a substance (solute) dissolves in a liquid (solvent) to produce a homogeneous system (solution).

solute sŏl′ūt: the dissolved substance in a solution.

solution (sô-lū′shŭn): a homogeneous mixture of a solid, liquid or gaseous substance.

solvent (sŏl′vênt): a liquid which dissolves another substance without any change in chemical composition.

specific gravity (spĕ-sĭf′ĭk grăv′ĭ-tē): the weight of a substance compared with that of an equal volume of another substance taken as a standard.

splash neutralizer (splăsh nū′trǎ-lī-zêr): a chemical agent capable of stopping the action of the cold waving solution and setting or hardening the hair in its new form.

spray gum (sprā gŭm): a sticky juice applied as a liquid going through the air in small drops.

spectrum (spĕk′trŭm): the band of rainbow colors produced by decomposing light by means of a prism.

stabilized (stā′bĭ-līzd): made stable or firm, preventing changes.

stabilizer (stā′-bĭ-lī-zêr): a retarding agent or a substance that counter-acts the effect of an accelerator; preserves a chemical equilibrium.

stable (stā′b'l): in a balanced condition; not readily destroyed or decomposed; resisting molecular change.

static electricity (stăt′ĭk ê-lĕk-trĭs′ĭ-tē): a form of electricity generated by friction.

steamer, facial (stēm′ẽr, fā′shâl): an apparatus, used in place of hot towels, for steaming the scalp or face.

stearic acid (stê-ăr′ĭk ăs′ĭd): a white fatty acid, occurring in solid animal fats and in some of the vegetable fats.

stripping (strĭp′ĭng): the removal of color from the hair shaft; bleaching; lightening; strong shampoos or soap removing some of the color from the hair is also known as stripping.

sulfite (sŭl′fīt): any salt of sulfurous acid.

sulfur, sulphur (sŭl′fŭr): a solid, non-metallic element, usually yellow in color; it is insoluble in water.

sulphide (sŭl′fīd): a compound of sulfur with another element or base.

sulphur: see sulfur.

sulphur bonds (sŭl′fŭr bŏndz): sulphur cross bonds, in the hair, which hold the chains of amino acids together in order to form a hair strand.

surface tension (sûr′fâs tĕn′shŭn): the tension or resistance to rupture possessed by the surface film of a liquid.

suspension (sŭs-pĕn′shŭn): a state of matter in which the solid particles are dispersed in, or distributed throughout a liquid medium; the particles in the medium are large but not large enough to settle to the bottom under the influence of gravity.

sweat (swĕt): see perspiration.

symbols: signs which identify.

symptom (sĭmp′tûm): a change in the body or its functions which indicates disease.

––––––––––––––– **T** –––––––––––––––

tartaric acid (tär′tâ-rĭk ăs′ĭd): a colorless crystalline acid compound.

tensile (tĕn′sĭl): capable of being stretched.

tension (tĕn′shŭn): stress caused by stretching or pulling.

terminology (tẽr-mĭ-nŏl′ô-jē): the special words or terms used in science, art or business.

tertiary (terminal) hair (tẽr′shê-â-rē hâr): the long, soft hair found on the scalp.

texture, hair (tĕks′tûr, hâr): the general quality as to coarse, medium or fine, and feel of the hair.

texture, skin (tĕks′tūr, skĭn): the general feel and appearance of the skin.

thallium (thă′lĭ-ûm): a bluish-white metallic element, the salts of which have been used for epilation; thallium is highly toxic to humans.

thio (thī′ō): see ammonium thioglycolate.

thioglycolic acid (thī-ō-glī′kô-lĭk ăs′ĭd): a colorless liquid or white crystals with a strong unpleasant odor, miscible with water, alcohol or ether; (used in permanent wave solutions, hair relaxers and depilatories).

tinting (tĭnt′ĭng): the process of adding artificial color to hair.

toluene diamine (tŏl′ū-ēn dī-ăm′ĭn): a colorless liquid, obtained from a coal tar product, used as a solvent and also in a drug designed to increase the amount of bile secreted.

toner (tōn′ẽr): an aniline derivative tint; a permanent penetrating type used primarily on bleached hair to achieve pale, delicate colors.

translucent (trăns-lū′sênt): somewhat transparent.

tyrosine (tī-rō′sĭn): an amino acid widely distributed in proteins, particularly in casein.

trypsin (trĭp′sĭn): an enzyme in the digestive juice secreted by the pancreas; trypsin changes proteins into peptones.

––––––––––––––– **U** –––––––––––––––

ultra-violet (ŭl′trǎ-vī′ô-lĕt): invisible rays of the spectrum which are beyond the violet rays.

unstable (ŭn-stā′b'l): liable to fade.

urea (ū-rē′ă): a diuretic; also employed externally in treating infected wounds; occurs as colorless to white crystals or powder; soluble in water.

urea peroxide (ū-rē′ă pĕr-ŏk′sīd): a combination of urea and peroxide in the form of a cream developer or activator; employed in hair tinting.

––––––––––––––––– V –––––––––––––––––

vacuum (văk′ū-ûm): a space from which most of the air has been exhausted.

valence (vâ′lĕns): the capacity of an atom to combine with other atoms in definite proportions.

vapor (vā′pĕr): the gaseous state of a liquid or solid.

virgin hair (vûr′jĭn hâr): normal hair which has had no previous bleaching or dyeing treatments.

viscid (vĭs′ĭd): sticky or adhesive.

viscosity (vĭs-kŏs′ĭ-tē): 1) resistance to change of form; 2) a resistance to flow that a liquid exhibits; 3) the degree of density, thickness, stickiness and adhesiveness of a substance.

viscous (vĭs′kûs): sticky or gummy.

visible rays (vĭz′ĭ-b′l rāz): light rays which can be seen; are visible to the eye.

––––––––––––––––– W –––––––––––––––––

wetting agent (wĕt′ĭng ā′jĕnt): a substance that causes a liquid to spread more readily on a solid surface, chiefly through a reduction of surface tension.

wrapping (răp′ĭng): winding hair on rollers or rods in order to form curls.